Drug Infusions in Anesthesiology

Second Edition

Drug Infusions in Anesthesiology

Second Edition

Editor
Robert J. Fragen, M.D.
Professor
Department of Anesthesia
Northwestern University Medical School
Chicago, Illinois

Lippincott - Raven
PUBLISHERS
Philadelphia • New York

**Lippincott-Raven Publishers, 227 East Washington Square,
Philadelphia, Pennsylvania 19106**

Made in the United States of America

Library of Congress Cataloging-in-Publication Data
Drug infusions in anesthesiology/editor, Robert J. Fragen.—2nd ed.
p. cm.
Includes bibliographical references and index.
ISBN 0-7817-0265-8
1. Intravenous anesthesia. 2. Intravenous therapy. I. Fragen, Robert J.
[DNLM: 1. Anesthesia, Intravenous. 2. Infusions, Intravenous.
WO 285 D794 1996]
RD85.I6D68 1996
617.9′62—dc20
DNLM/DLC
for Library of Congress

9 8 7 6 5 4 3 2 1

To my family

Ruth, Nathan, and Ronald
Joan
Daniel, Kathleen, Michael, and Patricia

Contents

Contributors

Michael J. Avram, Ph.D. *Associate Professor, Department of Anesthesia, Northwestern University Medical School, 303 E. Chicago Avenue, Chicago, Illinois 60611*

Honorio T. Benzon, M.D. *Professor, Department of Anesthesia, and Chief, Pain Management Service, Northwestern University Medical School, 303 E. Superior Street, Chicago, Illinois 60611*

Patrick K. Birmingham, M.D., F.A.A.P. *Assistant Professor, Department of Anesthesia, Northwestern University Medical School; and Children's Memorial Hospital, 2300 Children's Plaza, Chicago, Illinois 60614*

Robert J. Fragen, M.D. *Professor, Department of Anesthesia, Northwestern University Medical School, 303 E. Superior Street, Chicago, Illinois 60611*

Peter S. A. Glass, M.D. *Associate Professor, Department of Anesthesiology, Duke University Medical Center, P.O. Box 3094, Durham, North Carolina 27710*

Steven C. Hall, M.D. *Professor, Department of Anesthesia, Northwestern University Medical School; and Children's Memorial Hospital, 2300 Children's Plaza, Chicago, Illinois 60614*

Thomas K. Henthorn, M.D. *Associate Professor and Associate Chairman for Research, Department of Anesthesia, Northwestern University Medical School, 303 E. Chicago Avenue, Chicago, Illinois 60611*

Edward B. McKenzie, M.D. *Co-Director, Department of Cardiac Anesthesia, Staff Anesthesiologist, Durham County Medical Center, Durham, North Carolina 27706*

Mark F. Newman, M.D. *Assistant Professor, Department of Anesthesiology, Duke University Medical Center, P.O. Box 3094, Durham, North Carolina 27710*

Joseph G. Reves, M.D. *Professor, Department of Anesthesiology, Duke University Medical Center, P.O. Box 3094, Durham, North Carolina 27710*

Colin A. Shanks, M.D., Ch.B. *Professor, Department of Anesthesia, Northwestern University Medical School, 303 E. Chicago Avenue, Chicago, Illinois 60611*

Thomas E. Stanley III, M.D. *Assistant Professor, Department of Anesthesiology, The Heart Center, Duke University Medical Center, P.O. Box 3094, Durham, North Carolina 27710*

Preface

The Second Edition of *Drug Infusions in Anesthesiology* updates the material from the First Edition and adds a section on analgesic infusions for obstetric patients as well as a chapter on drug infusions for pediatric patients.

The important concepts of "equilibration time" and "context-sensitive halftime" are discussed in this new edition and their importance in understanding both initial dosing and recovery from infusion of various drugs given in the perioperative period is emphasized. "Context-sensitive halftime" also helps determine rational drug selection for infusions of different durations.

The increased interest in this field of anesthesia is exemplified by the formation of the Society of Intravenous Anesthesia which will hold its third biannual meeting this year in Europe and in the United States.

Since writing the First Edition of this book, software programs for "smart" pumps have been developed independently in California, Bonn, Germany, and Glasgow, Scotland. Currently, these are not commercially available and multidrug "smart" infusion pumps are still under development. Therefore, the field of intravenous anesthesia infusions has room to expand. Readers will find this book informative, practical, and helpful to their practice.

Robert J. Fragen

Acknowledgments

I heartily thank my colleagues who contributed chapters to this book; the staff at Lippincott-Raven Publishers for their help and patience while we wrote it; my wife, Joan, who watched me put in hours on the book that could have been leisure time spent with her and our family; and, finally, my chairman, Edward A. Brunner, M.D., Ph.D., who allowed time from clinical duties for book preparation. If the readers use the material to improve patient care, it was a worthwhile endeavor.

Drug Infusions in Anesthesiology

Second Edition

Drug Infusions in Anesthesiology, Second Edition,
edited by R. J. Fragen. Lippincott-Raven Publishers,
Philadelphia © 1996.

1

General Principles of Drug Infusions

Michael J. Avram

Department of Anesthesia, Northwestern University Medical School, Chicago, Illinois 60611

Since the early days of intravenous (IV) anesthesia, the importance of the method of drug administration in optimizing efficacy while minimizing toxicity has been well recognized. After the "short-acting barbiturates" were introduced in the early 1930s, they were often used in large doses as the sole anesthetic, sometimes with disastrous consequences (1). Perhaps the best-known consequences of this type of drug administration were the numerous anesthetic-related deaths of acutely hypovolemic casualties of Pearl Harbor, which led to the description of IV anesthesia as "an ideal method of euthanasia" (2). Fortunately, an accompanying anonymous editorial suggested that the method of drug administration, rather than the inherent toxicity of the drug, was responsible for the disastrous outcome (3). This suggestion was substantiated by an accompanying case report by Adams and Gray (4), in which they described the safe anesthetization of an acutely hypovolemic patient with "very small individual doses of pentothal sodium and a very small total dose."

Subsequent advances in the understanding of the dose-response relationship of IV anesthetics, the introduction of IV anesthetics with high elimination clearance, and the development of various drug infusion schemes and devices have made further optimization of the administration of IV anesthetics possible.

THE DOSE-RESPONSE RELATIONSHIP

Two types of dose-response relationships can be described, depending on the nature of the observed drug effect. Measures of drug effect can be quantal (i.e., nominal data, such as whether the patient is awake or asleep) or graded (i.e., interval data, such as percentage depression of baseline neuromuscular twitch). Representation of the cumulative frequency distribution of quantal responses as a function of the logarithm of the dose has a classically sigmoid shape (Fig. 1); the median effective dose (ED_{50}; e.g., MAC) provides information about the position of the log dose-cumulative frequency response curve along the abscissa. Log dose-graded response curves are also sigmoid in shape and linear from 20% to 80% of

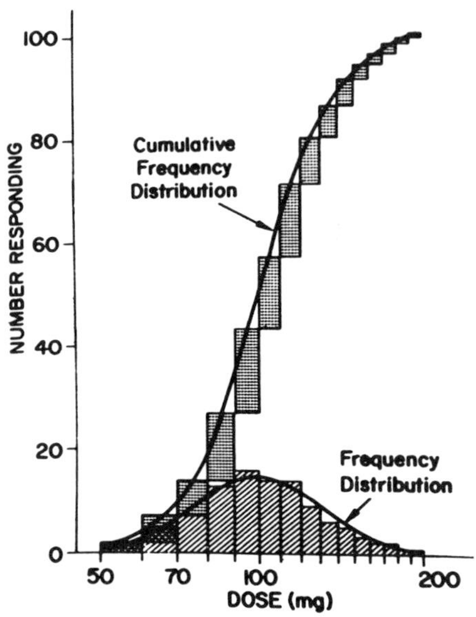

FIG. 1. Normal variability in quantal response to a dose of a drug may result in a log-normal frequency distribution (bars with diagonal lines). Expression of this log dose-quantal effect curve as a summation of the number of subjects responding at progressively larger doses results in a sigmoid cumulative frequency distribution curve (stippled bars). (From Ross and Gilman, ref. 5, with permission.)

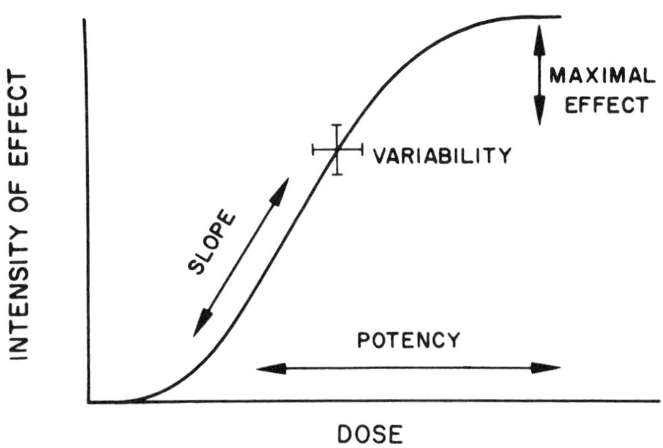

FIG. 2. The main features of the log dose-graded response curve are the maximal effect or efficacy of the drug and the position of the curve along the abscissa or the potency of the drug. The slope of this curve describes the relation between incremental changes in the dose and effect between 20% and 80% of the maximal effect. Individual variability in any of these features of the log dose-graded response relationship should be anticipated. (From Ross and Gilman, ref. 5, with permission.)

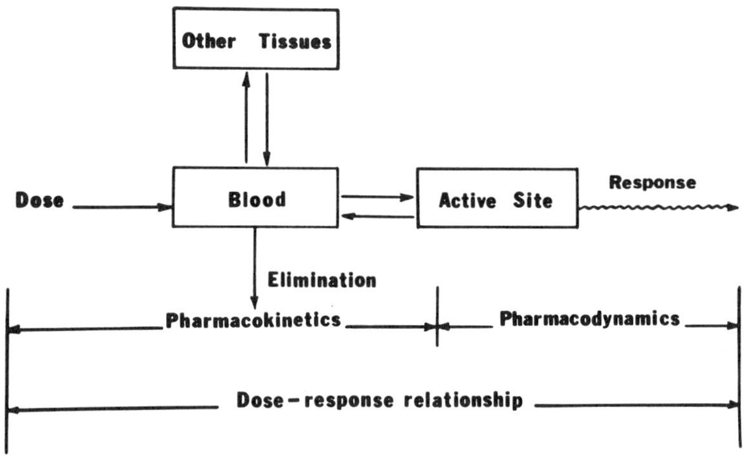

FIG. 3. The dose-response relationship for drugs that act by combining with receptors according to the laws of mass action can be subdivided into pharmacokinetics and pharmacodynamics. Pharmacokinetics describes the disposition of a dose of a drug in the body on the basis of the blood drug concentration versus time relationship, whereas pharmacodynamics describes the relationship between drug concentration at the active site (or effect compartment) and effect. (Adapted from Sheiner and Tozer, ref. 7, with permission.)

maximum effect (Fig. 2); drug potency is related to the position of this curve along the abscissa, whereas efficacy is related to the maximum effect of the drug. Variable frequency or intensity of response to a dose of a drug is a common clinical observation (Figs. 1 and 2) (5). Factors contributing to the variable response to a drug have been studied rigorously for thiopental sodium. Factors contributing to variability in induction dose requirements of thiopental include age, weight (or lean body mass), sex, and cardiac output (6).

The dose-response relationship for IV anesthetics consists of two phases: the pharmacokinetic phase and the pharmacodynamic phase (Fig. 3) (7). Pharmacokinetics describes the disposition (distribution and elimination) of a drug by the body, whereas pharmacodynamics characterizes the relationship between the concentration of the drug and the effect the drug exerts through interaction with receptors, enzymes, or other biological macromolecules according to the laws of mass action. The time to onset, duration, intensity, and variability of response to a dose of an intravenously administered anesthetic agent are affected by both its pharmacokinetics and pharmacodynamics.

PHARMACOKINETICS

Distribution

Physiological pharmacokinetic models provided the first insights into drug distribution (8,9). After IV administration, a drug mixes rapidly within the central blood pool and is distributed by blood flow and molecular diffusion throughout the tissues of the body according to their rate of perfusion, their affinity for the drug, and the relative concentration of the drug in the blood and tissues (Fig. 4). Highly perfused, relatively low-volume tissues such as the brain equilibrate rapidly with the high early blood concentrations observed after the rapid IV administration of lipid-soluble drugs, leading to the onset of effect of drugs acting on these tissues. Drug concentrations in the blood and highly perfused tissues then decrease rapidly as the drug is redistributed to the large reservoir of less well-perfused lean tissue such as muscle, terminating the effect of lipophilic drugs affecting the central nervous system. Despite its high affinity for lipophilic drugs, adipose tissue takes up drug slowly because of its poor perfusion; the amount of lipophilic drug

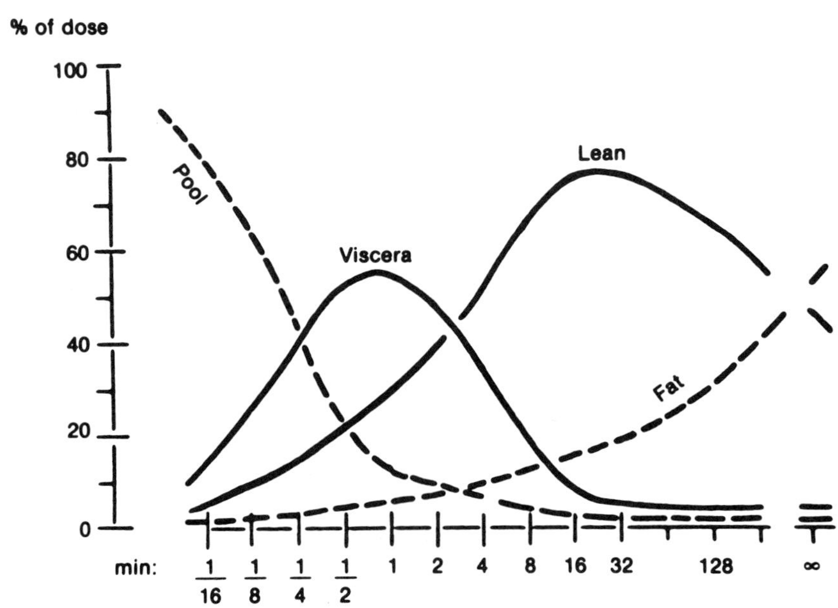

FIG. 4. The percentage of a rapidly administered dose of thiopental in the central blood pool, viscera, lean tissue, and fat as a function of time, assuming there is no elimination clearance. These data from a physiological pharmacokinetic model clearly illustrate the importance of thiopental distribution to the lean tissues for termination of its effect. They also illustrate the extremely slow distribution of drug to the poorly perfused adipose tissue and the minimal contribution of those tissues to termination of drug effect. (From Price et al., ref. 8, with permission.)

taken up by adipose tissue is insignificant until long after the effects of a single dose wane or long after an infusion is begun.

Because physiological models require extensive human data, they have largely been replaced by compartmental models (Fig. 5) which are based on the mathematical characterization of the blood drug concentration versus time relationship (Fig. 6) (10,11). The multiexponential equation describing the plasma drug concentration (C_p) at any time (t) during this relationship has the following general form:

$$C_p = \sum_{i=1}^{n} A_i e^{-\alpha t} \qquad [1]$$

where n is the number of exponential terms. From the coefficients (A_i) and exponents (α_i) of this relationship, compartmental volumes (V_i) intercompartmental clearances (Cl_{n1}, where $n>1$) and elimination clearance (Cl_E) (discussed below) are calculated (Fig. 5)(12).

In the compartmental kinetic model, drug that is injected intravenously is initially diluted within the central compartment (V_c or V_1), which includes blood and often highly perfused tissues. Almost instantaneously, the drug begins to equilibrate with other compartments; these are generally considered to be mathematical constructs that do not conform to definable tissues, although they are certainly influenced by the architecture of the body (10). The rate of equilibration with other compartments is determined by the intercompartmental clearance from V_1 to those compartments (Cl_{n1}, where $n>1$). Intercompartmental clearance depends on the

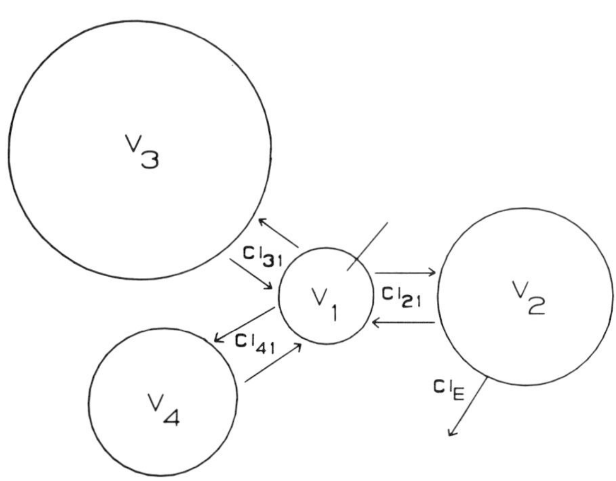

FIG. 5. A four-compartment model used to describe the disposition of thiopental after rapid IV administration (10). Drug is administered into volume 1 (V_1) and immediately begins to equilibrate with the peripheral compartments (V_2, V_3, and V_4) by intercompartmental clearance (Cl_{21}, Cl_{31}, and Cl_{41}). In this model, drug is irreversibly removed (Cl_E) from the system at V_2.

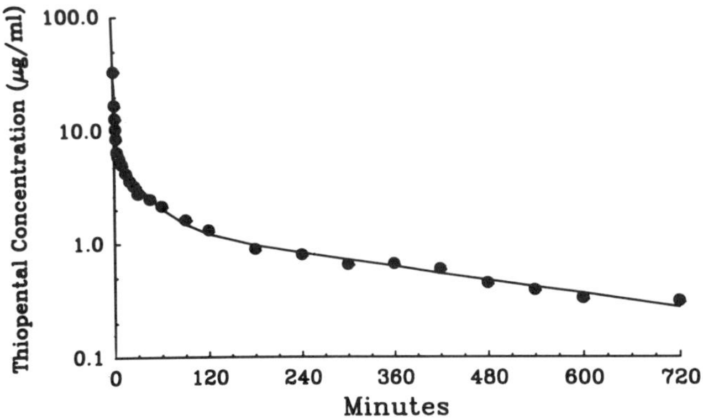

FIG. 6. The blood thiopental concentration versus time relationship after rapid IV drug administration to a representative patient. The measured thiopental concentrations in the blood (circles) are fit by computer to a quadriexponential equation (line) on which the compartmental model (Fig. 5) is based. (Data are from Henthorn et al., ref. 10). (From Fragen and Avram, ref. 11, with permission.)

blood flow to the tissues represented by the compartment and the physicochemical properties governing the rate of drug diffusion into tissues and has units of volume-per-unit time. Drug distribution is a dynamic process, governed by the laws of mass action, in which an equilibrium between blood and tissues is approached. After momentary equilibration between the blood and the rapidly equilibrating compartment is reached, there is a net movement of drug out of the compartment, which results in the redistribution of drug from the rapidly equilibrating compartment to the slowly equilibrating compartment. The total volume of distribution representing the theoretical volume that would be observed when all peripheral compartments are in equilibrium with V_1 is the steady-state volume of distribution (Vd_{ss}) and is the sum of the volumes of all compartments (1 to n). This estimate of total volume of distribution is similar to, but should not be confused with, the larger volume (Vd_{β}), which is calculated from the ratio of the dose (D) to the product of the area under the plasma drug concentration versus time curve (AUC) and the terminal slope of that curve (k_{el}), the elimination rate constant.

Clearance

Elimination clearance (Cl_E) is the irreversible removal of drug from the body; it is the sum of clearances by all mechanisms, including, principally, hepatic metabolism and renal excretion. Although Cl_E begins the moment a drug reaches its clearing organ or organs, it becomes the dominant factor in the plasma drug concentration versus time relationship only during the terminal phase of the curve—after the end of the rapid decline in plasma drug concentrations during the distribution and redistribution phases (Fig. 6). Thus, for most drugs, Cl_E is so slow relative to the distribution and redistribution of drugs that it contributes minimally to the termination of the effect of a single IV dose. However, its importance to termination of the effect of a drug given by infusion increases with the duration of the infusion.

The rate at which drug is eliminated by a clearing organ is a function of both blood flow to the organ (Q), which determines the rate of drug delivery to the organ, and the extraction ratio (E), the efficiency with which the clearing organ removes drug from the blood. Therefore, Cl_E can be affected by factors affecting blood flow to the clearing organ (or organs) or by the efficiency of the organ in removing the drug. Thus, hepatic elimination clearance (Cl_H) can be described by the following equation:

$$Cl_H = Q_H \cdot E_H \qquad [2]$$

Drugs cleared by the liver are classified on the basis of their hepatic extraction ratio (E_H)(13). Drugs with a high extraction ratio (E_H>0.7) have a Cl_H that varies only with Q_H because E_H is minimally affected by physiologic perturbations (flow-limited Cl_H). The Cl_H of low extraction ratio drugs (E_H<0.3) is independent of changes in Q_H because such changes are offset by opposite changes in E_H (capac-

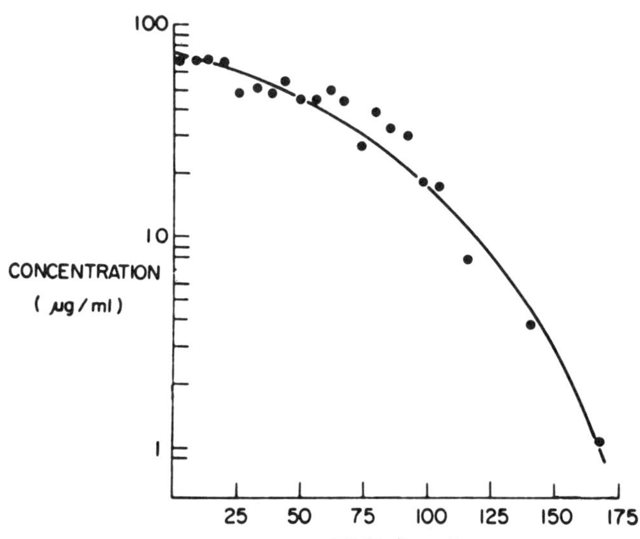

FIG 7. The blood thiopental concentration versus time relationship during the elimination phase after a 42-hr infusion of 40.2 g of the drug to a patient for cerebral resuscitation. These data illustrate nonlinear (Michaelis-Menten) elimination clearance resulting from administration of a large dose of the drug. Compare this elimination phase with the terminal phase for a standard dose of the drug in Fig. 6. (Modified from Stanski et al., ref. 14, with permission.)

ity-limited Cl_H); factors other than changes in Q_H may affect the E_H of these drugs. Factors producing changes in either Q_H or the E_H of drugs with intermediate extraction ratios ($E_H = 0.3$–0.7) can affect the clearance of these drugs.

Hepatic elimination clearance is principally by drug metabolism, which is an enzymatic process. As such, at low drug concentrations (i.e., for most drugs, at standard clinical doses administered as a bolus or a continuous infusion), there is a linear relationship between drug concentration and the rate of metabolism (i.e., a constant percentage of drug presented to the liver is metabolized). At high drug concentrations, the enzymes approach saturation and the rate of drug metabolism is not linearly related to drug concentration (i.e., a constant amount of drug is metabolized regardless of the amount of drug presented to the liver). Most drugs administered by bolus or infusion at standard doses are metabolized in a linear manner, but unpredictable metabolism is possible when large doses are administered (Fig. 7) (14).

Glomerular filtration, tubular secretion, and tubular reabsorption are the processes involved in renal clearance. Glomerular filtration depends on both renal blood flow and the efficiency with which the glomeruli filter the drug (the extraction ratio). Because of the autoregulation of renal blood flow, this flow is less variable than hepatic blood flow and, therefore, is less likely to be rate limiting in drug clearance. Because only unbound drugs are filtered, a slight decrease in the protein binding of an extensively (>90%) bound drug that is eliminated by glomerular filtration will significantly increase its glomerular filtration.

Elimination Half-Life

The elimination half-life ($t_{1/2\beta}$) is the time required for the amount of drug in the body to decrease by one-half. Elimination half-life is a dependent variable that is related directly to $V_{d\beta}$ and inversely to Cl_E:

$$t_{1/2\beta} = 0.693\, V_{d\beta}/Cl_E \qquad [3]$$

The elimination half-life can be estimated from the terminal slope of the plasma drug concentration versus time relationship (k_{el}):

$$t_{1/2\beta} = 0.693/k_{el} \qquad [4]$$

Because the effect of a standard dose of intravenously administered drug usually terminates during the redistribution phase of the plasma drug concentration versus time relationship, $t_{1/2\beta}$ provides no information about the time to termination of its effect. Even when multiple doses or continuous infusions of drug are given and a steady-state is approached, recovery is always faster than predicted from $t_{1/2\beta}$ (15).

Accumulation

Accumulation, or a progressive increase in the amount of drug in the body during multiple-dose or infusion regimens, will occur until a steady-state is achieved. At steady-state, all compartments are in equilibrium and there is no net distribution of administered drug because the dosing rate (I) exactly matches the Cl_E. The steady-state plasma drug concentration (C_{ss}) is predictable from these variables:

$$C_{ss} = I/Cl_E \quad [5]$$

The accumulation of drug in indifferent body tissues during an infusion was described as early as 1960 by Price (9), who correctly noted that the longer the duration of infusion, the less the dilutional capacity of these indifferent tissues upon termination of the infusion. As a result, after infusions of all but the briefest duration, recovery from an infusion is slower than it would be after rapid IV (bolus) administration.

Shafer and Varvel (16) formally analyzed the relationship between the duration of infusion and the time necessary to achieve given percentage decreases in targeted drug concentrations necessary to reach recovery (threshold) concentrations for fentanyl, alfentanil, and sufentanil. These simulations emphasized the importance of distributive characteristics of drugs to the termination of drug effect. Subsequent analysis by Youngs and Shafer (17) interpreted these results in straightforward pharmacokinetic terms. High elimination clearance always contributes to short recovery times. Large peripheral distribution volumes and high intercompartmental clearances enable sufficient drug redistribution to terminate drug effect relatively rapidly after brief infusions or when small decreases in concentrations are required. Conversely, large peripheral compartment volumes and high intercompartmental clearances return drug to the central compartment rapidly enough and long enough to prolong termination of drug effect after long infusions or when large decreases in concentrations are required. These insights provide a rational basis for selecting the best opioid for the anticipated duration of infusion, the expected intensity of stimuli, and the characteristics of the desired recovery (16,17).

Context-Sensitive Half-Time

Although the elimination half-life may be a basic pharmacokinetic variable for a drug, knowledge of the time required for the amount of drug in the body to decrease by half does not allow comparison of postinfusion drug characteristics because it only describes the decrease in drug concentration in the central compartment during the elimination phase. To rectify this, Hughes and colleagues (18) introduced the concept of context-sensitive half-time, the time required for the drug concentration in the central compartment to decrease by 50% after an infusion of a given duration (the context). This term is far more appropriate than the

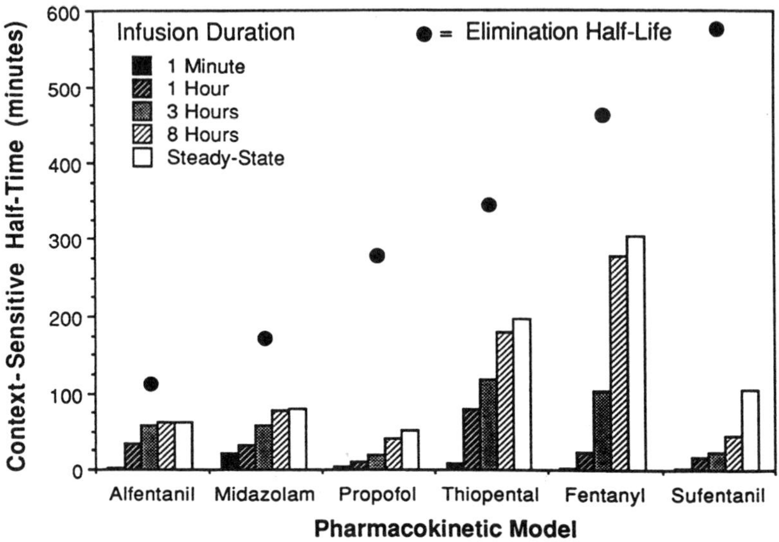

FIG. 8. Context-sensitive half-times for six IV anesthetic agents after infusions of various durations. Traditional elimination half-lives for the drugs are also indicated to allow comparison with the context-sensitive half-lives. Even the longest context-sensitive half-times (those after steady-state infusions) are significantly shorter than the elimination half-lives. (From Hughes et al., ref 18, with permission.)

elimination half-life for describing postinfusion drug kinetics because it is a simple variable reflecting the effects of the extent of drug accumulation during the infusion and the potential for drug redistribution after termination of the infusion in addition to the effect of elimination clearance. Youngs and Shafer (17) called the context-sensitive half-time the 50% decrement time to avoid confusion with elimination half-life and emphasized its description of a decrease in drug concentration in the central compartment (17).

The context-sensitive half-times for six commonly used anesthetic drugs after infusions of various durations ranging from 1 minute to steady-state are illustrated in Fig. 8 (18). The lack of relationship between the context-sensitive half-time and the elimination half-time is obvious from this figure.

The context-sensitive half-time or 50% decrement time should be used with the understanding that the time to terminate the drug effect may be less or more than the context-sensitive half-time if a decrease in drug concentration smaller or larger than 50%, respectively, is necessary to terminate the drug effect. In addition, the context-sensitive half-time cannot be extrapolated to predict times to smaller or larger decrements in drug concentration for a given infusion rate.

PHARMACODYNAMICS

The importance of the pharmacokinetic description of the drug concentration versus time relationship for a dose of a drug rests on the premise that there is a relationship between drug concentration and effect. This latter relationship is described by pharmacodynamics (19).

The relationship between steady-state plasma drug concentration (C) and graded drug effect (E) from no effect to the maximum effect (E_{max}) can be characterized by a sigmoid E_{max} pharmacodynamic model. This model uses the Hill equation:

$$E = \frac{E_{max} \cdot C^{\gamma}}{EC_{50}{}^{\gamma} + C^{\gamma}} \quad [6]$$

where γ is a variable influencing the slope and sigmoidicity of the curve and EC_{50} is the steady-state plasma drug concentration producing half the maximum effect. In the special case where $\gamma = 1$, the model is called the E_{max} effect model.

A pharmacodynamic model similar to the sigmoid E_{max} model for graded drug effect has been described for quantal drug response (20). This model describes

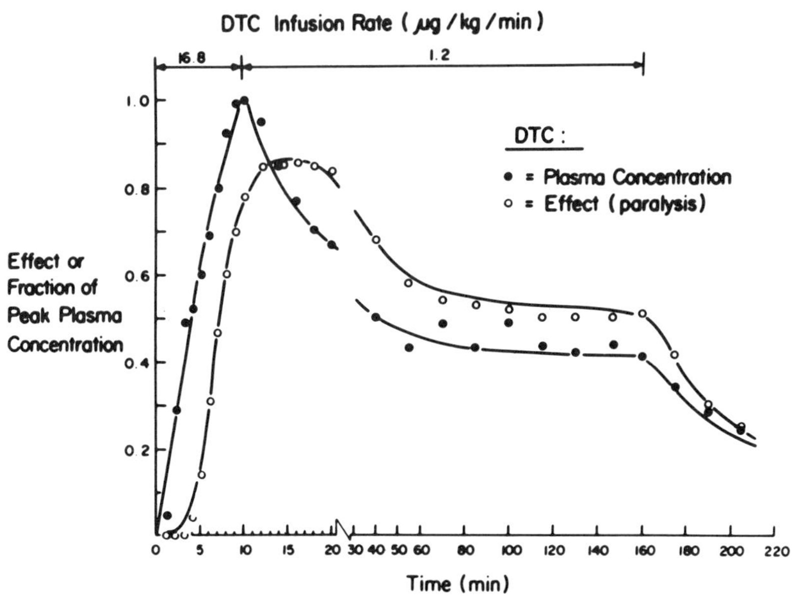

FIG. 9. The plasma D-tubocurarine (DTC) concentration versus time relationship during and after an infusion of the drug (closed circles) and the corresponding twitch height suppression (open circles) with a computer-generated fit of the data (solid lines). The delayed onset and offset of the effect of DTC is an illustration of counterclockwise hysteresis resulting from an equilibration delay between drug concentrations in the plasma and those at the effector site. (From Stanski et al., ref. 21, with permission.)

the probability of drug response (P) as a function of steady-state plasma drug concentration (C), the steady-state plasma drug concentration that produces a 50% probability of response (CP_{50}), and γ, as described above. Thus,

$$P = \frac{C^{\gamma}}{CP_{50}^{\ \gamma} + C^{\gamma}} \qquad [7]$$

COMBINED PHARMACOKINETIC-PHARMACODYNAMIC MODELS

Whereas pharmacodynamic models often describe the relationship between steady-state plasma drug concentrations and drug effect, steady-state drug concentrations are seldom observed in clinical anesthesia. For intravenously administered anesthetic agents, an equilibration delay often occurs between the drug concentrations in plasma and those at the effector site; hence there is a delayed onset of effect (this is called counterclockwise hysteresis) (Fig. 9) (21). Fortunately, the rate of equilibration between plasma and effector site, or biophase, is a first-order process. The time course of drug concentrations in the biophase can be predicted in a multicompartmental model on the basis of the time course of plasma drug concentrations and that of drug effect. The biophase drug concentrations are then used in the Hill equation instead of steady-state concentrations (Fig. 10) (21). From the combined pharmacokinetic-pharmacodynamic model, the rate constant characterizing the equilibration of drug in plasma with that at its

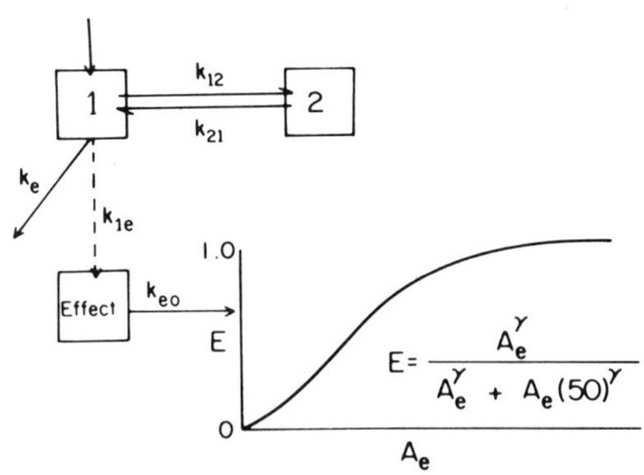

FIG. 10. A combined pharmacokinetic-pharmacodynamic model of D-tubocurarine (DTC). After infusion into the central compartment (1), DTC distributes to a tissue compartment (2), as determined by the transfer rate constants (k_{12} and k_{21}), while being cleared from the body, as determined by the elimination rate constant (k_e). The effect compartment is the biophase of drug effect, with the rate constants k_{1e} and k_{eo} determining the rate of onset and the rate of offset of effect. The sigmoidal steady-state plasma DTC concentration versus effect relationship can be described using these variables and the Hill equation (Eq. 6), which assumes the form in the figure because here $E_{max} = 1$. (From Stanski et al., ref. 21, with permission.)

site of action (k_{eo}) can be characterized, and from this the equilibration half-time for drug effect can be calculated:

$$t_{1/2keo} = \ln 2/k_{eo} \qquad [8]$$

The history of the central compartment drug concentration determines the history of drug concentration at the effect site. Therefore, different pharmacokinetic models predict different biophase drug concentration histories for a given k_{eo}, making k_{eo} model dependent (22). In addition, for a given pharmacokinetic model, more rapid equilibration between the central compartment and the biophase (i.e., a shorter $t_{1/2keo}$) is determined by a larger k_{eo} (22). Finally, the difference between the central compartment drug concentration and the effect site drug concentration is significant only after the drug is administered as a bolus or during brief infusions (17).

DRUG INFUSIONS

Drug infusions are optimally based on well-characterized pharmacokinetic and pharmacodynamic (e.g., effective plasma drug concentration) data. Individualization of an infusion regimen requires knowledge not only of the average kinetic data from well-designed and well-conducted studies but also of the variability of the data and the identifiable factors that contribute to the variability (i.e., the population pharmacokinetics). Two methods of estimating population pharmacokinetics are the standard two-stage method (STS) and the first-order method (FO) (23).

The first stage of the STS method of estimating population pharmacokinetics for a drug consists of the description of individual pharmacokinetic models for a relatively small number of subjects. Average pharmacokinetic variables and indexes of their variability are then calculated, and correlations of the individual variables with age, weight, sex, and so forth are sought in the second stage. Because the STS estimate of population pharmacokinetics is frequently based on data from a limited number of subjects, it may not identify the sources of pharmacokinetic variability as readily as does the FO method.

The FO method of estimating the population pharmacokinetics of a drug pools the plasma drug concentration versus time and dose administration data from a relatively large number of individuals. With these data and patient demographic data, this complex analysis produces a kinetic model with an estimate of not only intrasubject variability but also intersubject variability and the contribution of patient characteristics to that variability.

Drug infusions can be either open-loop or closed-loop regimens (24). Open-loop drug infusions make no formal allowance for individualizing the drug infusion on the basis of the patient's response. They are fixed regimens that are often based on conservative estimates of the effective plasma drug concentration and the pharmacokinetics of the drug. Although such drug infusions may produce effective drug concentrations in most patients, one should expect some patients to have plasma drug concentrations that are inadequate and others to have concentrations that are too high, resulting in a relatively prolonged drug effect on termination of the infusion.

Closed-loop infusion regimens are individualized to a patient's needs by feedback control of the infusion rate, which closes the loop (25). Such an infusion requires an unequivocal measure of drug effect that the infusion rapidly achieves and maintains; unequivocal measures of drug effect are not available for many of the drugs used by anesthesiologists. A computer, the anesthesiologist, or even the patient (e.g., in patient-controlled analgesia) monitoring the effect adjusts the rate at which the drug is being given, increasing the rate if the effect is too low, maintaining it if the effect is appropriate, or decreasing it if the effect is too high.

The longer an infusion is maintained, the closer the tissues of the body approach equilibrium with the concentrations of drug in the blood (i.e., steady-state). The closer the body is to steady-state, the less important is redistribution and the more important is elimination clearance to the termination of drug effect (compare Figs. 6 and 7). Therefore, drugs with a high elimination clearance are most suitable for administration by continuous IV infusion because the contribution of high elimination clearance to the offset of drug effect will facilitate rapid reversal of drug effect on termination of the infusion. Several drugs available for use in the practice of anesthesia have high or relatively high elimination clearances that make them suitable for administration by continuous IV infusion.

Open-Loop Infusions

A predictable and effective steady-state plasma drug concentration can be produced and maintained by a continuous, constant rate of IV infusion of sufficient duration. Rearrangement of Eq. 5 gives the infusion rate (I) necessary to produce the desired steady-state plasma drug concentration (C_{ss}) in the presence of a given elimination clearance (Cl_E). Thus,

$$I = C_{ss} \cdot Cl_E \qquad [9]$$

However, if only such an infusion were used, it would take a long time for the infusion to produce plasma drug concentrations within 10% of the desired concentrations. Infusion of a drug in this manner will not meet the needs of the anesthesiologist who must rapidly achieve and maintain effective drug concentrations.

The steady-state plasma drug concentrations determined by the infusion rate and the elimination clearance during a continuous, constant-rate infusion are not reached until the drug concentrations in the tissues of the body are in equilibrium with the concentration in the blood, that is, until drug distribution is complete.

TABLE 1. *Midazolam bolus and infusion calculation*[a]

Loading dose	$= C_{ss} \cdot Vd_{\beta}$
	$= 0.17$ μg/ml · 1600 ml/kg
	$= 270$ μg/kg or about 0.25 mg/kg
Infusion rate	$= C_{ss} \cdot Cl_{E}$
	$= 0.17$ μg/ml · 440 ml/min
	$= 75$ μg/min $= 4.5$ mg/hr

[a] Calculated using the method of Mitenko and Ogilvie (26) and data from Avram et al. (29)

Several practical methods of drug administration will produce effective drug concentrations rapidly and maintain them during and after the drug distribution phase. The simple combined bolus and infusion method of Mitenko and Ogilvie (26) rapidly produces effective plasma drug concentrations and maintains them until the infusion is terminated. The bolus or loading dose is the dose that would produce the desired plasma drug concentration if it achieved instantaneous equilibration throughout the tissues of the body:

$$\text{Loading dose} = C_{ss} \cdot V_{d\beta} \qquad [10]$$

The loading dose is administered concomitantly with the commencement of an infusion matched to the elimination clearance (Eq. 9). A potential disadvantage of this method is that plasma drug concentrations are high initially and remain high throughout the distribution phase because equilibration of the load-

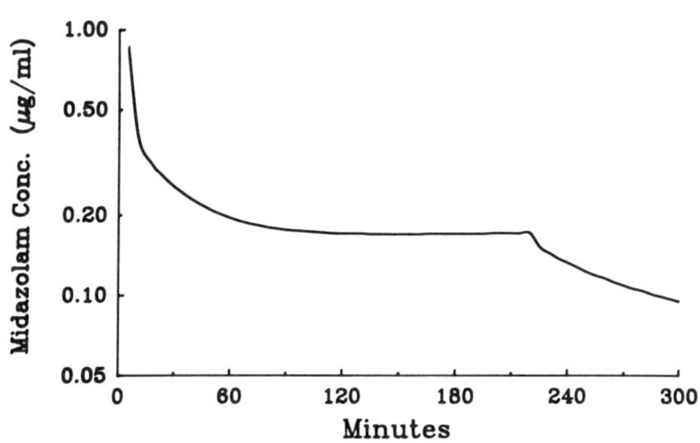

FIG. 11. A computer simulation of plasma midazolam concentration versus time relationship during and after 220 minutes of the bolus and infusion scheme calculated in Table 1. The loading dose is 0.25 mg/kg and the infusion rate is 4.5 mg/hr. Notice the extremely high early drug concentrations. This is characteristic of those seen in any Mitenko and Ogilvie infusion scheme (26) and is perfectly acceptable for a drug with a sufficiently large clinical margin of safety, such as midazolam, being infused for a sufficiently long time (more than 1/2 hr). (Based on data from ref. 29.)

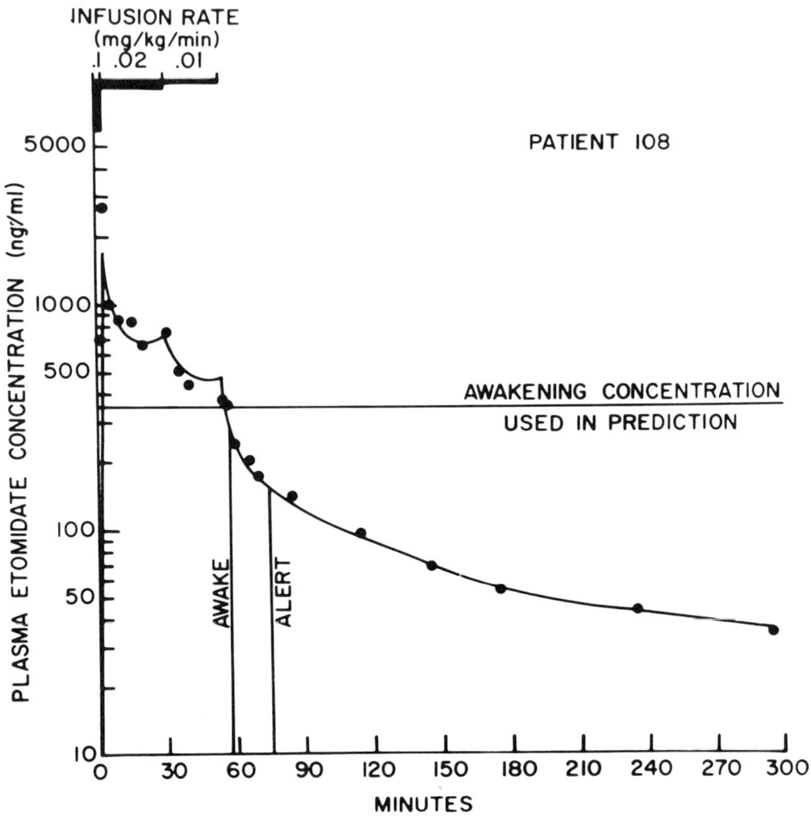

FIG. 12. A plasma etomidate concentration versus time relationship during and after a three-stage infusion of etomidate lasting nearly one hour. The infusion rates are as indicated on the figure. The infusion scheme was developed from computer simulations using published etomidate pharmacokinetics with the goal of maintaining effective plasma etomidate concentrations from the beginning of the infusion while avoiding the relatively long period of extremely high drug concentrations seen in a Mitenko and Ogilvie infusion scheme (see Fig. 11). (From Fragen et al., ref. 30, with permission.)

ing dose throughout the tissues is not instantaneous. As a result, the infusion method of Mitenko and Ogilvie (26) is appropriate only for drugs with high clinical margins of safety in the hands of anesthesiologists: for example, muscle relaxants (27,28) and midazolam (Table 1, Fig. 11) (29) but not for drugs such as thiopental, propofol, and alfentanil, which have relatively low clinical margins of safety.

An infusion regimen for a drug with a low clinical margin of safety must minimize initial plasma drug concentrations and side effects, yet maintain effective drug concentrations throughout the infusion (Fig. 12) (30). This can be accom-

TABLE 2. *Alfentanil bolus and infusion calculation*[a]

Loading dose	$= C_{ss} \cdot Vd_{\beta}$
	= 0.3 μg/ml · 380 ml/kg
	= 114 μg/kg!!!
	Note: The predicted dose for this drug is unsafe. It should be divided into 4–6 doses of 25 μg/kg given over 30 min.
Infusion rate	$= C_{ss} \cdot Cl_{E}$
	= 0.3 μg/ml · 32 ml/kg/min
	= 0.96 μg/kg/min or about 1.0 μg/kg/min

[a] Calculated using the method of Mitenko and Ogilvie (26) and data from Henthorn et al. (31) and Ausems et al. (20)

plished by choosing a smaller loading dose on the basis of the desired plasma drug concentrations and the relatively small initial volume of distribution rather than the total volume of distribution. Effective plasma drug concentrations can then be maintained during the distributive phase by using an intermediate infusion rate that matches elimination clearance and compensates for drug loss from the central to the peripheral compartments during the period of extensive drug distribution. The terminal infusion is matched to elimination clearance as before (Eq. 9). Alternatively, if the terminal infusion matched to elimination clearance (Eq. 9) is begun with the administration of the small loading dose, effective plasma drug

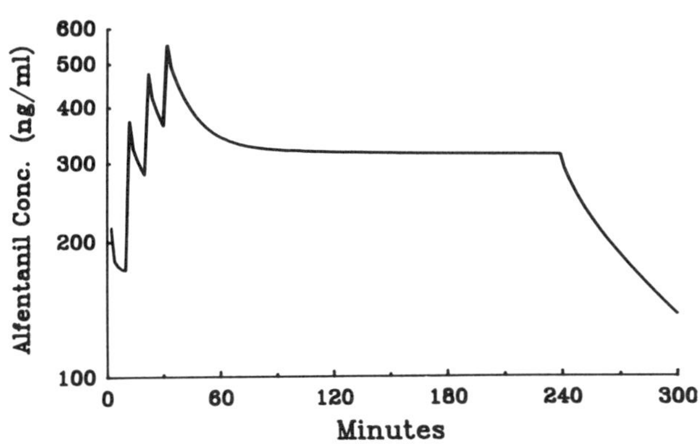

FIG. 13. A computer simulation of the plasma alfentanil concentration versus time relationship during and after four hours of the multiple bolus and infusion scheme calculated in Table 2. The "loading dose" of alfentanil is given as four doses of 25 μg/kg over 30 minutes and the infusion of 1.0 μg/kg/min is maintained from the beginning of drug administration. This approach to administering alfentanil clearly avoids excessively high drug concentrations but does not consistently achieve the target concentration until after the second dose is given. (Based on data from refs. 20 and 31.)

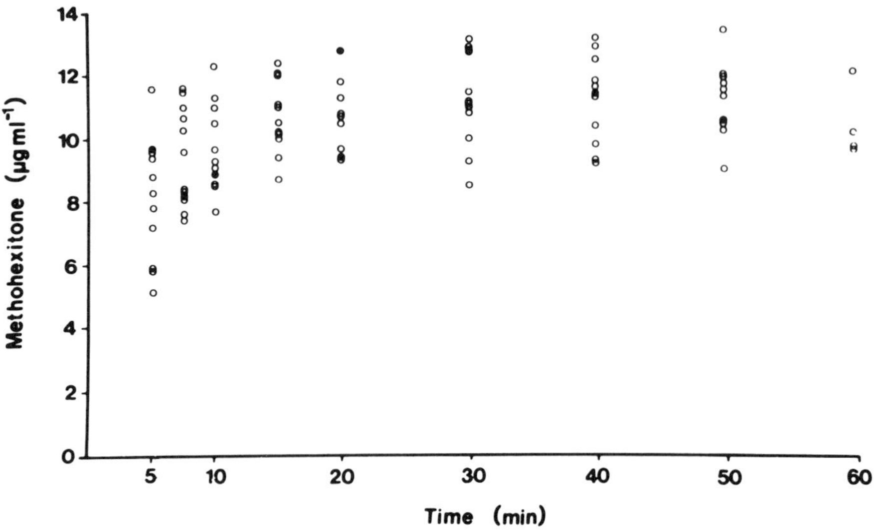

FIG. 14. Plasma drug concentration versus time relationships for 12 patients during an infusion of methohexital using the exponentially decreasing infusion rate method of Krüger-Thiemer (32). (The solid circles are coincident points.) This infusion was used with reasonable success to provide hypnosis as part of an anesthetic regimen that also included N_2O and fentanyl. (From McMurray et al., ref. 33, with permission.)

concentrations can be maintained during the period of extensive drug distribution by a brief series of small bolus doses (Table 2, Fig. 13) (20,31).

An ideal drug infusion regimen to achieve and maintain constant plasma drug concentrations rapidly was proposed by Krüger-Thiemer in 1968 (32). This regimen combines a loading dose with an exponentially decreasing infusion rate. The loading dose is designed to produce the desired plasma drug concentration after mixing within the initial distribution volume (V_1):

$$\text{Loading dose} = C_{ss} \cdot V_1 \qquad [11]$$

The exponentially decreasing infusion rate is matched not only to elimination clearance but also to drug distribution. For the simplest case of an infusion regimen based on a two-compartment pharmacokinetic model of drug being infused, the maintenance infusion is described by the following relationship:

$$I = C_{ss}(Cl_E + Cl_{12}e^{-k_{21}t}), \qquad [12]$$

where Cl_{12} is the intercompartmental clearance (Fig. 5), k_{21} is the rate constant from V_2 to V_1 and t is the duration of the exponential infusion. Krüger-Thiemer infu-

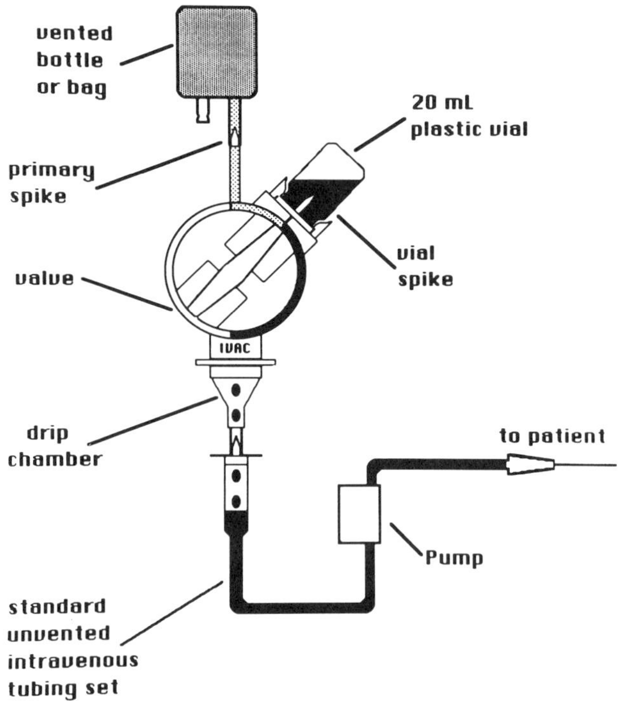

FIG. 15. An apparatus for administering an infusion at an exponentially decreasing rate, as described by Ambre et al. (34), who report that this apparatus is set up and used as easily as any standard IV infusion. (From Avram and Henthorn, ref. 35, with permission.)

sions of IV anesthetics have been successfully applied to IV anesthetics using a dilutional method of exponential drug delivery (Fig. 14) (33).

An inexpensive apparatus for administering an exponentially decreasing infusion that is as easy to set up and use as a standard IV infusion system has been described by Ambre and colleagues (Fig. 15) (34,35). Computer-controlled infusion pumps also can administer drugs on the basis of their pharmacokinetics. These pumps have algorithms based on approximations of pharmacokinetic differential equations that allow them to provide desired plasma drug concentrations on command (36–38). For drugs that equilibrate rapidly with the biophase (e.g., alfentanil), computer-controlled targeting of plasma drug concentrations may be appropriate. However, because of the disequilibrium between the plasma and the biophase after a loading dose or a change in infusion rate, targeting biophase concentrations for drugs that equilibrate more slowly with the biophase is more appropriate (17,39) (e.g., fentanyl, midazolam). Computer-controlled pump algorithms that allow rapid achievement and maintenance of stable drug concentrations

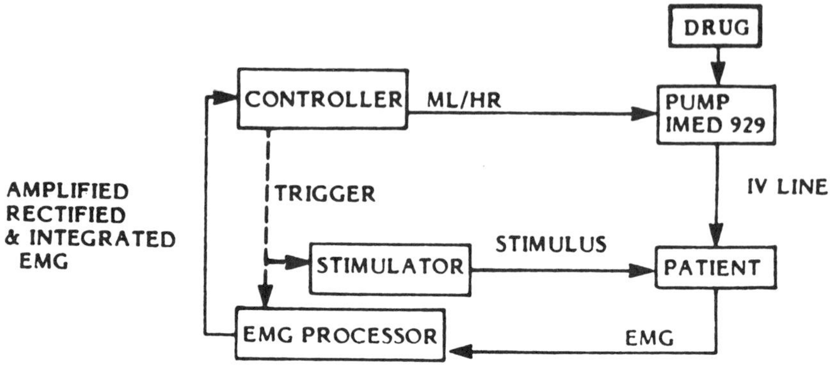

FIG. 16. A control system for a closed-loop infusion of muscle relaxants, as described by Ebert et al. (43). (From Ebert et al., ref. 43, with permission.)

at the effect site have been developed (40). Thus, computer-controlled infusion pumps have the ability to be for IV anesthetics what the vaporizer is for potent volatile anesthetics.

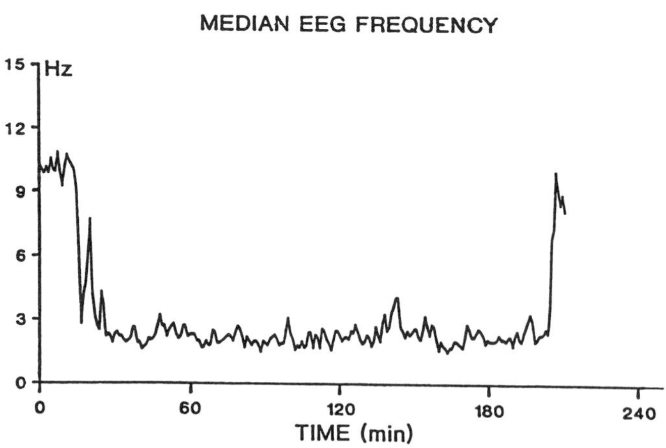

FIG. 17. The median EEG frequency versus time relationship recorded during a computer-based closed-loop infusion of methohexital. The feedback-controlled infusion was designed to maintain a median EEG frequency of 2–3 Hz in flunitrazepam-premedicated patients who also received fentanyl by infusion. (From Schwilden et al., ref. 45, with permission.)

Closed-Loop Infusions

Anesthesiologists can close the open-loop infusions described above by vigilantly monitoring the patient for signs of adequate response to the drug being infused or by anticipating the patient's needs and adjusting the infusion rate accordingly, just as they would adjust the concentration of a volatile anesthetic on the basis of a patient's needs. Such a variable rate infusion has been described for alfentanil (20,41,42).

Feedback control of drug infusions is also based on computer monitoring of a measure of drug effect and adjustment of the infusion on the basis of the monitored measurement. A diagram of such a control system is represented in Fig. 16. The measure of drug effect monitored in such a closed-loop drug infusion system may be unequivocal (e.g., the electromyogram [EMG] monitoring the effects of muscle relaxants) or equivocal (e.g., the electroencephalogram [EEG] monitoring the effect of hypnotics or narcotics). The EMG-based closed-loop infusion of muscle relaxants has been used successfully (43,44). The EEG-based infusion of a barbiturate was less successful in volunteers, especially if they were unstimulated (45), but it was used successfully in patients who were premedicated with flunitrazepam, were undergoing general surgery, and also received a narcotic by infusion (46) (Fig. 17). As the ability to monitor the effects of drugs that are clearly related to their contribution to anesthesia improves, computer-based closed-loop drug infusions are likely to represent an attractive method of drug administration (25).

USES OF INFUSIONS

Many drugs are available that have pharmacokinetic properties making them suitable for easily predictable administration by continuous IV infusion. Many of the general approaches to drug infusions described above and the commercial availability of infusion pumps make such administration practicable. A recently described pocket-calculator program (47) that estimates the plasma drug concentration at any time during and after a drug infusion can help anesthesiologists understand drug administration by infusion the way they understand the administration of inhalational anesthetics.

Continuous IV drug infusions can be used to produce sedation, hypnosis, analgesia, or muscle relaxation. Such infusions can be used together to produce total IV anesthesia, or they can be used selectively as adjuvants to nitrous oxide, the potent volatile anesthetics, or regional anesthetic techniques. They also have considerable utility in the postoperative period and critical care setting.

The advantages of continuous IV drug infusion techniques over intermittent dose administration are similar to the advantages of intermittent doses over the "industrial" dose administration described in 1943 (3,4). Continuous IV drug infusions use lower total doses than intermittent bolus techniques do, yet they provide better control of the effects of the drug (48). They allow optimum efficacy of the drug while minimizing drug toxicity and shortening recovery times.

ACKNOWLEDGMENTS

The author would like to thank Thomas K. Henthorn, MD, and Tom C. Krejcie, MD, for their assistance with the simulations and graphics.

REFERENCES

1. Dundee JW. Fifty years of thiopentone. *Br J Anaesth* 1984;56:211–213.
2. Halford FJ. A critique of intravenous anesthesia in war surgery. *Anesthesiology* 1943;4:67–69.
3. Editorial. The question of intravenous anesthesia in war surgery. *Anesthesiology* 1943;4:74–77.
4. Adams RC, Gray HK. Intravenous anesthesia with pentothal sodium in the case of gunshot wound associated with accompanying severe traumatic shock and loss of blood: report of a case. *Anesthesiology* 1943;4:70–73.
5. Ross EM, Gilman AG. Pharmacodynamics: mechanisms of drug action and the relationship between drug concentration and effect. In: Gilman AG, et al, eds. *Goodman and Gilman's The pharmacologic basis of therapeutics*. 7th ed. New York: Macmillan; 1985:35–48.
6. Avram MJ, Sanghvi R, Henthorn TK, Krejcie TC, Shanks CA, Fragen RJ, Howard KA, Kaczynski DA. Determinants of thiopental induction dose requirements. *Anesth Analg* 1993;76:10–17.
7. Sheiner LB, Tozer TN. Clinical pharmacokinetics: the use of plasma concentrations of drugs. In: Melmon KL, Morelli HF, eds. *Clinical pharmacology: basic principles in therapeutics*. New York: Macmillan; 1978:71–109.
8. Price HL, Kovnat PJ, Safer JN, Conner EH, Price ML. The uptake of thiopental by body tissues and its relation to the duration of narcosis. *Clin Pharmacol Ther* 1960;1:16–22.
9. Price HL. A dynamic concept of the distribution of thiopental in the human body. *Anesthesiology* 1960;21:40–45.
10. Henthorn TK, Avram MJ, Krejcie TC. Intravascular mixing and drug distribution: the concurrent disposition of thiopental and indocyanine green. *Clin Pharmacol Ther* 1989;45:56–65.
11. Fragen RJ, Avram MJ. Barbiturates. In: Miller RD, ed. *Anesthesia*. 4th ed. New York: Churchill Livingstone; 1994:229–246.
12. Gibaldi M, Perrier D. *Pharmacokinetics*. 2nd ed. New York: Marcel Dekker; 1982.
13. Wilkinson GR, Shand DG. A physiological approach to hepatic drug clearance. *Clin Pharmacol Ther* 1975;18:377–390.
14. Stanski DR, Mihm FG, Rosenthal MH, Kalman SM. Pharmacokinetics of high-dose thiopental used in cerebral resuscitation. *Anesthesiology* 1980;53:169–171.
15. Shafer SL, Stanski DR. Improving the clinical utility of anesthetic drug pharmacokinetics. *Anesthesiology* 1992;76:327–330.
16. Shafer SL, Varvel JR. Pharmacokinetics, pharmacodynamics, and rational opioid selection. *Anesthesiology* 1991;74:53–64.
17. Youngs EJ, Shafer SL. Pharmacokinetic parameters relevant to recovery from opioids. *Anesthesiology* 1994;81:833–842.
18. Hughes MA, Glass PSA, Jacobs JR. Context-sensitive half-time in multicompartmental pharmacokinetic models for intravenous anesthetic drugs. *Anesthesiology* 1992;76:334–341.
19. Holford NHG, Sheiner LB. Understanding the dose-effect relationship: clinical application of pharmacokinetic-pharmacodynamic models. *Clin Pharmacokinet* 1981;6:429–453.
20. Ausems ME, Hug CC, Jr., Stanski DR, Burm AGL. Plasma concentrations of alfentanil required to supplement nitrous oxide anesthesia for general surgery. *Anesthesiology* 1986;65:362–373.
21. Stanski DR, Ham J, Miller RD, Sheiner LB. Pharmacokinetics and pharmacodynamics of d-tubocurarine during nitrous oxide-narcotic and halothane anesthesia in man. *Anesthesiology* 1979;51:235–241.
22. Gentry WB, Krejcie TC, Henthorn TK, Shanks CA, Howard KA, Gupta DK, Avram MJ. Effect of in-

fusion rate on thiopental dose-response relationships: Assessment of a pharmacokinetic-pharmacodynamic model. *Anesthesiology* 1994;81:316–324.
23. Beal SL, Sheiner LB. Methodology of population pharmacokinctics. In: Garrett ER, Hirtz JL, eds. *Drug fate and metabolism methods and techniques*. Vol 5. New York: Marcel Dekker; 1985:135–183.
24. Vozeh S, Steimer JL. Feedback control methods for drug dosage optimisation: concepts, classification and clinical application. *Clin Pharmacokinet* 1985;10:457–476.
25. O'Hara DA, Bogen DK, Noordergraaf A. The use of computers for controlling the delivery of anesthesia. *Anesthesiology* 1992;77:563–581.
26. Mitenko PA, Ogilvie RI. Rapidly achieved plasma concentration plateaus, with observations on theophylline kinetics. *Clin Pharmacol Ther* 1972;13:329–335.
27. Shanks CA. Pharmacokinetics of the nondepolarizing neuromuscular relaxants: application to calculation of bolus and infusion dosage regimens. *Anesthesiology* 1986;64:72–86.
28. Shanks CA, Avram MJ, Fragen RJ, O'Hara DA. Pharmacokinetics and pharmacodynamics of vecuronium administered by bolus and infusion during halothane or balanced anesthesia. *Clin Pharmacol Ther* 1987;42:459–464.
29. Avram MJ, Fragen RJ, Caldwell NJ. Midazolam kinetics in women of two age groups. *Clin Pharmacol Ther* 1983;34:505–508.
30. Fragen RJ, Avram MJ, Henthom TK, Caldwell NJ. A pharmacokinetically designed etomidate infusion regimen for hypnosis. *Anesth Analg* 1983;62:654–660.
31. Henthorn TK, Avram MJ, Krejcie TC. Alfentanil clearance is independent of the polymorphic debrisoquin hydroxylase. *Anesthesiology* 1989;71:635–639.
32. Krüger-Thiemer E. Continuous intravenous infusion and multicompartment accumulation. *Eur J Pharmacol* 1968;4:317–324.
33. McMurray TJ, Robinson FP, Dundee JW, Ridell JG, McLean E. A method for producing constant plasma concentrations of drugs: application to methohexitone. *Br J Anaesth* 1986;58:1085–1090.
34. Ambre JJ, Smith-Coggins R, Belknap S, Nelson J. A technique for producing constant plasma drug concentrations. *Ann Intern Med* 1987;107:122.
35. Avram MJ, Henthorn TK. What's new in pharmacokinetics and pharmacodynamics? *Anesth Clin North Am* 1988;6(special issue):257–280.
36. Schwilden H, Schüttler J, Stoeckel H. Pharmacokinetics as applied to total intravenous anesthesia: theoretical considerations. *Anaesthesia* 1983;38:51–52.
37. Schüttler J, Schwilden H, Stoeckel H. Pharmacokinetics as applied to total intravenous anesthesia: practical implications. *Anaesthesia* 1983;38:53–56.
38. Shafer SL, Siegel LC, Cooke JE, Scott JC. Testing computer-controlled infusion pumps by simulation. *Anesthesiology* 1988;68:261–266.
39. Jacobs JR, Reves JG. Effect site equilibration time is a determinant of induction dose requirement. *Anesth Analg* 1993;76:1–6.
40. Shafer SL, Gregg KM. Algorithms to rapidly achieve and maintain stable drug concentrations at the site of drug effect with a computer-controlled infusion pump. *J Pharmacokinet Biopharm* 1992;20: 147–169.
41. Shafer A, Sung M-L, White PF. Pharmacokinetics and pharmacodynamics of alfentanil infusions during general anesthesia. *Anesth Analg* 1986;65:1021–1028.
42. Fragen RJ, Avram MJ, Henthorn TK, Asada A, Pemberton D, Correll T. Total intravenous anesthesia with propofol, alfentanil, and vecuronium for superficial surgery. *Anesth Analg* 1990;70:Sl12.
43. Ebert J, Caroll SK, Bradley EL, Jr. Closed-loop feedback control of muscle relaxation with vecuronium in surgical patients. *Anesth Analg* 1986;65:S44.
44. Ritchie G, Ebert JP, Jannett TC, Kissin I, Sheppard LC. A microcomputer based controller for neuromuscular block during surgery. *Ann Biomed Eng* 1985;13:3–15.
45. Schwilden H, Schüttler J, Stoeckel H. Closed-loop feedback control of methohexital anesthesia by quantitative EEG analysis in humans. *Anesthesiology* 1987;67:341–347.
46. Schwilden H, Stoeckel H. Effective therapeutic infusions produced by closed-loop feedback control of methohexital administration during total intravenous anesthesia with fentanyl. *Anesthesiology* 1990; 73:225–229.
47. Maitre PO, Shafer SL. A simple pocket calculator approach to predict anesthetic drug concentrations from pharmacokinetic data. *Anesthesiology* 1990;73:332–336.
48. White PF. Clinical uses of intravenous anesthetic and analgesic infusions. *Anaesth Analg* 1989;68: 161–171.

Drug Infusions in Anesthesiology, Second Edition,
edited by R. J. Fragen. Lippincott-Raven Publishers,
Philadelphia © 1996.

2

Intravenous Drug Delivery Systems

Peter S. A. Glass

Department of Anesthesiology, Duke University Medical Center, Durham, North Carolina 27710

For a drug to be effective, it must enter the body and reach the cellular or subcellular site of action. The way a drug is introduced into the body can be considered the drug delivery system. This chapter discusses drug delivery systems used by anesthesiologists to administer conventionally administered drugs by continuous intravenous (IV) infusion in the perioperative period.

HISTORIC DEVELOPMENTS

The impetus to administer drugs intravenously was provided when William Harvey, who, in *Exercitatio Anatomica de Motu Cordis et Sanguinis in Animalibus* (1628), published proof that venous blood was transported to the heart and from there to the other organs of the body via the arterial circulation (1). Christopher Wren in 1657 intravenously injected opium by means of quill and bladder into dogs and humans, rendering them unconscious. This was probably the first IV anesthetic. The first use of an intravenously administered drug to provide anesthesia for surgery was by Pierre-Cyprien Ore in 1874 using chloral hydrate.

Drug delivery systems for the administration of IV drugs have been vastly improved since the original quill and bladder. As a result of the development of the hypodermic needle by Frances Rynd and a functional syringe by Charles Pravaz, in 1853 Alexander Wood used a needle and syringe to administer a drug intravenously. This was a significant improvement over the original IV delivery device used by Wren. Present day syringes, catheters, and needles are descendants of these early devices.

Technological developments in the 20th century led to the next major advance in IV drug delivery systems: the introduction of infusion pumps that could accurately control the rate of drug administration. The development of microchip and computer technology led to the introduction of calculator and smart pumps. Calculator pumps are capable of automating simple calculations from information entered into them. Smart pumps solve complex mathematical equations to implement sophisticated administration schemes that could not be achieved manually by the user. Closed-loop controllers and pharmacokinetic model-driven infusion pumps are examples of smart pumps.

In contrast to the development of sophisticated pumps for IV drug delivery, systems to deliver traditional IV drugs by simple means noninvasively are also being developed. These include transdermal and transmucosal delivery of opiates and hypnotics.

Classically, IV anesthetics were given either as a large single dose or by multiple smaller intermittent doses for induction and maintenance of anesthesia. Recent studies indicate that IV anesthetics given by variable-rate continuous infusions provide several advantages over intermittent bolus administration. These include (1) greater hemodynamic stability, (2) fewer incidences of hemodynamic breakthrough and other signs of patient responsiveness, (3) reduced need for supplemental anesthetics or vasoactive drugs, (4) more rapid awakening, (5) decreased requirements for naloxone or for postoperative ventilatory support, (6) decreased incidence of side effects, and (7) lower total dose of drug given (2). In addition to the introduction of anesthetic drugs with properties ideal for administration by continuous infusion, there have been technological developments (e.g., infusion pumps) and conceptual developments (e.g., variable-rate continuous infusion) that will make drug delivery by IV infusion useful for anesthesiologists.

CONCEPTS FOR INTRAVENOUS DRUG DELIVERY

The goals of general anesthesia are to render the patient unconscious rapidly, maintain adequate anesthesia (irrespective of any surgical intervention), then allow a rapid recovery to the awake state. To achieve these goals, the therapeutic range of the drug must be known, the properties of the drug should provide a rapid onset and offset, and the drug should have a delivery system that can readily alter its concentration in the body. Over the past 30 years, we have gained a greater appreciation of the pharmacokinetic principles that determine onset and offset of IV drugs. Simultaneously, introduction of IV drugs that meet the above goals make the administration of IV anesthetics as convenient as administering volatile anesthetics.

Pharmacokinetics

Classically, texts on designing infusion schemes for IV anesthetics recommend calculating the initial loading dose as

$$\text{Loading dose} = Vd_1 \times Cp \quad [1]$$

and the maintenance infusion as

$$\text{Maintenance infusion} = Cp \times Cl, \quad [2]$$

where Vd_1 is the initial volume of distribution, Cp is the desired plasma drug concentration, and Cl is systemic clearance. This classic description of obtaining a target concentration with drugs having multicompartment pharmacokinetics is flawed because it does not incorporate the biophase or account for drug distribution when a drug's pharmacokinetics are best described by a two- or three-compartment model.

The Biophase

For IV anesthetics, the plasma is not the site of drug effect. Even if the precise concentration for the desired effect is known, calculating the loading dose according to Equation 1 would obtain the target plasma drug concentration, but the desired biophase concentration (and thus the effect) would not be achieved. The site at which a drug produces its effect is termed the biophase. For a drug to reach the biophase, it must distribute from the plasma/blood to the tissue of the biophase. While this occurs, the drug also distributes to other tissues. Thus, the loading dose necessary to produce the desired effect cannot be calculated using the initial volume of distribution (which includes primarily the blood volume), but rather should be calculated on the basis of the volume into which the drug has distributed when it equilibrates with the biophase (3). Also, the plasma concentration will be a measure of the effect only when the biophase and the plasma equilibrate. By continuously measuring the drug effect and its plasma concentration, it is possible to relate plasma concentration to the effect it produces in the biophase (4,5). Figure 1 illustrates the measurement of fentanyl concentrations following rapid infusion and the simultaneous measurement of the spectral edge of

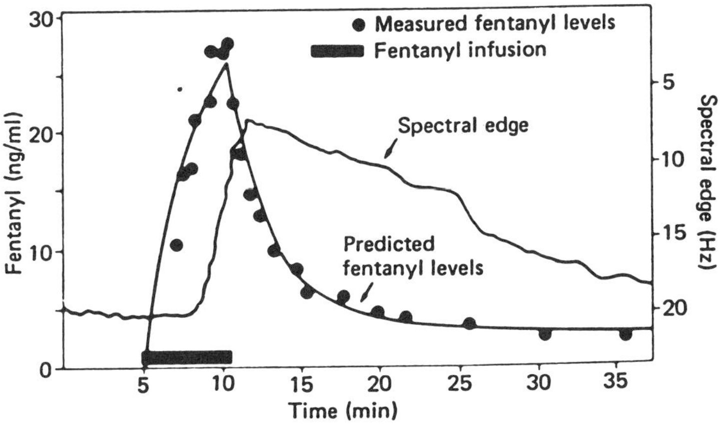

FIG. 1. The measured fentanyl concentration and its resultant effect on the spectral edge with respect to time following a brief infusion of fentanyl. (From Scott et al., ref. 5, with permission.)

TABLE 1. *Initial volume V_1 compared with the volume of distribution at the time of peak effect*

Drug	V_1 (liters)	% of peak concentration	^{Vd}peak effect (liters)
Fentanyl	12.70	17%	75.0
Alfentanil	2.19	37%	5.9
Sufentanil	17.80	20%	89.0
Propofol	6.70	18%	37.0

the EEG produced by these fentanyl concentrations. The rapid rise in plasma concentration is not paralleled by a similar change in the spectral edge, but there is hysteresis of this relationship. Furthermore, there is a time when the fentanyl concentration and the measure of effect are equal (i.e., where they cross). The area under the time-concentration curve up to this point represents the volume of distribution that incorporates the biophase. This can be measured as a percentage of the volume of distribution at steady state (Vd_{ss}) (3). The percentage of the Vd_{ss} that incorporates the biophase for several IV anesthetics is listed in Table 1. This volume of distribution is then used in Equation 1 to calculate the appropriate loading dose to achieve the desired concentration within the biophase.

When drug concentrations are plotted against effect following a bolus dose or a rapid infusion, a hysteresis loop rather than a linear relationship results (Fig. 2). The mathematical relationship (a time constant) that causes the hysteresis loop to collapse, thus providing a linear relationship between concentration and effect, is

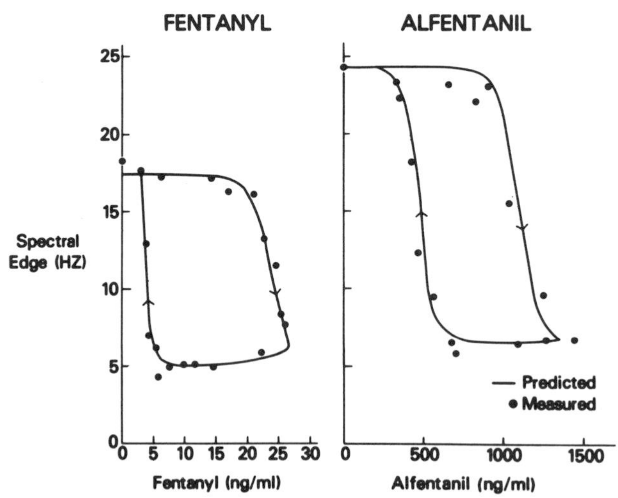

FIG. 2. The fentanyl and alfentanil concentration to the measured effect (EEG spectral edge) showing the hysteresis loop that occurs following a brief infusion of either drug. (From Scott et al., ref. 5, with permission.)

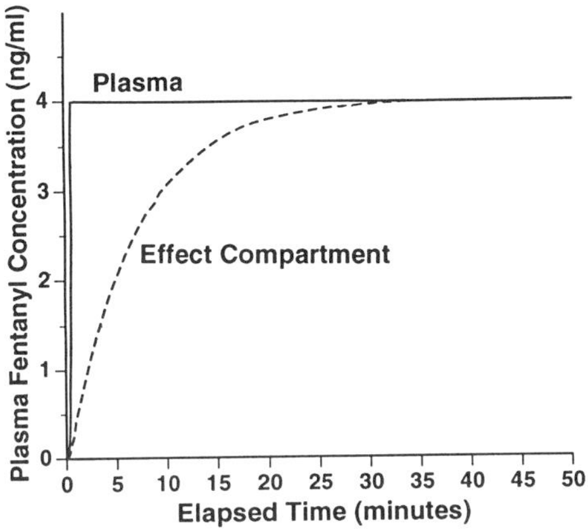

FIG. 3. Simulation of the rise in the effect site concentration of fentanyl when administered to maintain a constant plasma concentration.

termed the k_{e0}. The constant k_{e0} represents the equilibration rate of the drug between the plasma and the biophase. The $t_{1/2}$ k_{e0} is the time it takes for half of this equilibration to occur. For example, the $t_{1/2}$ k_{e0} for fentanyl is 4.7 minutes. If the plasma concentration of fentanyl were maintained constant at 4 ng/ml, then 4.7 minutes after the infusion were initiated the biophase concentration would be 2 ng/ml. It will take four half-lives (18.8 min) before the biophase and plasma concentration are almost equal (Fig. 3).

The time to peak effect following a bolus dose is a function of the drug's k_{e0} and its disposition (3). A drug with a brief $t_{1/2}$ k_{e0} will have a rapid onset to peak effect. It is important for clinicians to know the time to peak effect for each IV

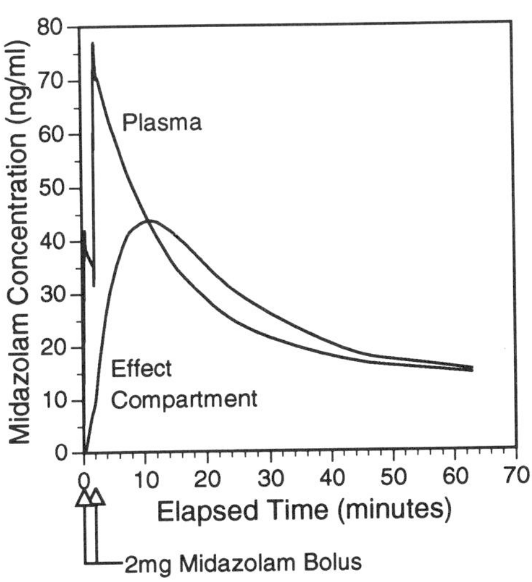

FIG. 4. Simulation of the resultant midazolam plasma and effect site concentration after two bolus doses of 1 mg of midazolam spaced 1 min apart. Note that although the plasma concentration has peaked, the effect site concentration and thus effect is still rising at the time of the second dose.

TABLE 2. *The $t_{1/2}k_{e0}$ and time to peak drug effect following a bolus dose*

Drug	Time to peak effect (min)	$t_{1/2}\ k_{e0}$ (min)
Fentanyl	3.6	4.7
Alfentanil	1.4	0.9
Sufentanil	5.6	3.0
Propofol	2.2	2.4
Thiopental	1.7	1.5
Midazolam	2.8	4.0
Etomidate	2.0	1.5

drug. For example, with a rapid sequence induction, it is desirable to use drugs with a rapid onset, such as thiopental (time to peak effect, 100 sec) and alfentanil (82 sec) so that loss of consciousness is rapid and both drug effects peak at the same time, ablating the response during laryngoscopy and endotracheal intubation. If fentanyl (216 sec) rather than alfentanil is administered at the same time as thiopental and succinylcholine, its effect will not be maximal at the time of the greatest stimulus (intubation), resulting in initial hypertension following laryngoscopy, then hypotension as fentanyl reaches its peak effect when stimuli are minimal. In addition, when giving IV drugs by intermittent bolus injection, the interval between doses must be of sufficient duration so that the peak drug effect is observed before the next dose is administered. This is illustrated in Fig. 4, where 2 doses of midazolam are given 1 minute apart (i.e., before the peak effect of the drug is observed). It can be noted from the figure that although the plasma concentration has peaked before the second dose, the effect has not and thus continues to rise. As a result, the second dose produces greater sedation than anticipated from the effect observed from the first dose. Knowledge of the k_{e0} allows for the rational choice of drugs used to provide anesthesia and for proper timing of their administration. The time to peak effect and k_{e0} values for IV anesthetics are listed in Table 2.

Multicompartment Models in Dosing Strategies

The infusion scheme from Equation 2 will maintain a precise plasma drug concentration if its decrease results only from drug clearance (i.e., the drug is a one-compartment drug: It is not distributed from the blood/plasma to other tissues). This is not true for any of the drugs used for anesthesia; thus, any infusion scheme must account for distribution of drug into peripheral tissues. Drugs that are distributed only in the blood or plasma can be considered contained in a single compartment and their pharmacokinetics can be described by a one-compartment model. As drugs are distributed to various other tissues from the blood/plasma (e.g., to muscle and fat), distribution occurs at different rates and the tissues contain different volumes of drug. Depending on how the body disposes of a drug, its pharmacokinetic parameters can be best described by a two- or three-compartment model. When designing an infusion scheme to maintain a target concentration in the plasma, the infusion scheme must replace drug lost from the plasma as a result of both its terminal clearance and its distribution to peripheral tissues. The infusion scheme to maintain a precise target concentration has been termed the BET scheme (6,7). B is the loading bolus dose as described above, E is the infusion to replace drug removed by its terminal elimination (clearance), and T is an exponentially declining infusion proportional to the rate of transfer of drug to peripheral tissues. Therefore, one begins with a high infusion rate and decreases it over time to maintain a stable plasma concentration. A typical example of a BET scheme used in daily practice is that of Roberts et al. (8) for propofol: an initial load of 2 mg/kg, followed by 70 ml/hr for 10 minutes, 55 ml/hr for another 10 minutes, and 40 ml/hr thereafter to maintain the blood propofol concentration at 3.5 μg/ml.

The pharmacokinetic processes within a two- or three-compartment model that determine the rate of decrease of drug concentration have recently been elucidated (3,9). The drug concentration in the plasma and the biophase is dependent on those processes adding drug to the body and disposing of drug within the body. When drug administration is terminated, the drug concentration in the plasma (and the biophase) will decrease as a result of both the irreversible elimination of drug from the body and the redistribution of drug from the plasma to peripheral tissues. Previously, the elimination half-life of a drug was thought to represent how

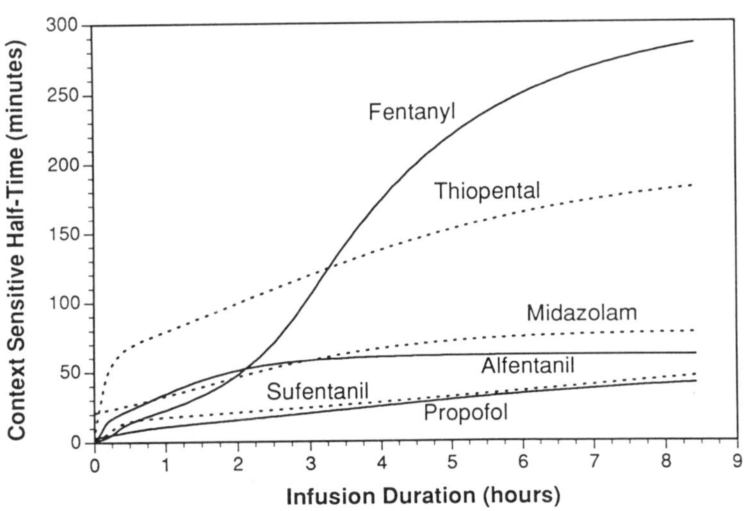

FIG. 5. Context-sensitive half-times as a function of duration of infusion derived from pharmacokinetic models of fentanyl, sufentanil, alfentanil, propofol, midazolam, and thiopental. (From Hughes et al., ref. 9, with permission.)

rapidly recovery from its effects occurred. Actually, the elimination half-life represents the terminal clearance of the drug, does not incorporate any redistribution of drug, and clearly provides no quantitative measure of how long it will take for the drug concentration to decrease by some percentage after the infusion. To estimate the time for a 50% decrease in drug concentration after an infusion designed to maintain a constant concentration, Hughes et al. (9) proposed the concept of "context-sensitive half-time." It is the time required for the plasma concentration of a drug to decrease by 50% for any given infusion duration (i.e., context sensitive to the duration of the infusion). Figure 5 illustrates the context-

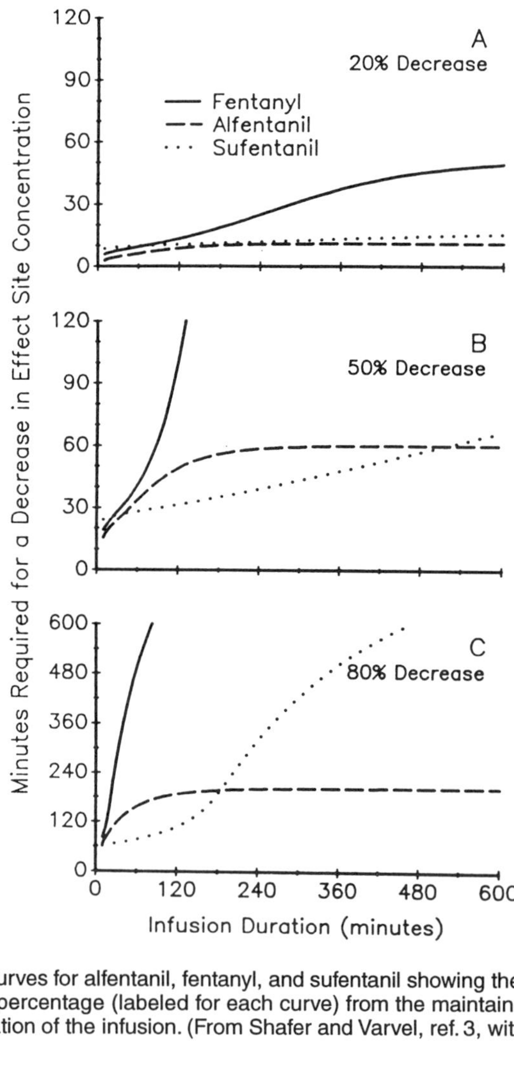

FIG. 6. Recovery curves for alfentanil, fentanyl, and sufentanil showing the time required for decreases of a given percentage (labeled for each curve) from the maintained effect site concentration after termination of the infusion. (From Shafer and Varvel, ref. 3, with permission.)

sensitive half-times of the most commonly used IV anesthetics. Also, pharmacokinetic simulations demonstrate that the time for a 20%, 50%, or 80% decrease in plasma drug concentration is not linear: i.e., a 20% decrease may take 5 minutes; a 50% decrease, 20 minutes; and a 80% decrease, 120 minutes (Fig. 6).

Apparently, for many clinical circumstances, a 50% decrease in plasma concentration is required from maintenance of anesthesia to the awake state and an 80–90% decrease is required to achieve readiness for discharge from the hospital. By estimating recovery times with this knowledge and using computer simulations, more appropriate drug choices can be made. For example, if a 50% decrease in opiate plasma concentration following an infusion of less than 6 hours is desired, sufentanil will provide the most rapid recovery (3). However, if the analgesic concentration needs to be maintained and only a 20% decrease is required, then fentanyl may be a better choice.

If a varying plasma concentration is administered, the context-sensitive half-time illustrated in Fig. 5 will no longer reflect the time for a 50% decrease in drug plasma concentration when the infusion is terminated. The time for a 50% (or any other percentage) decrease under these circumstances can still be computed if the precise infusion scheme is known. Even though the context-sensitive half-time illustrated in Fig. 5 is limited because of a narrowly defined set of circumstances (i.e., a constant concentration and a decrease of 50%), it still provides a better guide to recovery after the termination of an IV anesthetic infusion lasting a few hours than was previously estimated by the elimination half-life.

Pharmacodynamics

To provide effective anesthesia, the clinician is guided by the therapeutic range of the drug being administered. The concept of MAC (minimum alveolar concentration of a volatile anesthetic that would prevent purposeful movement following skin incision) was introduced initially to enable comparisons between volatile anesthetics at equipotent concentrations. MAC provides a measure of the therapeutic concentration of the anesthetic. For IV anesthetics, a similar concept is termed the Cp_{50}: the plasma concentration in equilibrium with the biophase that will prevent purposeful movement to a defined stimulus (10,11). With the possible exception of ketamine, no single drug provides all the components of anesthesia (i.e., hypnosis, analgesia, and amnesia). Thus, to provide an adequate state of anesthesia, hypnotics and analgesics are usually combined. The Cp_{50} for skin incision for many of the IV anesthetics combined with 60–70% nitrous oxide (N_2O) are presented in Table 3

Combinations of opiates and hypnotics are used for both induction and maintenance of anesthesia. Excellent studies have demonstrated the interaction of a variety of drug combinations that can be used to induce anesthesia. For loss of consciousness, the combination of a benzodiazepine and either an opiate or another hypnotic anesthetic results in a marked synergistic interaction (i.e., the dose

TABLE 3. *Steady-state concentrations for predefined effects*[a]

Drug	IC_{50}[b] (±SD)	Cp_{50} incision or painful stimulus (±SD)[c]	Cp_{50} LOC (±SD)[d]	Cp_{50} Spont Vent (±SD)[e]	50% reduction in isoflurane MAC	MEAC[f]
Alfentanil (ng/ml)	520 ± 123	241 ± 16		226 ± 10	50.0	10.0
Fentanyl (ng/ml)	6.9 ± 1.9	4.2		(3–4)	1.67	0.7
Sufentanil (ng/ml)	0.68 ± 0.31	(0.3–0.4)		(0.3–0.4)	0.145	0.04
Remifentanil (ng/ml)	14.7				1.8	
A3665 (ng/ml)	429 ± 313					
Thiopental (μg/ml)	17.9	39.8 ± 3.3	15.6 ± 1.1			
Propofol (μg/ml)		15.8	3.4			

[a] Values in parentheses are estimated by scaling to the alfentanil Cp_{50}.
[b] IC_{50} is the steady-state serum concentration in equilibration with the effect compartment that causes a 50% slowing of the maximal EEG.
[c] Cp_{50} skin incision is the steady-state plasma concentration in equilibration with the effect compartment that will prevent a somatic or autonomic response in 50% of patients.
[d] Cp_{50} LOC is the steady-state plasma concentration in equilibration with the effect compartment that provides absence of a response to a verbal command in 50% of patients.
[e] Cp_{50} Spont Vent is the steady-state plasma concentration in equilibration with the effect compartment that is associated with adequate spontaneous ventilation in 50% of patients.
[f] MEAC is the minimum effective plasma concentration providing postoperative analgesia.

of each drug required when used in combination is markedly less than that predicted from the doses required of each drug for the same effect when used alone (12–20). Opiates also tend to produce a synergistic interaction with other IV anesthetics for loss of consciousness, but the extent of this interaction is much less than with the benzodiazepines (13,21–24).

Reduction in MAC or Cp_{50} characterizes the interaction between opiates and anesthetics for the maintenance of anesthesia (Fig. 7) (24–29). The reduction of isoflurane MAC by fentanyl (25), sufentanil (28), alfentanil (27), and remifentanil (29) is remarkably similar to the reduction in Cp_{50} of propofol by fentanyl (24). Several important concepts for the administration of IV anesthetics can be derived from Fig. 7. First, the dose reduction of the anesthetic (isoflurane or propofol) by the opiate at low concentrations (within the range required to provide postoperative analgesia) is steep. Second, opiate concentrations equivalent to a fentanyl concentration of 3–4 ng/ml or greater reduce very little the concentration of propofol or isoflurane needed to provide adequate anesthesia; there is a ceiling effect of the opiate. This has several important clinical caveats for anesthetic techniques. If adequate anesthesia occurs when the opiate concentration is less than an equivalent of 3–4 ng/ml of fentanyl, the concentration of either the opiate or the anes-

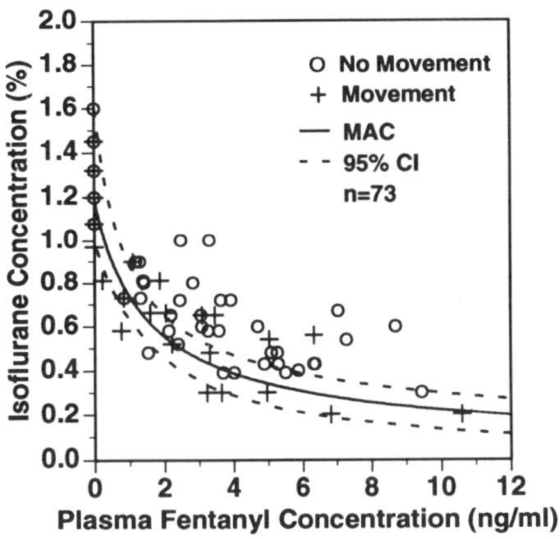

FIG. 7. The reduction of the MAC (minimum alveolar concentration that will prevent movement in 50% of patients following skin incision) of isoflurane by increasing concentrations of fentanyl that have equilibrated with the biophase. The 95% confidence interval is also shown. (From McEwan et al., ref. 25, with permission.).

thetic (hypnotic) drug can be increased to provide an adequate depth of anesthesia. If, however, the opiate concentration is more than an equivalent of 3–4 ng/ml of fentanyl, little is achieved by increasing the opiate concentration: it is better to increase the concentration of the anesthetic (hypnotic) drug. Opiate concentrations equal to 2 ng/ml fentanyl or higher, however, can cause clinically significant respiratory depression (30). Furthermore, the ceiling effect of the opiate occurs when the end-tidal concentration of isoflurane equals MAC_{awake} (0.4%) and for propofol at its $Cp_{50\ awake}$ concentration (3.3 μg/ml) (24,31). To avoid awareness under anesthesia when using an opiate plus a volatile anesthetic or propofol, it is advisable to maintain the volatile anesthetic above its MAC_{awake} value or propofol above its $Cp_{50\ awake}$ value of 3.3 μg/ml (i.e., an infusion rate of 80 μg/kg/min).

MANUAL INFUSION DEVICES

Although the syringe is the simplest device for IV drug delivery, maintaining any desired drug concentration with a syringe alone is impossible because of the effect of pharmacokinetics on dosing. It is better to deliver potent drugs such as anesthetics, analgesics, hypnotics, neuromuscular blockers, and vasoactive agents via an infusion using a device that is capable of providing an accurate and safe infusion rate. Initially, infusion devices were calibrated to control the rate of fluid flow and, secondarily, to control the drug infusion rate. Two basic systems are used to regulate fluid flow: gravimetric-controller or positive-displacement pumps.

Gravimetric Controller Pumps

A controller infusion device regulates the rate of flow caused by gravity. The simplest but least accurate such device is the CAIR clamp, in which the flow rate is altered by varying the radius of the infusion tubing. A CAIR clamp is attached to infusion tubing containing a drip chamber. The infusion rate can be calculated by knowing the volume of each drop and by tediously counting the drip rate. The Dial-a-Flo, a modification of the CAIR clamp, consists of a variable-orifice device within the infusion tubing. The fluid drip rate is marked on the variable orifice device. Flow is related to the radius of the tubing, the pressure difference across the orifice, and the viscosity of the fluid. Thus, the Dial-a-Flo allows only a crude estimate of flow rate, which is subject to change as the pressure difference across the orifice varies with the height of the fluid column as the fluid container empties. When only relative changes in infusion rates are important or when the dose response effect is relatively flat, a Dial-a-Flo is both cheap and effective. A more accurate infusion device is necessary for most of the drugs used by anesthesiologists.

More accurate controllers are nonvolumetric pumps that rely on drop counting to calculate the volume infused. They consist of a drop counter coupled to a device controlling the orifice of the infusion tubing. When the flow rate is set, the drop size is assumed to be constant and known. The drop counter counts the drop rate and, via a feedback mechanism, continuously adjusts the tubing orifice to maintain the specified drip rate. These pumps are capable of producing highly accurate flow rates. Their major source of error is that the volume of each drop is affected by the characteristics of the solution.

The drop rate can be controlled by one of several mechanisms: (1) a pincher-anvil that variably occludes or intermittently pinches the administration tubing to maintain a desired flow rate, (2) a rotary valve system that alters the radius and flow rate because flow is proportional to r^{-4}, (3) a magnetically coupled steel-ball valve where flow is controlled by intermittently creating an electromagnetic field that displaces the ball valve, and (4) a drip-chamber diaphragm valve that variably occludes the drip chamber by the diaphragm. Free flow may occur when the administration set is removed from the pump control mechanism. This is prevented in pumps utilizing a rotary valve or steel-ball valve. Controller pumps will generally have an air-in-line detection device because they can entrain air.

Positive Displacement Pumps

Nonvolumetric (drop counting) or volumetric positive-displacement pumps, as implied, positively displace fluid and thus are capable of pumping against pressure. Their basic pumping mechanisms are either peristaltic or piston action. Peristaltic pumps use either a wobble plate, a linear mechanism, or a rotary mechanism. Infusion pumps with a piston mechanism use either a to-and-fro or a screw motion to drive the piston. Depending on the particular pumping mechanism, the pump will use either a special administration set or standard syringes and IV tubing for fluid administration. Because they can pump against pressure, positive-displacement pumps must be carefully designed to prevent infusion of air or large infiltrations of tissue. A wide range of accurately delivered infusion rates is needed for IV drugs during anesthesia. Because positive-displacement pumps provide these requirements more readily than do gravimetric controllers, they are used most often for continuous IV delivery of anesthetic drugs.

Calculator Pumps

There are both essential (Table 4) and desirable features (Table 5) of infusion pumps that optimize drug delivery during the perioperative period (32). Present-day infusion pumps generally include all the essential features listed in Table 4. Manufacturers are now trying to provide the features listed in Table 5, especially the introduction of calculator pumps. The basic microchip technology for infusion devices to do simple arithmetic calculations has been present in most instruments for many years. Marketing anesthetic agents (e.g., alfentanil, propofol) for continuous infusion provided the impetus to develop infusion devices with calculator features that markedly simplify their administration by continuous infusion. Calculator pumps contain mechanisms that allow the user to set the drug infusion rate in terms of dose/weight/time. A microprocessor in the pump calculates the actual infusion rate in volume/time according to the concentration of the drug entered by the user and the patient's weight. Drug infusion rates are simply adjusted by either altering a dial or entering the new infusion rate desired. This increases the convenience of infusion pumps for IV anesthetic drug delivery and minimizes human error in calculating infusion rates manually. By entering the drug concentration and the patient's weight, bolus doses entered in dose/weight can also be given with a calculator pump. The pump calculates the bolus volumes and then infuses it at the maximum rate of the pump. Several suitable calculator pumps are commercially available.

In addition to making infusion pumps smarter, tremendous strides are being made to reduce their size so that three or four pumps can be combined into a single unit that is not much bigger than a current single pump. An infusion pump suitable for perioperative use should be able to administer a muscle relaxant, a hypnotic, and an opiate.

TABLE 4. *Essential features for infusion devices*

1. Electrical safety
2. Air detection
3. Occlusion alarm—time to alarm <3 min
4. Maximum infusion pressure <250 mmHg
5. Flow rate accuracy of ±2%
6. Prevention of free flow
7. Continuous flow (i.e., minimal intermittent flow)
8. Function unaffected by electromagnetic field

From Glass et al., ref. 32.

TABLE 5. *Desirable features for infusion pumps*

1. Versatility
   a. Choice of bolus or infusion mode
   b. Internal calculator for choice of dosing scheme
   c. Adaptable for use with all anesthetic drugs
   d. Choice of infusion rates from 0–1500 with 0.1-ml/hr resolution in the range 0–100 ml/hr and 1-ml/hr resolution in the range 100–1500 ml/hr
   e. Choice of up to 4 separate channels with no possibility of backflow or drug mixing proximal to the IV cannula
2. Light weight
3. Automatic priming of administration set
4. Clear display of drug administered and infusion rate
5. Simple protocols for initiation or change of infusion rates
6. Digital interface for record keeping or external automated control
7. Automated drug recognition
8. Alarm for tubing disconnect

From Glass et al., ref. 32.

MANUAL INFUSION SCHEMES

To obtain appropriate drug concentrations, two pharmacokinetically based schemes can be used to administer a manual infusion. These are either the BET scheme (6) or the approach proposed by Wagner (33). To compensate accurately for the processes of drug disposition that occur during an infusion, the BET scheme (as described above) is most appropriate. The BET scheme can be strictly accomplished only by using a computer-controlled device. Wagner proposed a two-stage infusion scheme that is more practical to deliver manually and is readily implemented with a calculator pump. The Wagner approach provides an initial rapid infusion to fill the volume of distribution followed by a maintenance infusion rate determined by the targeted central-compartment drug concentration and its clearance. The initial infusion rate in the Wagner method is based on a nomogram that is rarely available to the clinician. More commonly, the Wagner approach is modified to base the initial loading infusion on either the volume of distribution of the central compartment or the volume of distribution at steady state. If the initial loading dose is calculated from the volume of distribution of the central compartment, the desired plasma level will transiently be obtained but then decrease below this level during redistribution (Fig. 8). Either the BET scheme or the Wagner approach can obtain appropriate initial drug concentrations. Table 6 provides a Wagner-type approach to obtain clinically relevant target concentrations of the commonly used anesthetics. Many factors such as age, sex, concomitant disease, or drug interactions can alter either the individual's pharmacokinetics or pharmacodynamic response or both. Therefore, any infusion must ultimately be titrated to each individual's requirements.

The approaches discussed above are based on linear pharmacokinetic models. If an infusion rate for a given drug is administered to provide a steady-state blood

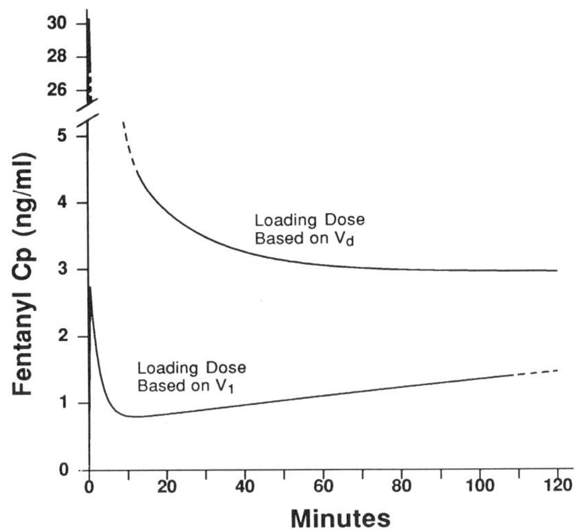

FIG. 8. Computer simulation of the plasma drug concentration resulting from an initial loading dose based either on the initial volume of distribution (central compartment) or on the volume of distribution at steady state.

concentration x, when the drug is given at twice this rate, the resultant steady-state concentration will be 2x. If an increase in blood concentration of double the initial concentration is desired, the infusion rate must be doubled. By increasing only the infusion rate, it will take several elimination half-lives to obtain the new, desired concentration. Thus, a loading bolus dose should be given first. Again, redistribution must be accounted for by providing either a larger loading dose or an exponentially decreasing infusion.

TABLE 6. *Manual infusion schemes when combined with 66% nitrous oxide*[a]

	Anesthesia		Sedation or Analgesia	
Drug	Loading dose ($mg \cdot kg^{-1}$)	Maintenance infusion $mg \cdot kg^{-1} \cdot min^{-1}$	Loading dose $mg \cdot kg^{-1}$	Maintenance infusion $mg \cdot kg^{-1}$
Alfentanil	50–150	0.5–3.0	10–25	0.25–1.0
Fentanyl	5–15	0.03–0.10	1.5–3	0.01–0.03
Sufentanil	1–2.0	0.006–0.02	0.15–0.3	0.002–0.007
Methohexital	1000–2000	50–150	500–1000	10–50
Ketamine	1000–2000	10–50	500–1000	10–20
Propofol	1000–2000	80–150	250–1000	10–50
Midazolam	50--150	0.25–1.0	20–100	0.25–1.0

[a] Following the loading dose, an initially high infusion rate to account for redistribution should be used and then titrated to the lowest infusion rate that will maintain adequate anesthesia or sedation. For sedation, the loading dose is given over 5–10 min and is adjusted according to the patient's response. For anesthesia, midazolam must be administered in combination with an opiate.

Calculator pumps greatly simplify the administration of drugs by infusion. For the optimal control of drug administration, smart pumps capable of either pharmacokinetic model-driven infusion (when the physiological endpoint is not easily measured) or closed-loop adaptive control (when the physiological variable is easily measured) are needed.

AUTOMATED DRUG DELIVERY

Automated drug delivery implies that some form of electronic or mechanical instrumentation performs dose-rate adjustments independent of human intervention in contrast to the manual devises described above (34). The desired target drug concentration or clinical response is still chosen by the clinician. Preprogrammed dosing of either the bolus or infusion is the simplest form of automated drug delivery. This consists of a preprogrammed infusion that is usually calculated to provide a single target blood or effect concentration that is automatically implemented by the microprocessor in the pump. Preprogrammed devices are limited in their application for IV anesthetic drugs because they do not allow the user to vary the target concentration. Generally, two methods may be applied for automated target anesthetic drug delivery: either model-based (a form of open loop control) or closed-loop.

Terms and Definitions

Both model-based and closed-loop systems require a set point (Fig. 9). The set point is the quantifiable endpoint, the plasma concentration or percentage T1 (1 of twitch of a train of four) of the EMG related to the clinical objective (e.g., level of anesthesia, neuromuscular blockade). Accordingly, the set point is the target value that the automated control system tries to control. The feedback signal is

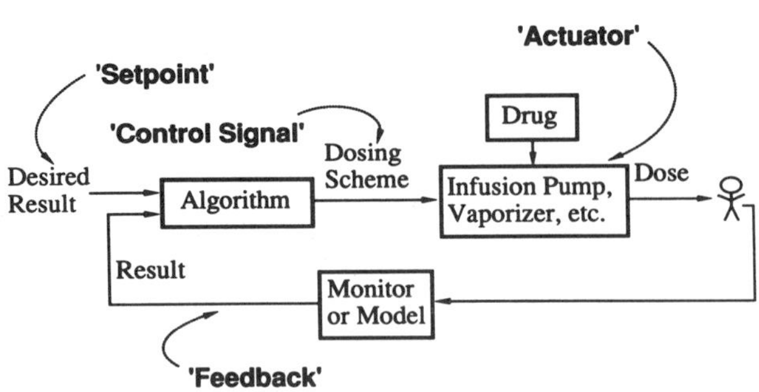

FIG. 9. The components of an automated drug-delivery system. (From Reves et al., ref. 34, with permission.)

the actual measured concentration value (e.g., percentage T1 of the EMG) or the simulated concentration value (e.g., predicted plasma concentration from pharmacokinetic simulation) that results from the automated delivery process.

Although closed-loop is the ideal means of automated drug delivery, there is not always a measurable feedback signal. Therefore, model-based drug delivery provides an important alternative in circumstances when the feedback signal cannot be measured and an appropriate model is available. A mathematical equation that simulates the process that produces the set point provides the model. Consequently, the accuracy of any model-based control system depends on how well the model represents the process under control. The control signal, which for automated drug delivery is the dosing scheme, is generated by a set of instructions known as an algorithm. An algorithm is ordinarily designed to keep the control variable as close as possible to the set-point value. The set point and feedback values, in turn, act on the algorithm to generate the control signal. The control signal directs the actuator, producing the intervention necessary to obtain the set point (i.e., it delivers the dosage regimen prescribed by the algorithm to the patient). This intervention results in a new feedback control signal, and the process repeats itself to maintain the target value. In an adaptive control system, the algorithm is altered or adapted to the individual's unique response to the intervention produced by the actuator. For example, in a closed-loop system to control blood pressure, the algorithm may prescribe an increase in the infusion of sodium nitroprusside of 1 μg/kg/min when the blood pressure exceeds 5 mmHg above the target. Although this may generally be an appropriate prescription, a change of this magnitude may cause a much greater drop in blood pressure in a sensitive individual than is desired. An adaptive controller will, after experience with the patient, learn the patient's sensitivity and change the algorithm so that the control signal (dosing scheme) results in an intervention by the actuator that brings the feedback signal closest to the target.

Pharmacokinetic Model-Driven Drug Infusion

There is no known measure or combination of measures that can be used to provide a quantifiable monitor of anesthetic depth that is constant between drugs or patients. The drug concentration at the site of action governs the degree of pharmacological effect (35), causing a strong relationship between anesthetic depth and the steady-state plasma blood concentration or partial pressure of the anesthetic agent. This relationship enables the definition of MAC for each inhalational agent (36) and Cp_{50} (10), respectively, for each IV anesthetic. Because of this relationship between depth of anesthesia and partial pressure, the calibrated vaporizer was developed to enhance the delivery of the potent inhaled anesthetics for anesthesia. Because the blood concentration of IV anesthetics is related to the desired effect, delivering anesthetic drugs to a concentration rather than by a dose rate also may improve their administration.

Pharmacokinetics is the science of calculating concentration from drug dose. Complex mathematical formulas can be calculated rapidly, accurately, and repeatedly by computer. Pharmacokinetic model-driven drug infusion consists of an infusion device controlled by a computer containing the pharmacokinetic parameters necessary to calculate the dosing scheme to produce a physician-specified plasma drug concentration. Thus, pharmacokinetic model-driven drug infusion devices are for IV anesthesia what calibrated vaporizers are for inhalational anesthesia. A basic understanding of the pharmacokinetic principles and the mathematical concepts used by the computer will help users of the device.

Principles

Computerized pharmacokinetic model-driven drug delivery stems from the understanding that a pharmacokinetic model can be used to predict the plasma drug concentrations that result from any administration scheme at any time. The operative word here is predict. No mathematical model, however sophisticated, can fully characterize the nonlinear, time varying, chaotic processes that determine drug disposition. If the plasma drug concentration resulting from a dose regimen can be predicted, one can invert the process and use the pharmacokinetic model to predict the dose regimen necessary to achieve a specified plasma-drug concentration profile. In outpatient medicine, this may take the form of "take one tablet twice daily." In IV anesthesia, the result may be infusion rates that change several times each minute for the duration of the anesthetic. When a computerized instrument is used to compute and implement the dosing scheme, the result is computerized pharmacokinetic model-driven drug delivery. Such devices applied to IV drug infusion are called CACI, an acronym for computer-assisted continuous infusion coined by Alvis et al. (37), who constructed the first such instrument used clinically in the United States. The same process is also called TCI or target-controlled infusion.

Given a fully parameterized linear, time-invariant, two- or three-compartment pharmacokinetic model, several approaches can determine the infusion rates required as a function of time to achieve the target plasma drug concentrations specified as a function of time. The BET dosing scheme discussed earlier was the first algorithm proposed for computerized pharmacokinetic model-driven drug delivery and is widely used. In 1968 Kruger-Thiemer (38) described the infusion regimen theoretically required to achieve rapidly and maintain a constant plasma concentration of an intravenously administered drug, the kinetics of which are described by a two-compartment model. Clearly, these complex dosing regimens, which require infusion rates that change continuously as a function of time until steady state is achieved, cannot be computed or implemented manually.

More than a decade after publication of Kruger-Thiemer's classic article, as personal computers became commonplace, Schwilden et al. (6) interfaced a microcomputer to an infusion pump and demonstrated clinical application of the BET infusion scheme. They wrote a software program using the theorem of su-

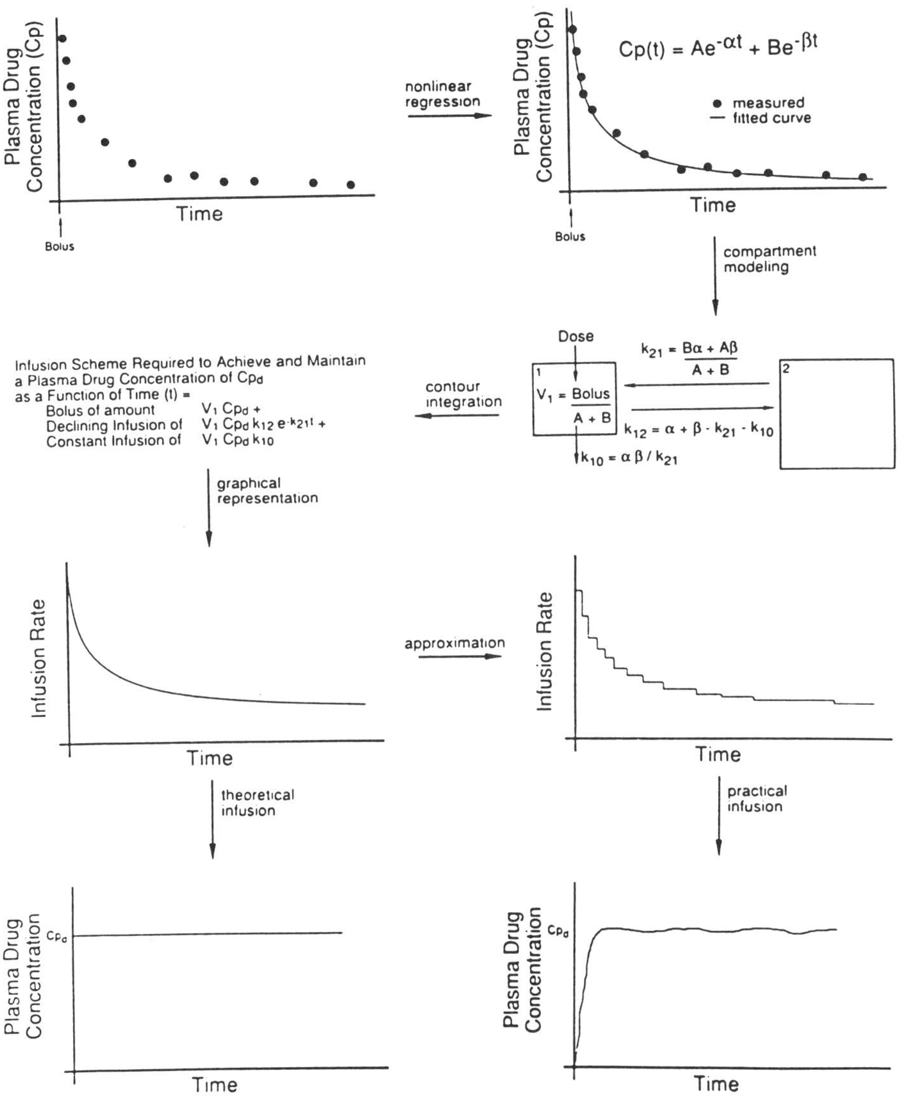

FIG. 10. Steps involved in pharmacokinetic model-driven infusion. Typically, pharmacokinetic models are derived from experiments in which plasma drug concentrations are measured at intervals following bolus administration of the drug. Nonlinear regression is used to fit a mono-, bi-, or triexponential curve to the resulting concentration versus time data. There is an algebraic relationship between the exponential decay curves and a one-, two-, or three-compartment pharmacokinetic model. The BET infusion scheme is derived from the two-compartment model using contour integration. A BET infusion results in the maintenance of a constant specified plasma drug concentration. Practical implementation of the BET scheme using real infusion pumps and infusion rates that change only at discrete intervals of time results in a plasma-drug concentration profile that approximates that resulting from a BET infusion.

perposition to compute and implement BET infusion regimens in real time to obtain plasma drug concentrations specified by the anesthesiologist. The BET infusion regimen is now just one of several algorithms that are used to effect pharmacokinetic model-driven infusion of anesthetic drugs through automated drug delivery devices. All of these algorithms are derived by manipulating a pharmacokinetic model, expressed as either the multiexponential equations or compartment models described previously, to calculate the infusion rates required to obtain the theoretically desired plasma drug or biophase concentrations.

Figure 10 demonstrates the BET scheme for a three-compartment model. Note that this regimen achieves and maintains only a single set-point plasma drug concentration. The superposition theorem must be added to these equations if the objective is titration of the set point. Also, these equations are derived analytically and, as a result, specify infusion rates of infinitely fine resolution that vary continuously as a function of time. In designing these algorithms, it is necessary to consider the physical limitations of the infusion device. It is impossible to implement the BET or any other analytically derived scheme precisely because the infusion rates generated by these instruments (1) have an upper limit (e.g., 999 ml/hr), (2) have finite resolution (e.g., integer values in ml/hr), and (3) can be changed only at finitely small intervals of time. Inspired by the BET concept, investigators subsequently proposed and used CACI algorithms that inherently realized superposition and that explicitly considered the electromechanical limitations of the infusion device (37,39,40). All of these algorithms result in infusion

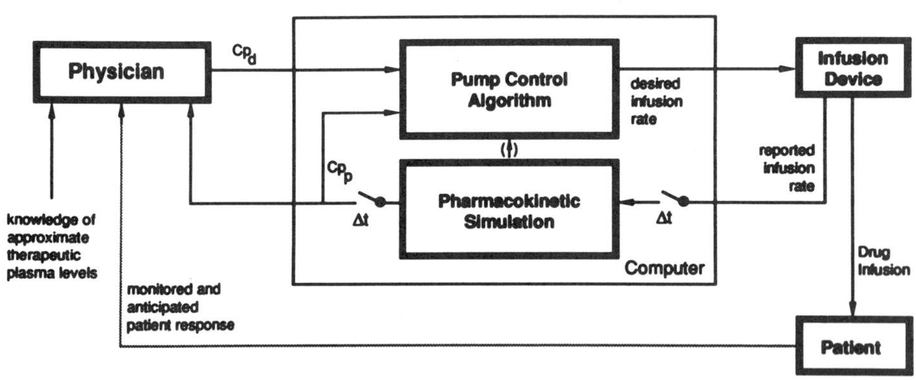

FIG. 11. Schematic illustration of the authors' approach to pharmacokinetic model-driven drug delivery. In this computer-assisted continuous infusion (CACI) device, the physician enters the desired plasma drug concentration (Cp_d). An infusion-device control algorithm uses a pharmacokinetic model for the drug being infused to determine what the infusion rate should be for the next infusion interval (e.g., 10 sec). The infusion device delivers drug to the patient, and the infusion rate is fed into a simulation of the pharmacokinetic model to compute the current predicted plasma drug concentration (Cp_p). The stated variables computed in the simulation are available to the algorithm. On the basis of monitored and anticipated patient response, knowledge of approximate therapeutic plasma drug concentrations (e.g., Cp_{50}), and on Cp_p, the physician can titrate Cp_d as necessary.

rate profiles that approximate the BET scheme. The BET equations provide the exact analytical solution toward the goal of maintaining a constant central compartment drug concentration in a multicompartmental model.

Each prototype pharmacokinetic model-driven infusion device has been implemented somewhat differently, but all of them are conceptually similar. Each consists of a microcomputer interfaced with a drug infusion pump, with a novel software program written by the investigators to implement the model-driven infusions (Fig. 11). The algorithm implemented by the CACI device makes express use of pharmacokinetic simulations to determine the infusion rates required to achieve set-point plasma drug concentrations. In using the device, the anesthesiologist specifies a target plasma or effect-site drug concentration via a computer keyboard (Fig. 12). This target concentration is based on knowledge of the pharmacokinetic-dynamic relationship of the drug and the desired effect, as well as on the individual patient's responses. The infusion rate required to achieve the target concentration at the beginning of each 9-second interval is calculated either directly (exact solution) or by interpolation. For interpolation, a numerical simulation of a pharmacokinetic model of the drug being infused is performed to determine what the plasma drug concentration would be at the end of that interval if no drug was infused (infusion rate, 0 ml/hr) during that interval. This process is repeated using an arbitrary positive infusion rate other than zero. Based on the linearity of the pharmacokinetic model, interpolation is performed with the results

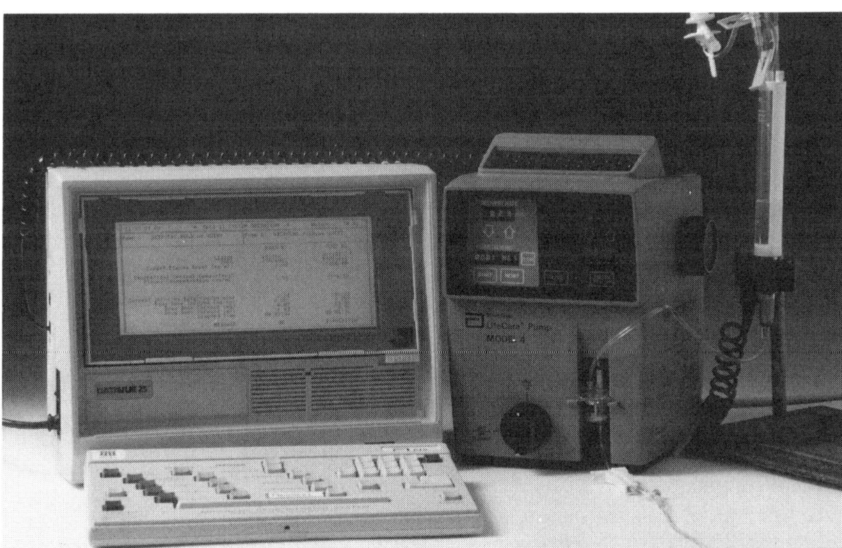

FIG. 12. The CACI system used at Duke University Medical Center. It consists of a laptop computer electronically linked to an infusion pump. The desired drug plasma or effect site concentration is entered with the keyboard.

of these two test simulations to determine the infusion rate required to achieve the desired concentration. The result is then clipped and rounded to match the upper and lower limits and the resolution of the infusion device; it is then transmitted electronically to the infusion device for use during that 9-second interval. At the end of the interval, the rate actually used by the device is transmitted back into the pharmacokinetic model so that the simulation can be updated to reflect the actual drug administration. During a significant error condition such as occlusion of the IV cannula, the infusion pump automatically stops and alerts the user to the specific error condition. This information is transmitted to the host computer's pharmacokinetic simulation, and the infusion algorithm automatically compensates for the period of interrupted drug delivery once the problem is corrected.

Just as it is unnecessary to have detailed knowledge of the physics of volatile gases to use a calibrated vaporizer skillfully to administer an inhalational anesthetic, expert knowledge of differential equations and pharmacokinetic computations is not required for efficacious use of a CACI device. Although the prototype CACI device now in use consists of a personal computer interfaced with an off-the-shelf infusion pump, most contemporary CACI systems do not differ that much. It is anticipated that commercial devices will implement CACI by enhancing the software and user interface of a standard infusion pump. To use CACI, a burette or other drug reservoir is filled with drug at a specified concentration. The pumping chamber and IV tubing are primed with this infusate. The physician uses the computer keyboard or the device keypad to indicate the drug to be infused, the patient's weight, and other demographic data that are relevant to the set of pharmacokinetic parameters programmed into the device. Thereafter, the set-point concentration of the IV agent is adjusted or titrated in a manner analogous to titration of the inspired concentration of an inhalational agent. Unlike a calibrated vaporizer, most CACI infusion algorithms automatically "overpressurize" to obtain the set-point plasma drug concentration as rapidly as possible. In other words, the infusion algorithm inherently compensates for the distribution time constants. Also, unlike delivery of inhalation agents, where elimination is uniformly rapid, the rate at which lower plasma concentrations of IV drugs are obtained depends on both the mode of drug clearance from the blood and the extent of drug distribution to the tissues. Therefore, the time when the infusion should be discontinued to achieve appropriate recovery varies from drug to drug and, temporarily, as a function of duration of operation (i.e., context-sensitive half-time). To help the clinician make the decision regarding when to stop the infusion, the CACI device can incorporate a forward simulation to continuously or periodically compute the amount of time required for the theoretical plasma drug concentration to decrease to the estimated recovery concentration.

CACI provides the clinician with a smart pump that enables delivery of IV drug to the desired concentration. This contrasts with even the most sophisticated calculator pumps that deliver drugs according to an infusion rate. Since the pharmacodynamic effect is related more to effect site concentration than to drug dose, CACI should improve IV drug delivery during anesthesia.

Clinical Evaluation

To evaluate CACI devices clinically, two important questions must be answered: (1) How well does the device perform (i.e., What is its predictive accuracy)? and (2) Does a CACI device improve the administration of IV drugs? Because neither question is completely answered, they are the focus of current research.

The sources of inaccuracy with pharmacokinetic model-driven devices include the software, the hardware, and variability of pharmacokinetics from patient to patient (Fig. 13).

Inaccuracy in the software results from both the program calculating the infusion rates and the actual pharmacokinetic parameters used for each drug. The program that is calculating infusion rates can be tested against computer simulation programs and should not be a source of error. Any inaccuracy caused by the infusion program can, in practice, be discounted because it should be corrected before the device is used for patients. Therefore, the major cause of inaccuracy (i.e., a difference between the concentration predicted by the computer and the actual measured concentration) is the difference between the patient's kinetics and those implemented in the computer program. Pharmacokinetics is usually defined from a relatively small population of people of similar age and weight and is calculated as the average of the group. They differ markedly from author to author for the same drug. This is a problem because the rate constants and the central-compartment volume used in pharmacokinetic model-driven devices are generally taken from the published literature. Thus, patient-to-patient variability, acute pharmacokinetic changes, and the many assumptions made in deriving a pharmacokinetic model in the first place preclude the possibility of consistently achieving accuracy when using such automated drug delivery devices regardless of how "good" a particular set of coefficients may be. For clinical use, however, it is not essential

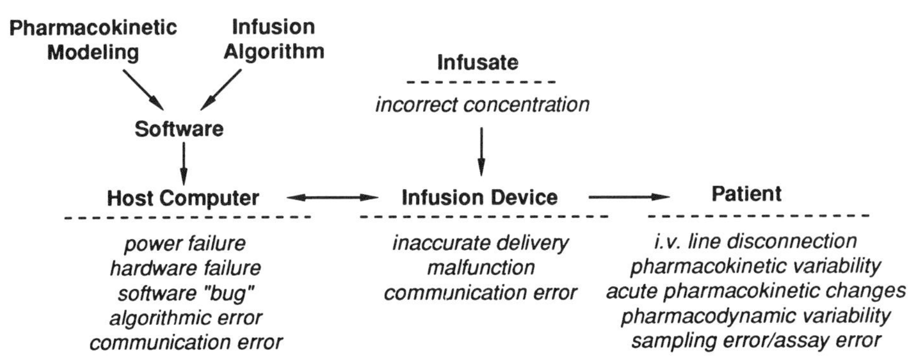

FIG. 13. Sources of error between the plasma concentration, as predicted by the pharmacokinetic model-driven infusion system, and the measured plasma drug concentration. (From Shafer and Gregg, ref. 55, and Glass et al., ref. 94, with permission.)

to have precise concentrations; instead, it is necessary that automated drug delivery achieve plasma concentrations within a defined range. Therefore, the question is: Do the kinetic parameters entered into the system sufficiently reflect those of the population so that the IV agents can be efficiently titrated to provide the optimal outcome for the patient?

Optimization of Target-Controlled Drug Delivery

The performance of computer-controlled drug administration must be interpreted in terms of the clinician's therapeutic expectations. Possible goals include accurately producing a desired concentration in the plasma, titrating the plasma drug concentration precisely, producing the desired drug effect, and producing the desired time course of the drug effect. Over the last decade, investigators have addressed each of these goals and refined the performance of automated drug delivery devices.

The ability of automated drug delivery to achieve and maintain a selected target concentration rapidly is a logical measure of its performance. The difference between the measured and the target concentrations can be expressed in several ways. The simplest way is to plot the target and measured concentrations of each sample in each patient and observe the variation from the line of identity (Fig. 14) (30). This is usually called the performance error: the difference between the mea-

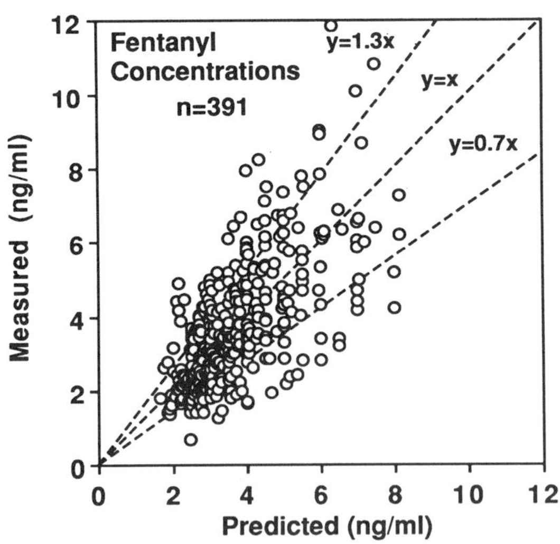

FIG. 14. Plot of the measured to the predicted concentration of fentanyl administered via CACI in 24 patients. The solid line represents the line of identity: i.e., the target concentration is equal to the measured. The dashed lines represent a bias of ±30%. (From Glass et al., ref. 30, with permission.)

sured and the target concentration as a percentage of the desired target [i.e., (target-measured)/target x 100%]. The median absolute performance error (MDAPE) is the median of the absolute value of all performance errors. The MDAPE is commonly used as a measure of the inaccuracy of an automated drug-delivery device. A MDAPE of 0 is perfect performance, whereas a MDAPE of 20% means that half of the plasma concentrations will be within 20% of the target and half will be outside that range.

It is unreasonable to expect all performance errors to be 0%. However, it would be desirable if positive and negative errors offset each other so that the median performance error (MDPE) of an automated drug delivery device were 0%. The MDPE does not indicate the range of performance errors because positive and negative performance errors offset each other, but it does indicate whether the plasma concentrations achieved with the device tend to overshoot the desired target (+MDPE) or undershoot the desired target (–MDPE).

The performance may be abnormally distributed. To demonstrate the variability of the pharmacokinetic set, the 10th, 50th (median), and 90th percentiles of the prediction error for each patient are calculated, and a cumulative probability curve for the population being studied is constructed (Fig. 15) (30). The same can be done for the absolute performance error. Bias is the median of the median individual performance errors. Precision is defined as the dispersion of the 10th to 90th percentile of the population median-performance error.

A number of parameter sets have been published for most of the drugs used in anesthesia. Selection of the proper parameter set influences the performance of a pharmacokinetic model-driven infusion. Because the optimal pharmacokinetic set is unknown, the "best" pharmacokinetic set is the one that produces the best accuracy. There are different approaches to obtaining the "best" pharmacokinet-

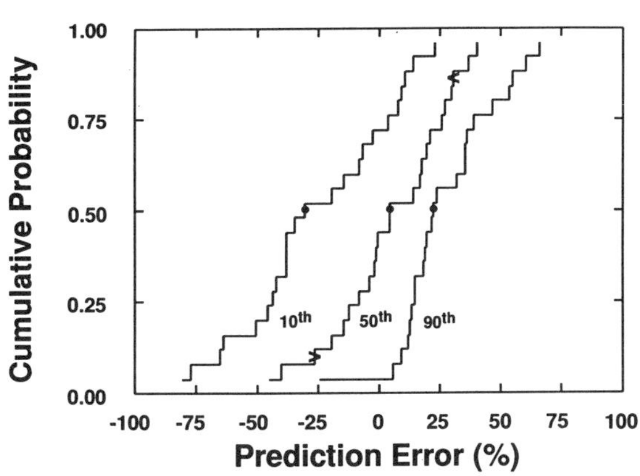

FIG. 15. The cumulative probability of the 10th, 50th, and 90th percentile of the median performance error of fentanyl administered via CACI in 24 patients. (From Glass et al., ref. 30, with permission.)

ic set. First, a purely retrospective evaluation can be done. This implies using a set of published pharmacokinetics in the CACI device and measuring actual blood levels at various times. The delivered infusion rates are simultaneously recorded. Subsequently, any set of pharmacokinetic values can be used with the known infusion rates to provide new predicted blood levels (41). For each pharmacokinetic set, accuracy can be calculated using the measured samples to determine the performance error, absolute performance error, and precision. The "best" pharmacokinetic set is the one that gives the best predictive accuracy.

By recording the infusion profile and measuring drug concentrations at predetermined times, a new set of pharmacokinetic parameters that more accurately defines the population investigated can be determined using one of several programs designed to calculate pharmacokinetic parameters (42). These programs seek the pharmacokinetic set that best fits the measured values for all the patients. The optimal pharmacokinetic parameters for fentanyl still have a median residual error of 21% when retrospectively tested against the same group of patients. This represents the limit imposed by pharmacokinetic variability on the possible performance of any fentanyl parameter set for dosing a similar adult population. In other words, it is unlikely that any fentanyl pharmacokinetic parameter set will produce less than 21% MDAPE. Crankshaw and colleagues (43,44) adopted an immediately prospective method to obtain the optimal infusion profile for a CACI type device. Although an infusion rate is used rather than a pharmacokinetic set, the infusion profile is based on the drug efflux from the central compartment and results in a bi- or triexponential equation that is the result of transfer functions used in other CACI devices. To achieve the optimal infusion profile, an error-correcting iterative approach is used whereby an infusion is administered and the drug concentration is measured. The resultant efflux at each sampling interval is calculated to produce a new infusion profile that will be used for the next set of patients. This is repeated until the optimal infusion profile is obtained. Although Crankshaw and colleagues calculated an optimal infusion profile, the process they used to obtain this value is similar to that used by Shafer et al. (42) to obtain their optimal pharmacokinetic set. However, the approach of Crankshaw's group was prospective, whereas Shafer et al.'s best fit was calculated retrospectively.

Unfortunately, the investigators who tried to establish an optimal pharmacokinetic set or infusion profile analyzed the results of their predictive accuracy of the set with the best fit differently. Nevertheless, some interpretation of this data can be made. The bias of the pharmacokinetic set should not be significantly different from zero. When the pharmacokinetic set is optimal, there should be, on the average, no over- or underestimation. The value of the mean absolute-prediction error is less easily stated. A review of the work of several authors suggests that it would be difficult in an average population to reduce the mean absolute prediction error below 20–30%. Schüttler et al. (45) stated that adequate clinical performance is achieved when a CACI device is used if the bias is less than 10–20%, the MAPE is 20–30%, and a maximal prediction error in any single sample is less than 50–60%.

The pharmacokinetic parameters of fentanyl (30,42), alfentanil (45–48), and propofol (45,49,50) have been evaluated in CACI devices during their administration to general surgical patients. In all instances, the resultant accuracy of the pharmacokinetic sets have been close to optimal. It is hoped that with greater use of CACI devices, the "best" pharmacokinetic values for all the anesthetic drugs will be defined.

There are two approaches to further improving the accuracy of a CACI device: use of a closed-loop system and use of the more practical population-specific kinetics (51). Population pharmacokinetics establishes sets of values that are altered by the specific physiological variables of height, weight, age, and sex. Pathological disease also can be incorporated to improve accuracy for an individual patient. Small changes in the pharmacokinetic set caused by minor physiological differences are less likely to improve the accuracy. If interpatient variability is 30% and the difference in the pharmacokinetic set resulting from the use of the population specific pharmacokinetic parameters is 20%, some individuals may have a pharmacokinetic set that is represented more closely by the original set than by the parameters derived from the population specific set. At present, few drugs used during the perioperative period have established population pharmacokinetic sets. Maitre et al. (52) retrospectively showed that their population pharmacokinetic sets for alfentanil improved accuracy. In prospective studies using this population pharmacokinetic set, variable accuracy has been demonstrated by different investigators. In Leiden, Lemmens et al. (48) found that this set of population pharmacokinetic parameters provided excellent accuracy in their patient group. In contrast, Raemer et al. (53) found that the same pharmacokinetic parameters resulted in a significant bias and a small absolute error in prediction and precision. This implies that inaccuracy resulting from interpatient variability, produced by population specific differences in their pharmacokinetic sets, may be reduced by the use of population-specific pharmacokinetics in CACI devices. However, the optimal pharmacokinetic set for each population subset needs to be established before accuracy will truly be improved.

Use of a pharmacokinetic loop implies that the drug concentration is measured on-line in real time and is used to revise the pharmacokinetic model continuously for the patient during ongoing drug administration. Although on-line drug analysis for IV anesthetics is unavailable at present, it is possible to achieve rapid analysis of the plasma concentration of certain compounds (e.g., lidocaine). One can recalculate individual pharmacokinetic parameters from one or two measured blood concentrations during target-controlled drug delivery. These parameters are then fed into the target control device and new infusion rates are calculated. Multiple practical and theoretical problems must be overcome before implementing such a system. Technological developments are rapidly providing methods and devices that can quantitatively measure a limited number of nonanesthetic drugs within minutes. The pharmacokinetic set used in the CACI device includes volumes of distribution and intercompartmental constants, including elimination. Samples taken early during the infusion will more accurately describe the central compartment volume and the intercompartmental constants that are responsible for redistribution. These samples will not, however, give an accurate estimate of elimination, which is best defined once redistribution nears completion (i.e., when a steady state is obtained). The major determinants of drug disposition during an anesthetic are the central compartment volume and the intercompartmental constants involved in redistribution. Therefore, early samples may prove to be useful. In a retrospective study, Maitre et al. (54) tested whether bayesian forecasting from a single sample or multiple samples could improve accuracy following alfentanil administration. A single plasma sample of alfentanil at 60 minutes improved overall accuracy, but bayesian forecasting in some individuals resulted in pharmacokinetic sets with greater inaccuracy. Hill's work (47) demonstrated an intrapatient variability of 20%. This variability may be greater during anesthesia and surgery as blood flow, organ metabolism, and fluid shifts are in a state of flux and may markedly affect an individual's pharmacokinetics during a brief period of time. Thus, when using a CACI device, one cannot assume that altering an individual's pharmacokinetics on-line will result in greater predictive accuracy. However, both investigators and industry can be expected to pursue actively closed-loop pharmacokinetic adaptive control.

In the absence of rapid assays for anesthetic drugs, the obvious method of reducing variability is to observe the drug effect and adjust the target to a concentration that produces the desired effect. By knowing the rate constant k_{e0}, one can model the concentration at the site of drug effect. Figure 16A shows the plasma fentanyl concentrations that could theoretically be obtained over the course of a brief operation. Figure 16B shows the fentanyl concentrations at the effect site for the same anesthetic shown in Fig. 16A. Even if the pump produced precisely the concentrations shown in Fig. 16A (i.e., it performed perfectly), the lag between the concentration in plasma and at the site of drug effect would, at best, produce a slurred response because of the equilibration delay between the plasma and the effect site. Several pharmacokinetic model-driven infusion devices now simultaneously display both the plasma and the effect site concentrations (55,56). These devices permit the clinician to target he concentration in the effect site rather than in plasma to make titration more precise by permitting the clinician to coordinate target concentration and observed drug effect.

The EEG has been used as a continuous measure of drug effect when determining k_{e0} values. The EEG may not be a measure of anesthesia for all the drugs. It also is impossible to measure (at least in humans) the concentration of drug in the biophase. Although the concept of using the k_{e0} to provide an appropriate effect compartment concentration is correct, it is important to test these values to ensure that they truly reflect the equilibration rate between plasma concentration and observed anesthetic effect. Several studies support the published values for the k_{e0} of both thiopental and propofol. Avram et al. (57) investigated the relationship between the dose of thiopental and population pharmacokinetics that produced loss of consciousness. Jacobs and Reves (58) were able to demonstrate that

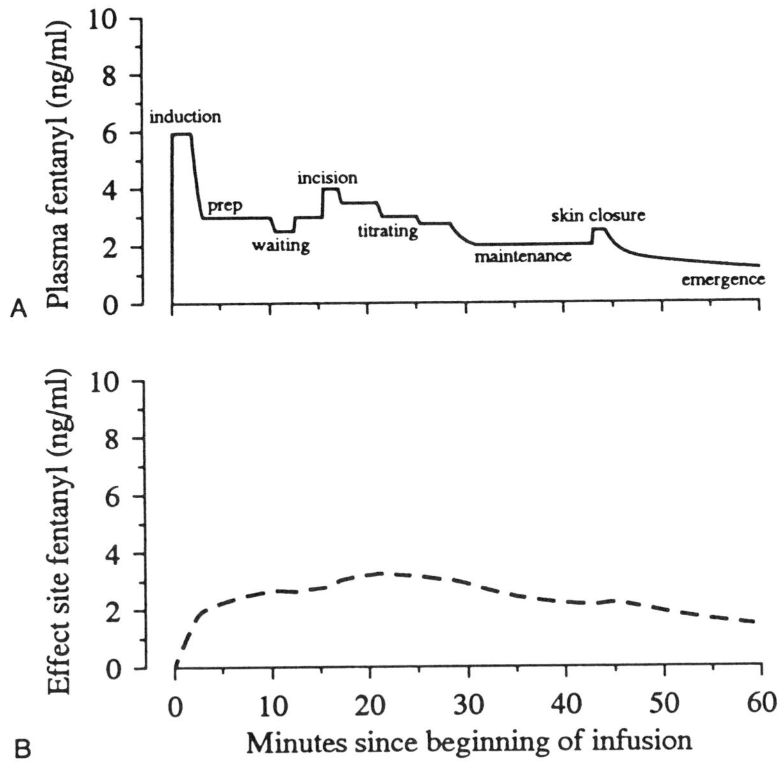

FIG. 16. A: Simulated plasma fentanyl concentrations over time for a brief anesthetic showing the rapid rise and fall and impression of precise titration that can be created by a target-controlled drug-delivery device. **B:** The effect site concentrations for the same anesthetic course, demonstrating that precise control of plasma concentration does not necessarily translate into precise control at the site of drug effect. (Adapted from Shafer and Gregg, ref. 55.)

if the k_{e0} value for thiopental was incorporated into their model, the dose that produced loss of consciousness in 50% of patients resulted in an effect compartment concentration of thiopental that was consistent with a previously demonstrated concentration that resulted in loss of consciousness in 50% of patients (59). Another study by the same group investigated the relationship between infusion rate and dose to loss of consciousness (57). Because of equilibration with the effect compartment, the dose for loss of consciousness varied as expected according to the infusion rate. When previously published k_{e0} values were incorporated into a simulation model, the dose predicted and the dose actually needed to achieve loss of consciousness were the same for each infusion rate, thus confirming a correct k_{e0} value. Even though the k_{e0} is based on the EEG, it represents the rate of equilibration between the plasma and the biophase.

Summary

Automated drug-delivery devices appear to achieve and maintain desired plasma concentrations with an expected error of about 20–30% of the target. Although reanalysis of pharmacokinetic parameters following automated drug delivery results in a reduction in the median error of closer to 20% in adults and possibly lower in children, as described by Shafer et al. (42) for fentanyl and Marsh et al. (50) for propofol, biological variability sets a limit on the expected accuracy of these devices. More accurate performance could be obtained with bayesian feedback using rapid intraoperative assays, but this is unavailable for the IV drugs used in anesthetic practice. However, the equilibration delay between the plasma and the effect site may make excessive focus on plasma concentrations unwarranted. Instead, learning about the pharmacokinetic/pharmacodynamic characteristics of the specific patient by titrating to a readily measured drug effect appears to be the most promising method of optimizing the performance of automated drug-delivery devices to the clinical needs of the individual patient.

A recent development for CACI drug delivery is the addition of an effect compartment to the pharmacokinetic model. This allows delivery of the IV anesthetic to a desired effect compartment (brain) concentration. Although it was initially emphasized that a strict relationship exists between drug concentration and anesthetic effect, this only holds true once blood and brain concentrations equilibrate. To overcome the juggling required because of hysteresis, the k_{e0} values (rate constant linking plasma and drug effect site) obtained from kinetic-dynamic modeling with an EEG can be used in CACI devices to administer the IV anesthetic to an effect compartment concentration.

Clinical Use

Ultimately, it is the performance during clinical use that is of greatest importance to the practicing clinician's acceptance of target-controlled drug delivery. To maintain a stable anesthetic state, one must always titrate drugs to provide an effective concentration. This depends on both the choice of the drug and the administration system. The evaluation of the technique requires a comparison between automated drug-delivery devices and manual methods of administration with the same drug and between automated drug delivery of IV anesthetics and inhalational anesthetics. Numerous studies have evaluated automated drug-delivery devices for the administration of IV anesthetics during both brief and complex surgery in children and adults and for short-term sedation, prolonged sedation (days), and chronic pain management. Unfortunately, few comparative studies have been done on automated drug-delivery devices versus manual delivery systems.

When pharmacokinetic model-driven delivery of alfentanil was compared to bolus dose administration (60), automated drug delivery produced fewer incidences of muscular rigidity, hypotension, and bradycardia on induction. With automated drug delivery, there was a greater percentage of anesthesia time within ±15% of the desired blood pressure and heart rate, and less naloxone was required during surgery for adequate ventilation. Pharmacokinetic model-driven infusion of fentanyl during cardiac surgery resulted in greater hemodynamic control, with fewer additional drug interventions and significantly fewer episodes of either hypo- or hypertension compared to bolus dose administration (37). A small study that compared manual administration with pharmacokinetic model-driven infusion of alfentanil resulted in similar anesthesia maintenance and recovery (61). A study of double-blind manual administration was compared with a pharmacokinetic model-driven infusion in a small group of patients undergoing cardiac surgery (62). In both methods, the drugs (one containing a placebo) were titrated at the same time with the aim of maintaining hemodynamic control. The greatest difference between the two methods was that more variability in drug plasma concentrations was observed in the manual group. This implies that pharmacokinetic model-driven infusion is able to maintain drug concentrations within a narrower therapeutic range—a particular advantage with drugs having a narrow therapeutic window. Although target-controlled delivery was at least equal to manual drug delivery, there were no real outcome measurements in this study. Thus, the need remains to establish which of the theoretical benefits to patients will be realized with model-based target-controlled delivery over manual delivery of IV drugs.

Pharmacokinetic model-driven infusion of propofol compares favorably to thiopental/isoflurane anesthesia for general surgery lasting several hours (63). Induction maintenance and recovery are similar between the two groups, implying that when appropriately administered, IV anesthesia can be equal to inhalational anesthesia in providing the objectives of anesthesia.

In noncomparative studies, pharmacokinetic model-driven infusions were used to administer propofol, midazolam, thiopental, alfentanil, and fentanyl for a variety of anesthetic techniques, including N_2O narcotic anesthesia, supplementation of volatile anesthetics, total IV anesthesia, sedation for monitored anesthesia care, regional anesthesia, or ICU sedation. In all these studies, irrespective of the accuracy obtained, hemodynamic stability and recovery met clinical expectations (32). These studies targeted plasma/blood concentrations. Although one can target the effect site for possibly better results, no reports of clinical outcomes when the effect site is targeted have been published.

Pharmacokinetic model-driven infusion can also provide sedation either in the ICU or for monitored anesthesia care. Target-controlled delivery can rapidly provide a desired state of sedation that can be maintained by varying the target concentration without causing significant cardiorespiratory compromise (32).

Automated drug delivery is for IV drugs what the calibrated vaporizer is for inhalational anesthetic agents. Like the vaporizer, pharmacokinetic model-driven infusion facilitates drug delivery on the basis of plasma or biophase concentration rather than on drug dosage. Just as there is variability in the uptake of volatile anesthetic agents, there will be predicted-to-actual differences in the plasma concentrations obtained by using pharmacokinetic model-driven infusion. An inspired halothane concentration of 1% results in an end-tidal concentration that is some fraction of 1%. Using pharmacokinetic model-driven infusion to maintain a fentanyl concentration in plasma of 3 ng/ml should result in plasma concentrations that hover around 3 ng/ml. However, if the pharmacokinetic model does not adequately describe the disposition of fentanyl in a particular patient, variations in the plasma concentration may result. This is a disadvantage of pharmacokinetic model-drive infusion. To achieve the desired effect concentration quickly, the model algorithm inherently and continuously calculates the required infusion rates. This is an advantage over both manual infusion techniques and the analogous situations with the delivery of inhalation anesthetics using the calibrated vaporizer because it is unnecessary to calculate a loading dose or to use overpressurization, respectively. Finally, the time-varying stresses of surgery and the variability in the patient's response require the anesthesiologist to titrate the administration of the potent inhalational anesthetics using the calibrated vaporizer for drug delivery. These same factors plus pharmacokinetic variability require vigilant titration of the infusion of IV anesthetic drugs when the drugs are given by automated drug delivery.

In addition to their importance for the clinical administration of IV anesthetics, target-controlled drug-delivery devices are extremely important for research. They can define equipotency between IV drugs as well as the physiological responses to IV drugs when they reach a steady concentration and equilibrate with their effect site. They enable interactions involving IV drugs as well as pharmacokinetic or dynamic differences produced by different physiological conditions to be clearly defined. Closed-loop target delivery will also enable unbiased and more precise comparisons between drugs. Target-controlled delivery can prospectively test pharmacokinetics and ultimately provide the most suitable pharmacokinetic parameters for infusion of IV drug in any given population. As a research tool, automated drug delivery has already made a major impact on anesthetic administration.

The introduction of several new IV anesthetic agents stimulates the use of IV anesthesia in clinical practice. The devices used to administer IV anesthesia are also undergoing an evolution. The introduction of infusion pumps designed specifically for continuous IV anesthetic drug delivery should further enhance IV anesthesia. "Calculator" pumps facilitate manual means of continuous IV drug administration. Although a major step forward for IV drug delivery, these pumps fall short of enabling the clinician to titrate drug concentration to drug effect. Automated drug delivery, however, provides this ability. Pharmacokinetic model-driven infusion has several theoretical advantages over manual infusion systems: for example, further improvements in hemodynamic control and a more predictable rapid awakening. The actual advantages of automated drug delivery of IV anesthetics over manual methods, or in comparison to inhalational anesthetics, are not yet fully established. Currently available pharmacokinetics used with pharmacokinetic model-driven infusion are adequate but not optimal for clinical use. Controlled studies with large patient populations are needed to establish fully its ultimate role in the clinical practice of anesthesia. Its mere convenience, however, should allow the clinician to choose the appropriate anesthetic drug on the basis of its characteristics rather than on the basis of the convenience of the administration device.

Closed-Loop Drug Delivery and Automatic Feedback Control Systems

Automatic mechanical feedback systems were first used by James Watt in the 18th century to control the speed of steam engines. Electronic systems were developed in the 1930s and 1940s to control aircraft and ships, giving birth to the subdivision of electrical engineering known as "control theory," which is basically the science of accurate indirect electronic control of a measured parameter. The basic building block of control theory is the "proportional controller," illustrated in generic terms in Fig. 17. Here, a measured value of a parameter (the "output") is arithmetically subtracted from the desired value (the "set point"), producing a difference value (the "error"). This error signal drives some device (the "prime mover") to decrease the error (i.e., "negative feedback"). Thus, the system tends toward an equilibrium where the set point is equal to the output and the error signal is zero. If the set point or output is subsequently changed, the system automatically corrects the situation. Proportional controllers are simple in concept, but perform poorly when there is an appreciable delay in the response of the prime mover. Then they tend to overcorrect and oscillate. This limitation led to the development of the "proportional derivative" (PD) controller, which generates an error signal based not only on the difference between the set point and the output but also on the time rate of change of this difference. In principle, a PD controller will detect the condition in which the error signal is rapidly approaching zero, then slow the corrective action of the prime mover. PD controllers perform well in servomechanical applications, but a slight limitation exists whenever the output is biased by a constant factor such as a mechanical load. In this

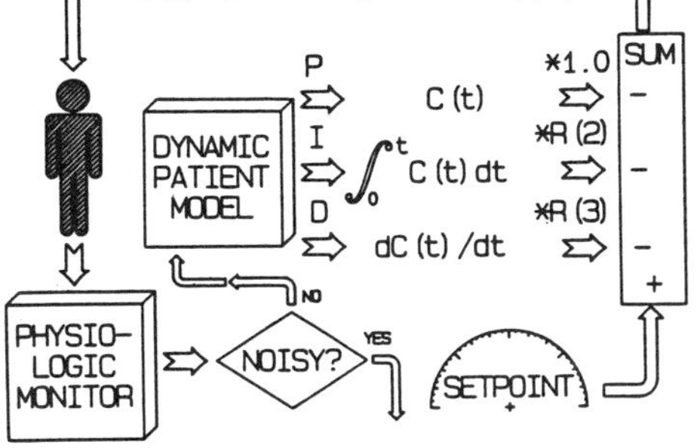

FIG. 17. PID controller incorporating an internal pharmacodynamic model and noise filter for reliable control of a physiologic variable.

situation, the PD controller comes into equilibrium with a small constant error that exactly balances the effect of the load. Frequently, the error is small enough to be negligible, but it can often be corrected by adding a third component of the time integral of the error, forming a "Proportional-Integral-Derivative" (PID) controller. The integral component corrects for the constant error and forces the output to be exactly equal to the set point. Applied control theory in the form of the PID controller is essential to the operation of much of modern electronic and mechanical equipment.

Since applied control theory works well in electronic applications, an obvious extension would be the automatic control of drug administration based on objectively measured patient response. Closed-loop control is an example. Several formidable difficulties arise in practical situations, however, because physiologic drug response (1) is nonlinear and exhibits hysteresis, (2) varies with time, (3) varies from subject to subject, and (4) exhibits an absolute time delay that also varies with time and individual. These factors limit the performance of simple PID controllers in physiologic applications since the differential equations resulting from a comprehensive system analysis are generally so complex that they are unsolvable except by numerical approximation techniques. Although virtually every successful closed-loop drug-delivery scheme that has been reported involves a PID controller, extensive empirical modifications and "tuning" are required before a practical device that is capable of adequate performance of different subjects can be developed. Common empirical modifications include limitation or elimination of the integral component, variable proportional gain as the error increases, and continuous dynamic automatic optimization of parameters: so-called "self-tuning" or "adaptive" controllers.

All closed-loop physiologic control systems incorporate several essential elements (Fig. 17). A reliable monitor is essential for efficient and safe performance, and it is often the limiting component of the system. Although monitoring is fairly routine for blood pressure or muscle relaxation, it can be extremely difficult for continuously measuring serum glucose for automatic insulin administration. The requirement to monitor possible adverse effects can likewise be a simple or complex problem, depending upon the drug. A logical filter for noise (Fig. 17), is generally required to eliminate improper operation from spurious input. Impressive computer hardware was developed in the 1980s with the advent of sophisticated, inexpensive microprocessors and memory. As a result, the currently available technology allows elegant and complex programming to be contained within an arbitrarily small package. Infusion pumps have become smaller, more sophisticated, and more reliable, so hardware itself is seldom a limiting factor in performance.

Systems for the automatic delivery of drugs based on negative feedback from pharmacological effects were developed and reported as early as 1950. A controller system administered anesthetic gasses intraoperatively using blood pressure as the controlled parameter. Although the system was large and awkward because of the technology of the times, it worked well. Other successful automatic drug-administration systems were subsequently tested and described, but clinical applications were limited before microprocessors were developed. Thus, small and reliable devices that lack the numerous problems associated with analog controllers can be used.

Several authors (64–66) tested and described automatic infusions of muscle relaxant using the electrically evoked response of skeletal muscle in both animals and humans. Although sophisticated self-tuning controllers are available for this purpose, the most successful devices incorporate fairly simple modifications of standard PID.

The IVAC Titrator, specifically designed to administer nitroprusside for blood pressure control in humans, was the only commercially available automatic feedback drug-delivery system available in the United States. Extensive clinical trials conclusively demonstrated its outstanding and consistent performance in automatically maintaining desired blood pressure (67,68). Despite these positive results, the IVAC Titrator was withdrawn from the market.

Closed-loop systems have been used for the administration of IV anesthetics. Schüttler et al. (69), using median EEG frequency and a pk/pd link, provided closed-loop anesthesia in volunteers with methohexital (69). Following their success in volunteers, they used this closed-loop system to provide anesthesia for surgical patients with a variety of anesthetic drugs (70,71). In their system, a predetermined infusion rate of opiate is administered, and the hypnotic infusion rate is altered by the closed-loop system because, at analgesic concentrations, the opiate has a minimal effect on the median EEG frequency. To insure that an adequate anesthetic state is maintained during periods of minimal surgical stimulation, a continuous nociceptive stimulus is continuously applied via the system to the patient. Kenny et al. (72) successfully used a closed loop system based on auditory evoked potentials. They administered the opiate at a preset infusion rate and adjusted the propofol infusion by the servosystem. These examples indicate that closed-loop anesthesia is a possibility. This would be the ideal drug-delivery system to administer IV anesthetics. However, the relationship between drug concentrations versus EEG/auditory-evoked potentials versus anesthetic state (i.e., level of awareness and recall) has not been fully elucidated because the number of patients, varying drug combinations, and types of surgical procedures have been limited. Also, no comparative studies have been done on closed-loop delivery versus other methods of drug delivery to demonstrate its advantages. Therefore, more work is needed to evaluate its clinical utility.

Almost without exception, automatic drug administration with a well-designed control algorithm and safety features outperforms, or at least equals, an average human operator accomplishing the same task. Countless skilled medical and nursing hours could be saved by the widespread application of closed-loop systems for muscle relaxants, vasoppressors, maintenance fluids, and anesthetic drug administration in the future.

OTHER DELIVERY SYSTEMS USED FOR INTRAVENOUS DRUG DELIVERY

Drugs can be given via inhalational, oral, IV, intramuscular, transmucosal, or transdermal routes. Providing a rapid onset of drug effect and improving bioavailability during anesthesia are reasons to administer a drug intravenously. During the preoperative and postoperative periods, however, drug onset and bioavailability may be less critical. During these periods, parenteral administration may be less desirable and the oral route may be unavailable. As a result, there is an interest in delivering opioids and hypnotics by either the transdermal or transmucosal route.

Transdermal Drug Delivery

The skin is generally considered to be a protective layer against the environment and relatively impervious to absorption of substances through it. Because of its high lipid content, lipophilic substances can be absorbed systemically through the skin. This leads to the development of patches for transdermal drug delivery for a limited number of drugs (73). Sebel et al. (74) demonstrated that the highly potent and lipid-soluble opioids, fentanyl and sufentanil, can be sufficiently absorbed through the skin to provide analgesic concentrations. This stimulated the development of fentanyl transdermal therapeutic systems for commercial use. The Alza patch, illustrated in Fig. 18, consists of an adhesive surface to insure optimal skin contact, a rate-limiting membrane, a drug reservoir, and backing. Transfer of drug across the dermis into the general circulation can be highly variable. The rate-limiting membrane is placed in the patch so that the membrane, rather than the dermis, is the rate-limiting step for drug transfer into the general circulation. Thus, the variability resulting from absorption through the dermis is minimized.

The transfer of drug from the patch to the circulation results in markedly different pharmacokinetics compared with any other delivery route (75). Initially, drug diffuses passively through the stratum corneum and epidermis and into the dermis. Once drug enters the dermis, it is removed to the general circulation via passive transfer to the cutaneous microcirculation. The rate of transfer into the circulation rises as the concentration in the dermis increases. Because transfer into the dermis is largely constant, transfer from the dermis to the circulation will subsequently behave like a continuous infusion and a steady fentanyl plasma concentration will be obtained. However, the time to reach this steady-state concentration will be longer than when the drug is infused intravenously. Once the patch is removed, a depot of fentanyl that remains within the dermis will continue to deliver drug into the circulation; the result is a markedly prolonged half-life. The differences between a continuous IV infusion of fentanyl at 50 μg/hr versus a patch estimated to deliver 50 μg/hr is illustrated in Fig. 19. The elimination half-life of fentanyl increases from 4–8 hours to 15–19 hours when delivered with a a transdermal patch (75).

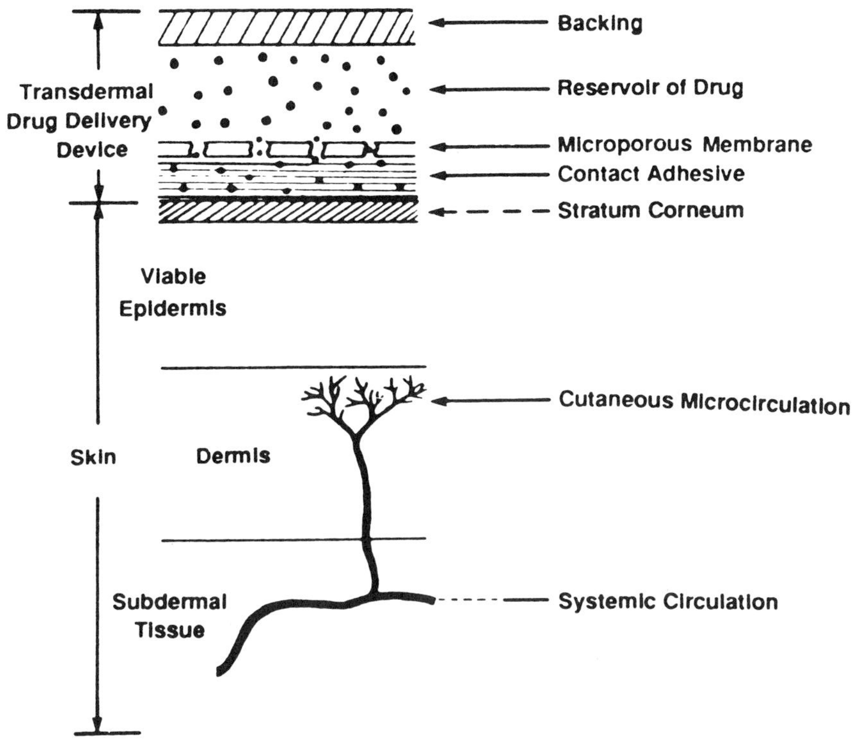

FIG. 18. A schematic representation of the Alza TTS Fentanyl Patch. (From Varvel et al., ref. 75, with permission.)

The delivery rate of the patch varies according to the size of the patch. Alza produces patches of various sizes. Gourlay et al. (76) defined 0.6 ng/ml with a range of 0.2–1.2 ng/ml as the minimum effective analgesic concentration of fentanyl for postoperative pain relief (76). A continuous infusion of fentanyl of 25 μg/hr to 125 μg/hr would be needed to obtain a steady-state fentanyl plasma concentration within this range.

The advantages and disadvantages of transdermal drug delivery are presented in Table 7. The major advantage is the ability to administer a drug noninvasively as a continuous infusion. Because a patch does not deliver directly into the circulation, the ability to rapidly achieve a desirable drug concentration or vary that concentration is limited. This is important because an analgesic level is needed immediately after surgery and the therapeutic concentration varies not only from patient to patient, but also within individual patients, depending on their level of activity. Thus, a transdermal patch that can alter the drug concentration more acutely may be needed to obtain optimal pain control. Fentanyl has a relatively narrow therapeutic range; therefore, if the patient develops respiratory depression, it may

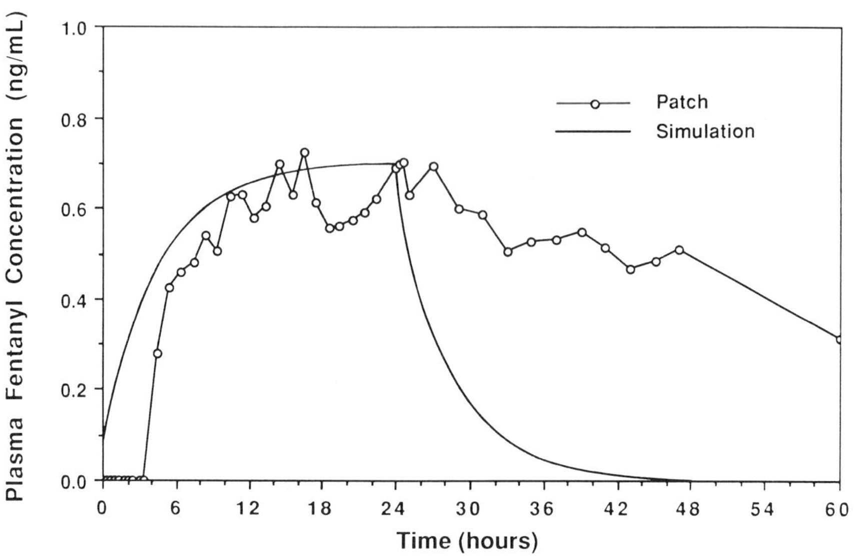

FIG. 19. A comparison between a computer simulation of a 50 μg/hr intravenous infusion and the measured fentanyl levels following the application of a 50 μg/hr transdermal fentanyl patch.

be prolonged because of the slow elimination of fentanyl even after the patch is removed. On the other hand, because the rate of rise of the fentanyl concentration will be slow, any sign of respiratory depression can be noted early and the patch can be removed. Consequently, the greatest use of transdermal fentanyl delivery will be treatment for chronic pain, where rapid fluctuations in fentanyl concentration are unnecessary but continuous noninvasive delivery of an analgesic will be a great advantage. The level of postoperative pain, changes continually. In addition, the concentration of fentanyl achieved from the combination of that delivered from the patch and that given intraoperatively may be inadequate initially and excessive later, with the very real possibility of clinically significant respiratory depression.

Fentanyl transdermal patches are passive drug-delivery systems because drug passes through the skin according to the concentration gradient between the patch and the systemic circulation and the resistance provided by the dermis. As noted above and in Chapter 7, the optimal means of providing postoperative analgesia is self-titration by the patient. The present transdermal system provides a change in concentration that is too slow to be effective for self-titration. A more active delivery system would be preferable. Iontophoresis produces active transfer of drug across the skin. Work on iontophoretic delivery of anesthetic or analgesic compounds is limited, although analgesic levels of morphine were obtained with an iontophoretic patch (77). More recently, iontophoresis potentiated the transfer

TABLE 7. *Advantages and disadvantages of a transdermal fentanyl patch*

Advantages	1. Provides a simple and convenient mode of drug delivery. 2. Allows a more precise control over plasma drug concentrations than does intermittent dosing. 3. Reduces the amount of drug needed daily to achieve a therapeutic effect by avoiding first-pass loss. 4. Avoids variability of gastrointestinal absorption. 5. Provides an alternative route when oral administration is not practical. 6. Provides a parenteral route without the inconvenience of intravenous infusions or intramuscular injections. 7. Allows delivery to be altered by changing the size of the patch.
Disadvantages	1. Long lag time between placing the patch and reaching therapeutic levels. 2. Concentration cannot be altered rapidly. 3. Patients cannot interact with the system to titrate themselves to achieve the plasma concentration that is effective for them. 4. Extremely long elimination time can be a problem if an overdose occurs.

of sufentanil across the skin, and lidocaine placed into an iontophoretic patch rendered the underlying skin anesthetized within a few minutes.

Transmucosal Drug Delivery

Using the transmucosal route for delivery of anesthetic drugs is not new. For many years, barbiturates were given transrectally to children to induce anesthesia. There is increasing interest in transmucosal delivery because the oral and nasal mucosal membranes provide a large and efficient surface area for absorption of drugs into the circulation.

Transmucosal drug delivery offers many of the same advantages that transdermal drug delivery does (Table 7). However, it is likely to be used as a complement to other routes of drug administration. Transdermal delivery enables prolonged administration with minimal patient interaction. Transmucosal drug delivery is less suitable for prolonged administration but provides rapid drug absorption to quickly achieve therapeutic concentrations. Transmucosal drug administration tends to be more interactive with the patient, enabling titration to a desired effect. Rapid absorption into the circulation is explained by the large surface area for drug transfer, the rich mucosal blood supply, and the absence of a mucosal drug depot (78). Because there is no drug depot within the mucosa, the pharmacokinetic characteristics of a drug are similar to those with parenteral administration. Absorption and elimination of a transmucosally delivered dose of fentanyl are illustrated in Fig. 20 (79). These are in contrast with the absorption and elimination characteristics of the transdermal delivery of fentanyl illustrated in Fig. 19.

The vehicle for transmucosal drug delivery is variable. Solutions, tablets, sprays, and "lollipops" have been used. Most of the potent opiates, hypnotics, and IV anesthetics have been administered via the transmucosal route. Oral transmucos-

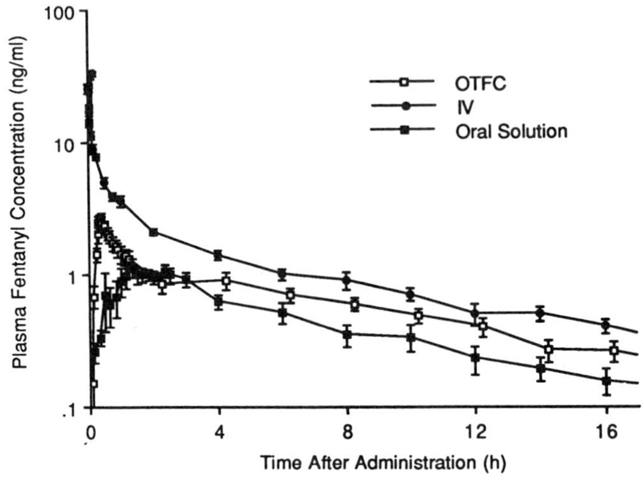

FIG. 20. The resultant plasma concentrations after the administration of fentanyl citrate at a dose of 15 μg/kg given either intravenously via a swallowed oral solution or by means of oral transmucosal (OTFC) administration. The inset shows the first 90 min in detail. (From Streisand et al., ref. 79, with permission.)

al fentanyl citrate (OTFC) (78), nasal transmucosal sufentanil (80), and midazolam provide effective premedication for children.

OTFC is used primarily for premedication in children. It comes in doses of 200 μg, 300 μg, and 400 μg. Because of its rate of absorption and its rate of equilibrium between plasma concentration and the biophase, transmucosal delivery of fentanyl citrate can produce a relatively rapid onset of a therapeutic effect that will last for several hours. Absorption occurs over 10–15 minutes with high peak plasma concentrations. However, as the k_{e0} for fentanyl is small (i.e., it slowly moves into the biophase) and redistribution is extensive the peak effect concentrations with doses of 15μg/kg are unlikely to exceed therapeutic concentrations. Also, because the fentanyl absorbed is extensively distributed by the time the peak concentration is reached, little further distribution will occur and the rate of decrease of drug concentration in the biophase will be close to the elimination half-life of fentanyl (i.e., 4–6 hr). Stanley et al. (81) first described the use of fentanyl "lollipops" in children as a nonthreatening way to produce analgesia and sedation with limited side effects. The initial doses of fentanyl within the OTFC of 0.5 mg and 1 mg delivered 5–20 μg/kg. The bioavailability of fentanyl from the OTFC is 50%, with absorption occurring through both the oral and gastric mucosa. Absorption is influenced by rate of sucking, saliva production, pH of the mouth, and the amount of saliva swallowed. Maximal concentrations of fentanyl after a 15 μg/kg unit were 2.8 ±1ng/ml and occurred 23 ± 3 minutes after administration. The elimination half-life of fentanyl is the same after IV or OTFC administration, indicating minimal sequestration of fentanyl into the buccal mucosa (79).

Subsequent studies evaluated the safety and efficacy of OTFC as a pediatric premedicant and showed that it was effective in producing preoperative sedation and anxiolysis within 20 minutes of administration (82–86). Various dosages were studied. High-dose OTFC (20–25 μg/kg) produced significantly more side effects than did a conventional premedicant of oral meperidine, diazepam, and atropine (78). These authors concluded that high doses of OTFC were unacceptable. A lower dose of 10–15 μg/kg was as effective as the higher dosage for producing drowsiness and anxiolysis. Nonetheless, the incidence of side effects was similar between the various doses. The most common side effect was pruritis (incidence, 60–100%), but was not viewed as troublesome. Unfortunately, the incidence of nausea and vomiting was 22–65%. One study, using high doses of OTFC, also reported a 30% incidence of vomiting before induction. Gastric volumes have increased in children receiving OTFC preoperatively compared with children receiving no premedication. The increase in gastric volume was statistically significant, but the increase was small (7–8 ml). Prophylactic droperidol, 50 μg/kg IV, does not significantly decrease postoperative nausea and vomiting following OTFC administration. Although respiratory depression is a serious adverse effect of opioid administration, the incidence of clinically important ventilatory impairment can be limited by keeping the dose lower than 15 μg/kg. Thus, OTFC is an appealing, safe, and effective premedicant for children, but it is associated with a high incidence of nausea and vomiting.

OTFC was also suggested as a treatment for "breakthrough" cancer pain (87,88). In an open-label study of 10 patients with advanced cancer pain, OTFC was found to be safe, effective, and provide a relatively quick onset of analgesia (88). As anticipated, a lower incidence of opioid side effects was observed in this population. In children with malignancy, OTFC was used before diagnostic procedures were performed (89). With a dose of 12.5 μg/kg, OTFC was effective in decreasing the pain felt by children 7–18 years old. Children aged 3–6 years had inadequate control; these assessed their pain as a 9 on a 10-point scale. OTFC was also evaluated for both postoperative pain control and breakthrough pain in patients on chronic pain regimens. OTFC, 10 μg/kg titrated to effect, provided 4–6 hours of effective postoperative analgesia for a variety of surgical procedures. One can use transmucosal administration of fentanyl to supplement a transdermal patch, thus providing all the advantages of patient-controlled analgesia but through noninvasive means. Drug abuse by the lay public is potentially a major disadvantage of transmucosal delivery of potent anesthetic/analgesic drugs.

Intranasal sufentanil was evaluated in both children and adults. Because it is highly lipid soluble and potent, small volumes of sufentanil produce clinically significant effects. In adults, 10 μg doses of nasal sufentanil produced a median onset of sedation within 10 minutes that waned by 60 minutes (90). Within 20 minutes after administration, nearly 80% of the patients experienced significant drowsiness (sedation). A higher dosage of 20 μg also was used in this study but was no more effective. In contrast to OTFC, the side effects with intranasal sufentanil were limited. The most common one was a brief period of dizziness in 16%

of the patients. A second study comparing IV and 15 μg of intranasal sufentanil as premedication for adults found a 78% bioavailability, with a peak concentration of 0.08 ng/ml at 10 minutes (91). The onset of sedation with IV sufentanil was more rapid than after intranasal administration. However, by 20 minutes, the degree of sedation and the plasma sufentanil levels were similar between the two groups. No intergroup differences in sedation were observed between 20 minutes and 60 minutes after drug administration. Effective preoperative sedation with a relatively quick onset was achieved with this dose. Again, the most common side effect was dizziness, which was experienced by three of nine patients receiving intranasal sufentanil. In adults, no clinically significant respiratory depression occurred with intranasal administration, whereas significant decreases in PaO_2 occurred in patients given IV sufentanil.

Because nasally administered sufentanil is a rapid, noninvasive method of achieving effective preoperative sedation, its use in the pediatric population is especially appealing. Henderson et al. (80) evaluated the safety and efficacy of 1.5–4.5 μg/kg of intranasally administered sufentanil in children aged 5 months to 7 years. Compared with placebo, sufentanil facilitated the separation of children from parents. Within 10 minutes of its administration, 75–86% of the children were willing to separate calmly from their parents. Children given sufentanil also required less postoperative analgesia. However, significant changes in ventilatory compliance during induction of anesthesia were noted in 50% of the children given sufentanil. This effect was dose related. One patient in the group that received 3 μg/kg required succinylcholine, oxygen, and positive pressure ventilation to treat a marked decrease in pulmonary compliance and arterial oxygen saturation. One episode of preoperative emesis also was reported.

A more recent study compared the safety and efficacy of intranasal sufentanil and intranasal midazolam as preinduction agents (92). Although both drugs were effective preinduction sedatives, 2 μg/kg of sufentanil was associated with a significant incidence of decreased chest-wall compliance and decreased arterial-oxygen saturation. Nearly one-fourth of the sufentanil-treated children experienced a PaO_2 of less than 90%, and 37% of the children were difficult to ventilate. Clearly, the sufentanil doses used for adults were much lower than were those for children. Higher doses of the potent opioid agonists are known to produce rigidity. Thus, although sufentanil is an effective preinduction agent, its use requires careful monitoring, especially in the pediatric population. Whether lower doses of intranasal sufentanil are effective but safer in this age group remains to be investigated.

There is limited experience with intranasal fentanyl for the management of postoperative pain. Striebel et al. (93) demonstrated that intranasal fentanyl could provide analgesia similar to IV fentanyl. Administration of intranasal fentanyl could be titrated to individual patients' needs, similar to what is done routinely with the IV route. Intranasal fentanyl was accepted well by the patient.

Intranasal and transmucosal midazolam were investigated for premedication in children. Both routes provided highly effective sedation in children and allowed atraumatic separation from parents and smoother induction of anesthesia. Absorption by both routes is relatively rapid, with peak concentration at 5–10 minutes and peak effect at 10–15 minutes. The dose for transmucosal oral midazolam is 0.1–0.2 mg/kg. Because the drug has a bitter taste, it is usually mixed with some form of sweetener. The dose for intranasal administration also is 0.1–0.2 mg/kg. Appreciation of this highly effective means of drug delivery is likely to increase its use during the perioperative period.

CONCLUSION

Anesthesiologists need a safe and effective means of delivering drugs to obtain a desired physiological state. For the inhalational anesthetics, delivery devices meeting these criteria are well known. Until recently, the administration of IV drugs was largely limited to needle and syringe. This is rapidly changing because of technological advances and the clinician's desire to infuse IV drugs. In the future, pharmacokinetic drug delivery, closed-loop drug delivery, and noninvasive delivery systems will have a marked impact on the everyday practice of anesthesiology. Familiarity with these devices will help to simplify the administration of IV anesthetic agents and ultimately improve patient outcomes.

REFERENCES

1. Corssen G, Reves J, Stanley T. *Intravenous anesthesia and analgesia.* Philadelphia: Lea and Febiger; 1988.
2. Jacobs J, Glass P, Reves J. Opioid administration by continuous infusion. In: Fg E, ed. *Opioids in anesthesia II.* London, UK: Butterworth & Co.; 1990: 248.
3. Shafer SL, Varvel JR. Pharmacokinetics, pharmacodynamics, and rational opioid selection. *Anesthesiology* 1991;74:53–63.
4. Sheiner LB, Stanski DR, Vozeh S, Miller RD, Ham J. Simultaneous modelling of pharmacokinetics and pharmacodynamics: application to d-tubocurarine. *Clin Pharm Ther* 1979;25:358–371.
5. Scott JC, Ponganis KV, Stanski DR. EEG quantitation of narcotic effect: the comparative pharmacodynamics of fentanyl and alfentanil. *Anesthesiology* 1985;62:234–241.
6. Schwilden H, Schüttler J, Stoekel H. Pharmacokinetics as applied to total intravenous anaesthesia: theoretical considerations. *Anaesthesia* 1983;38(Suppl):51–52.
7. Schüttler J, Schwilden H, Stoekel H. Pharmacokinetics as applied to total intravenous anaesthesia: practical implications. *Anaesthesia* 1983;38(Suppl):53–56.
8. Roberts F, et al. Induction and maintenance of propofol anaesthesia: a manual infusion scheme. *Anaesthesia* 1988;43(Suppl):14–17.
9. Hughes MA, Glass PSA, Jacobs JR. Context-sensitive half-time in multicompartment pharmacokinetic models for intravenous anesthetic drugs. *Anesthesiology* 1992;76:334–341.
10. Ausems ME, Hug CC Jr, Stanski DR, Burm AGL. Plasma concentrations of alfentanil required to supplement nitrous oxide anesthesia for general surgery. *Anesthesiology* 1986;65:362–373.
11. Glass PSA, Doherty M, Jacobs JR, Goodman D, Smith LR. Plasma concentration of fentanyl, with 70% nitrous oxide, to prevent movement at skin incision. *Anesthesiology* 1993;78:842–847.
12. Vinik HR, Bradley EL, Kissin I. Midazolam-alfentanil synergism for anesthetic induction in patients. *Anesth Analg* 1989;69:213–218.
13. Short TG, Plummer JL, Chui PT. Hypnotic and anaesthetic interactions between midazolam, propofol and alfentanil. *Br J Anaesth* 1992;69:162–167.
14. Short TG, Chui PT. Propofol and midazolam act synergistically in combination. *Br J Anaesth* 1991; 67:539–545.

15. Short TG, Galletly DC, Plummer JL. Hypnotic and anaesthetic action of thiopentone and midazolam alone and in combination. *Br J Anaesth* 1991;66:13–19.
16. Tverskoy M, Fleyshman G, Bradley EL, Kissin I. Midazolam-thiopental anesthetic interaction in patients. *Anesth Analg* 1988;67:342–345.
17. Tverskoy M, Fleyshman G, Ezry J, Bradley EL, Kissin I. Midazolam-morphine sedative interactions in patients. *Anesth Analg* 1989;68:282–285.
18. Tverskoy M, Ben-Shlomo I, Ezry J, Fleyshman G. Midazolam acts synergistically with methohexitone for induction of anaesthesia. *Br J Anaesth* 1989;63:109–112.
19. Kissin I, Vinik, HR, Castillo R, Bradley EL. Alfentanil potentiates midazolam induced unconsciousness in subanalgesic doses. *Anesth Analg* 1990;71:65–69.
20. Kissin I, Vinik HR, Bradley EL Jr. Midazolam potentiates thiopental anesthetic induction in patients. *J Clin Anesth* 1991;3:367–370.
21. Kissin I, Mason JO, Bradley EL. Morphine and fentanyl hypnotic interactions with thiopental. *Anesthesiology* 1987;67:331–335.
22. Telford RJ, Glass PSA, Goodman D, Jacobs JR. Fentanyl does not alter the "sleep" plasma concentration of thiopental. *Anesth Analg* 1992;75:523–529.
23. Vinik HR, Bradley EL, Kissin I. Alfentanil does not potentiate hypnotic effect of propofol. *Anesth Analg* 1991;72:S308(abst).
24. Smith C, McEwan AI, Jhaveri R, Wilkinson M, Goodman D, Smith LR, Canada AT, Glass PSA. The interaction of fentanyl on the CP_{50} of propofol for loss of consciousness and skin incision. *Anesthesiology* 1994;81:820–828.
25. McEwan AI, Smith C, Dyar O, Goodman D, Glass PSA. Isoflurane MAC reduction by fentanyl. *Anesthesiology* 1993;78:864–869.
26. Sebel PS, Glass PSA, Fletcher JE, Murphy MR, Gallagher C, Quill T. Reduction of the MAC of desflurane with fentanyl. *Anesthesiology* 1992;76:52–59.
27. Westmoreland CL, Sebel PS, Gropper A. Fentanyl or alfentanil decreases the minimum alveolar anesthetic concentration of isoflurane in surgical patients. *Anesth Analg* 1994;78:23–28.
28. Brunner MD, Braithwaite P, Jhaveri R, McEwan AI, Goodman DK, Smith LR, Glass PSA. The MAC reduction of isoflurane by sufentanil. *Br J Anaesth* 1994;72:42–46.
29. Kapila A, Lang E, Glass PSA, Sebel P, Shlugman D. MAC reduction of isoflurane by remifentanil. *Anesthesiology* 1994;81:A378(abst).
30. Glass PSA, Jacobs JR, Smith RL, Ginsberg B, Quill TJ, Bai SA, Reves JG. Pharmacokinetic model-driven infusion of fentanyl: assessment of accuracy. *Anesthesiology* 1990;73:1082–1090.
31. Vuyk J, Engbers FHM, Lemmens HJM, Burm AGL, Vletter AA, Gladines MPRR, Bovill JG. Pharmacodynamics of propofol in female patients. *Anesthesiology* 1992;77:3–9.
32. Glass PSA, Shafer SL, Jacobs JR, Reves JG. Intravenous drug delivery systems. In: Miller R, ed. *Anesthesia*. New York: Churchill Livingstone; 1944:389–416.
33. Wagner JG. A safe method for rapidly achieving plasma concentration plateaus. *Clin Pharmacol Ther* 1974;16:691–700.
34. Reves JG, Jacobs JR, Glass PSA. *Automated drug delivery in anesthesia.* ASA Refresher Course in Anesthesiology 1991;19:127–137.
35. Holford NHG, Sheiner LB. Understanding the dose-effect relationship: clinical application of pharmacokinetic-dynamic models. *Clin Pharmacokinet* 1981;6:429–453.
36. Eger EI, Saidman LJ, Brandstater B. Minimum alveolar anesthetic concentration: a standard of anesthetic potency. *Anesthesiology* 1965;26:756–763.
37. Alvis JM, Reves JG, Govier AV, Menkhaus PG, Henling CE, Spain, JA Bradley, E. Computer assisted continuous infusions of fentanyl during cardiac anesthesia: comparison with a manual method. *Anesthesiology* 1985;63:41–49.
38. Kruger-Thiemer E. Continuous intravenous infusion and multicompartment accumulation. *Eur J Pharmacol* 1968;4:317–324.
39. Shafer SL, Siegel LC, Cooke JE, Scott JC. Testing computer-controlled infusion pumps by simulation. *Anesthesiology* 1988;68:261–266.
40. Jacobs JR. Algorithm for optimal linear model-based control with application to pharmacokinetic model-driven drug delivery. *IEEE Trans Biomed Eng* 1990;37:107–109.
41. Glass PSA, Goodman DK, Ginsberg B, Reves JG, Jacobs JR. Accuracy of pharmacokinetic model-driven infusion of propofol. *Anesthesiology* 1989;71:A277(abst).
42. Shafer SL, Varvel JR, Aziz N, Scott JC. The pharmacokinetics of fentanyl administered by computer controlled infusion pump. *Anesthesiology* 1990;73:1091–1102.

43. Crankshaw DP, Boyd MD, Bjorksten AR. Plasma drug efflux—a new approach to optimization of drug infusion for constant blood concentration of thiopental and methohexital. *Anesthesiology* 1987;67:32–41.
44. Crankshaw DP, Karasawa F. A method for implementing programmed infusion of thiopentone and methohexitone with a simple infusion pump. *Anaesth Intens Care*;1989:496–499.
45. Schüttler J, Kloos S, Schwilden H, Stoeckel H. Total intravenous anaesthesia with propofol and alfentanil by computer-assisted infusion. *Anaesthesia* 1988;43(Suppl):2–7.
46. Ausems ME, Stanski DR, Hug CC. An evaluation of the accuracy of pharmacokinetic data for the computer assisted infusion of alfentanil. *Br J Anaesth* 1985;57:1217–1225.
47. Hill HF. Pharmacokinetic tailoring of computer-controlled alfentanil infusions: current problems, potential solutions. In: Kroboth PD, Smith RB, Juhl RP, eds. *Pharmacokinetics and pharmacodynamics: current problems, potential solutions. Vol. 2.* Cincinnati: Harvey Whitney Books; 1988:157–166.
48. Lemmens HJM, Bovill JG, Burm AGL, Hennis H. Alfentanil infusion in the elderly. *Anaesthesia* 1988;43:850–856.
49. White M, Kenny GNC. Intravenous propofol using a computerised infusion system. *Anaesthes* 1990; 45:204.
50. Marsh B, White M, Morton N, Kenny GN. Pharmacokinetic model driven infusion of propofol in children. *Br J Anaesth* 1991;67:41.
51. Maitre PO, Vozeh S, Heykants J. Population pharmacokinetics of alfentanil: the average dose-plasma concentration relationship and interindividual variability in patients. *Anesthesiology* 1987;66:3–12.
52. Maitre PO, Ausems ME, Vozeh S, Stanski DR. Evaluating the accuracy of using population pharmacokinetic data to predict plasma concentrations of alfentanil. *Anesthesiology* 1988;68:59–67.
53. Raemer DB, Buschman A, Varvel JR. The prospective use of population pharmacokinetics in a computer driven infusion system for alfentanil. *Anesthesiology* 1990;73:66.
54. Maitre PE, Stanski DR. Bayesian forecasting improves the prediction of intraoperative plasma concentrations of alfentanil. *Anesthesiology* 1988;69:652–659.
55. Shafer SL, Gregg K. Algorithms to rapidly achieve and maintain stable drug concentrations at the site of drug effect with a computer controlled infusion pump. *J Pharmacokinet Biopharm* 1992;20: 147–169.
56. Jacobs JR, Williams EA. Algorithm to control "effect compartment" drug concentrations in pharmacokinetic model-driven drug delivery. *IEEE Trans Biomed Eng* 1993;40:993–999.
57. Avram MJ, Sanghvi R, Henthorn TK, et al. Determinants of thiopentone induction dose requirements. *Anesth Analg* 1993;76:10–17.
58. Jacobs JR, Reves JG. Effect site equilibration time is a determinant of induction dose requirement. *Anesth Analg* 1993;76:1–6.
59. Hung, OR Varvel JR, Shafer SL, Stanski DR. Thiopental pharmacodynamics II: quantitation of clinical and electroencephalographic depth of anesthesia. *Anesthesiology* 1992;77:237–244.
60. Ausems ME, Vuyk J, Hug CC, Stanski DR. Comparison of a computer-assisted infusion versus intermittent bolus administration of alfentanil as a supplement to nitrous oxide for lower abdominal surgery. *Anesthesiology* 1988;68:851–861.
61. Glass PSA, Jacobs J, Alvis M, et al. Computer assisted continuous infusion of alfentanil during noncardiac anesthesia: a comparison with a manual method. *Anesthesiology* 1986;65:A546(abst).
62. Theil DR, Stanley TE Ill, White WD, et al. Midazolam and fentanyl continuous infusion anesthesia for cardiac surgery: a comparison of computer-assisted vs. manual infusion systems. *J Cardiothorac Vasc Anesth* 1993;7:300.
63. Glass PSA, Ginsberg B, Hawkins ED, et al. Comparison of sodium thiopental/isoflurane to propofol (delivered by means of a pharmacokinetic model-driven device) for the induction, maintenance, and recovery from anesthesia. *Anesthesiology* 1988;69:A575(abst).
64. Ritchie G, Ebert JP, Jannett TC, Kissan I, Sheppard LC. A microcomputer based controller for neuromuscular block during surgery. *Ann Biomed Eng* 1985;13:3–15.
65. DeVries JW, Ros HH, Booij LH. Infusion of vecuronium controlled by a closed-loop system. *Br J Anaesth* 1986;58:1100–1103.
66. Jaklitsch RR, Westenskow DR. A model-based self-adjusting two-phase controller for vecuronium-induced muscle relaxation during anesthesia. *IEEE Trans Biomed Eng* 1987;34:583–594.
67. Cosgrove DM, Petre JH, Waller JL, Roth JV, Shepherd C, Cohn LH. Automated control of postoperative hypertension: a prospective, randomized, multicenter study. *Ann Thorac Surg* 1989;47:678–683.
68. Sheppard LC, Computer control of the infusion of vasoactive drugs. *Ann Biomed Eng* 1980;8:431–444.
69. Schwilden H, Schüttler J, Stockel H. Closed-loop feedback control of methohexital anesthesia by quantitative EEG analysis in humans. *Anesthesiology* 1987;67:341.

70. Schwilden H, Stoeckel H, Schüttler J. Closed-loop feedback control of propofol anaesthesia by quantitative EEG analysis in humans. *Br J Anaesth* 1989;62:290–296.
71. Schwilden H, Stoeckel H. Effective therapeutic infusions produced by closed-loop feedback control of methohexital administration during total intravenous anesthesia with fentanyl. *Anesthesiology* 1990; 73:225–229.
72. Kenny GNC, Davies FW, Mantzardis H, Fisher AC. Closed-loop control of anesthesia. *Anesthesiology* 1992;77:A328(abst).
73. Shaw JE, Theeuws F. Transdermal dosage forms. In: Presscott LF, Nimo WS, eds. *Rate control in drug therapy*. Edinburgh: Churchill Livingstone; 1985.
74. Sebel PS, Barrett CW, Kirk CJC, Heykants J. Transdermal absorption of fentanyl and sufentanil in man. *Eur J Clin Pharmacol* 1987;32:529–531.
75. Varvel JR, Shafer SL, Hwang SS, Coen PA, Stanski DR. Absorption characteristics of transdermally administered fentanyl. *Anesthesiology* 1989;70:928–934.
76. Gourlay GK, Kowalski SR, Plummer JL, Cousins MJ, Armstrong PJ. Fentanyl blood concentration analgesic response relationship in the treatment of postoperative pain. *Anesth Analg* 1988;67:329–337.
77. Ashburn MA, Stephen RL, Petelenz TJ, Hoffman AA. Controlled iontophoretic delivery of morphine HCI for post-operative pain relief. *Anesthesiology* 1988;69:A348(abst).
78. Nelson PS, Streisand JB, Mulder SM, Pace NL, Stanley TH. Comparison of oral transmucosal fentanyl citrate and an oral solution of meperidine, diazepam, and atropine for premedication in children. *Anesthesiology* 1989;70:616–621.
79. Streisand JB, Varvel JR, Stanski DR, et al. Absorption and bioavailability of oral transmucosal fentanyl citrate. *Anesthesiology* 1991;75:223–229.
80. Henderson JM, Brodsky DA, Fisher DM, Brett CM, Hertzka RE. Preinduction of anesthesia in pediatric patients with nasally administered sufentanil. *Anesthesiology* 1988;68:671–675.
81. Stanley TH, Leiman BC, Rawal N, et al. The effects of oral transmucosal fentanyl citrate premedication on preoperative behavioral responses and gastric volume and acidity in children. *Anesth Analg* 1989;69:328–335.
82. Ashburn MA, Streisand JB, Tarver SD, et al. Oral transmucosal fentanyl citrate for premedication in paediatric outpatients. *Can J Anaesth* 1990;37:857–866.
83. Feld LH, Champeau MW, van Steennis CA, Scott JC. Preanesthestic medication in children: a comparison of oral transmucosal fentanyl citrate versus placebo. *Anesthesiology* 1989;71:374–377.
84. Streisand JB, Stanley TH, Hague B, van Vreeswijk H, Ho GH, Pace NL. Oral transmucosal fentanyl citrate premedication in children. *Anesth Analg* 1989;69:28–34.
85. Friesen RH, Lockhart CH. Oral transmucosal fentanyl citrate for preanesthetic medication of pediatric day surgery patients with and without droperidol as a prophylactic anti-emetic. *Anesthesiology* 1992;76:46–51.
86. Goldstein-Dresner MC, Davis PJ, Kretchman E, Siewers RD, Certo N, Cook DR. Double-blind comparison of oral transmucosal fentanyl citrate with oral meperidine, diazepam, and atropine as preanesthetic medication in children with congenital heart disease. *Anesthesiology* 1991;74:28–33.
87. Ashburn MA, Fine PG, Stanley TH. Oral transmucosal fentanyl citrate for the treatment of breakthrough cancer pain: a case report. *Anesthesiology* 1989;71:615–617.
88. Fine PG, Marcus M, DeBoer AJ, Van der Oord B. An open label study of oral transmucosal fentanyl citrate (OTFC) for the treatment of breakthrough cancer pain. *Pain* 1991;45:149–153.
89. Schechter NL, Weisman SJ, Rosenblum, et al. Sedation for painful procedures in children with cancer using the fentanyl lollipop: a preliminary report. In: Tyler DC, Krane EJ, eds. *Advances in pain research therapy*. New York: Raven Press; 1990:209–214.
90. Vercauteren M, Boeckx E, Hanegreefs G, Noorduin H, Bussche GV. Intranasal sufentanil for pre-operative sedation. *Anaesthesia* 1988;43:270–273.
91. Helmers JH, Noorduin H, Van Peer A, Van Leeuwen L, Zuurmond WWA. Comparison of intravenous and intranasal sufentanil absorption and sedation. *Can J Anaesth* 1989;36:494–497.
92. Karl HW, Keifer AT, Rosenberger JL, Larach MG, Ruffle JM. Comparison of the safety and efficacy of intranasal midazolam or sufentanil for preinduction of anesthesia in pediatric patients. *Anesthesiology* 1992;76:209–215.
93. Striebel HW, Pommerening J. Intranasal fentanyl for pain management: patient's assessment. *Anesthesiology* 1992;77:A853(abst).

Drug Infusions in Anesthesiology, Second Edition, edited by R. J. Fragen. Lippincott-Raven Publishers, Philadelphia © 1996.

3

Infusions of Intravenous Anesthetics

Robert J. Fragen

Department of Anesthesia, Northwestern University Medical School, Chicago, Illinois 60611

Intravenous (IV) anesthetic agents include the potent sedative hypnotic drugs propofol, midazolam, etomidate, methohexital, and thiopental and the dissociative drug ketamine. They can be used as components of "balanced" anesthesia with nitrous oxide (N_2O), analgesics, and muscle relaxants; with analgesics and muscle relaxants for total IV anesthesia (TIVA); as sedatives or hypnotics for patients undergoing local or regional anesthesia; and for sedation for diagnostic procedures and in the intensive care unit (ICU). The trend in anesthesiology is to administer drugs that have a rapid onset of effect and a short duration of effect so that recovery will occur soon after the patient no longer needs the effect and drug administration is stopped. Table 1 compares the pharmacokinetic properties of these drugs (1).

Although the purpose of this chapter is not to discuss the pharmacology of each drug thoroughly, the chapter will concentrate on the factors that are important for administration of the drugs by continuous infusion. A more complete pharmacological profile is available in several other texts (2–4). However, two concepts mentioned in Chapter 1 will be discussed regarding their relationship to IV anesthetics. These concepts relate to drug properties that are desirable for drugs used by IV infusion.

The first concept is "equilibration time" (k_{e0}): the time from injection of a drug into the blood until it has a therapeutic or maximal effect at its site of action (5). It is a determinant of induction dose requirements. Equilibration time should be as rapid as possible so that the effects of the initial dose are seen soon after injection; otherwise, it is tempting to give another dose to speed the onset time. This action may result in a drug overdose with resultant side effects. It also means that the bolus dose given during anesthetic maintenance will have a fast effect to correct the reason the bolus dose was given (e.g., "light" anesthesia). All the IV anesthetics except midazolam and ketamine have a rapid equilibration time approaching 1 minute or less. Because the equilibration time, or onset time, may be influenced by the rate of injection, it is important, when comparing different studies, that they use the same injection rates (6). Also, when comparing the onsets of effect of different IV anesthetic agents within the same study, the differences in their equili-

TABLE 1. *The pharmacokinetics of IV anesthetic agents (mean)*

Drug	Vd_{ss} (1/kg)[a]	Elimination clearance (ml/kg/min)	t ½ b (hr)[b]	Protein binding (%)	Minimum effective concentration (μg/ml)
Propofol	2.8	59.4[c]	0.9	97	1.10
Midazolam	1.1	7.5	2.7	94	0.16
Etomidate	2.5	17.9	2.9	77	0.31
Ketamine	3.1	19.1	3.1	12	0.64
Methohexital	2.2	10.9	3.9	73	10.00
Thiopental	2.3	3.4	12.0	83	19.20

Modified from Fragen and Avram, ref. 1, with permission.
[a] Vd_{ss}, volume of distribution at steady state.
[b] t 1/2 b, elimination half-life.
[c] Whole blood clearance vs. plasma clearance for the other drugs.

bration times, if they exist, should be considered in the study design; otherwise, some results will be predictable from the differences in equilibration time. The k_{e0} values of thiopental induction doses are shown in Fig. 1. Figure 2 shows the relationship between k_{e0} and thiopental drug concentrations after a 312 mg dose injected over 30 seconds.

The second concept is the "context-sensitive half-time" (7), the time for the plasma concentration (and presumably the concentration at the site of action) to

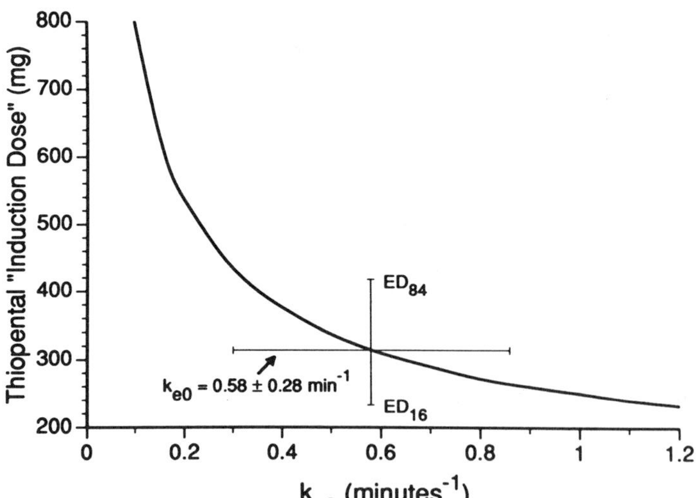

FIG. 1. Relationship between apparent thiopental "induction dose" and effect site equilibration time (as quantified by k_{e0}). Induction doses were determined by the amount of time required for a thiopental infusion to produce an effect compartment concentration of at least 17 μg/ml. The thin vertical line represents a determined ED_{16} to ED_{84}. The thin horizontal line is centered at k_{e0} = 0.58 min^{-1}. (From Jacobs and Reves, ref. 5, with permission.)

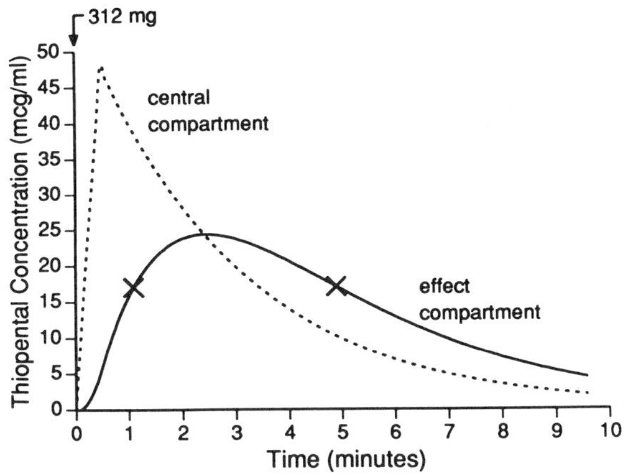

FIG. 2. Kinetic-dynamic simulation of the central and effect compartment thiopental concentrations that result from administering 312 mg over 30 sec. The presumed threshold for loss of consciousness (effect compartment thiopental concentration of 17 μg/ml) is indicated by the Xs. (From Jacobs and Reves, ref. 5, with permission.)

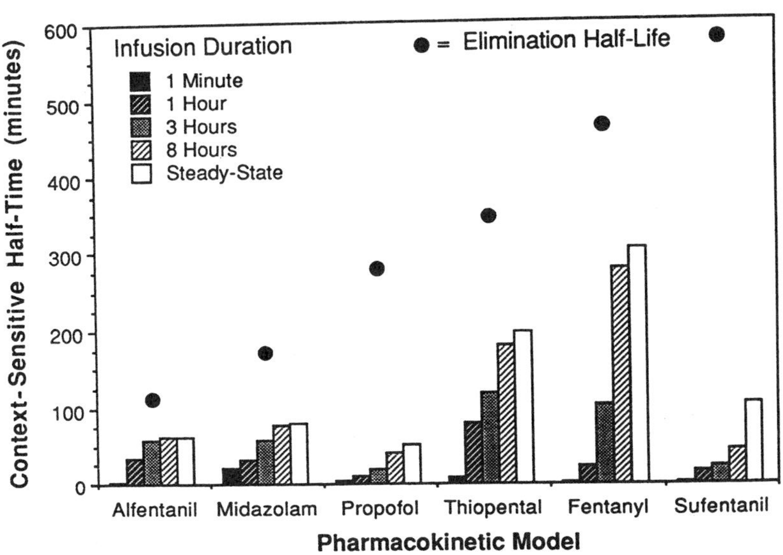

FIG. 3. Context-sensitive half-times (bars) for each of the pharmacokinetic models after terminating a 1-min, 1-hr, 3-hr, 8~-hr, or infinitely long (i.e., to steady state) BET-type infusion shown relative to the elimination half-life (dots) computed from each model. (From Hughes et al., ref. 7, with permission.)

decrease by 50% related to the duration of infusion for a drug fitting a multi-compartmental model. The context-sensitive half-times for midazolam, propofol, thiopental, and three opiates, as well as their elimination half-lives, are shown in Fig. 3. These two half-times (half-lives) are unrelated. When therapeutic doses are given for fairly brief operations, the context-sensitive half-time is mainly related to redistribution. Both redistribution and elimination contribute to the context-sensitive half-time for longer infusions. It is important to keep the effect site concentration fairly close to recovery values because recovery can be prolonged if the concentration has to decrease by more than 50%

PROPOFOL

The pharmacology of propofol will be discussed more thoroughly than that of the other IV hypnotics because propofol is the best hypnotic drug available for administration by continuous infusion. It has a large volume of distribution, is readily cleared by the liver and by extrahepatic sites (8), and has a rapid equilibration time and the most favorable context-sensitive half-time. Propofol (2,3-diisopropyl

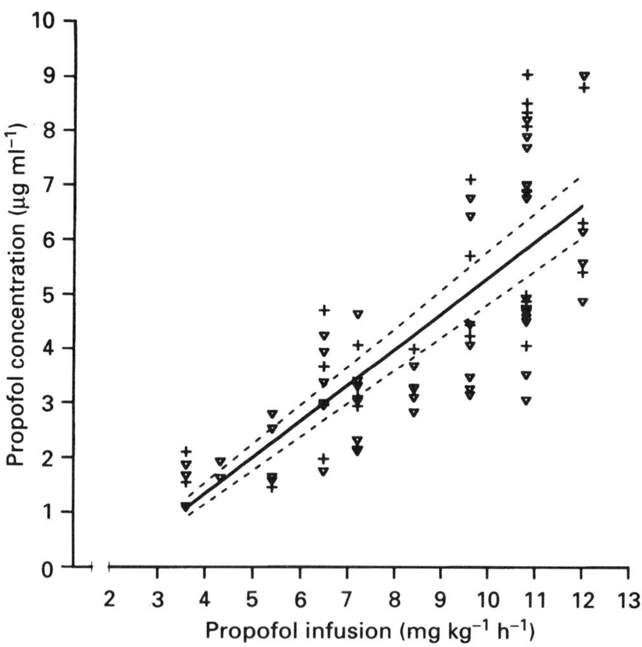

FIG. 4. Relationship at 30 min (▲) and 45 min (+) between the whole blood propofol concentration and dose (final infusion rate) for patients receiving a range of infusion rates of propofol. Propofol concentration (y) is given by the linear regression: $y = 0.67$ (propofol dose)–1.32 ($R^2 = 0.62$). Dashed lines represent ±7.3% coefficient of variation either side of the regression line (----). (From Forrest et al., ref. 14, with permission.)

phenol) is prepared as a 1% solution in a milky-white emulsion consisting of 10% soybean oil, 2.25% glycerol, and 1.2% purified egg phosphatide (9). People who are allergic to eggs should be able to take propofol because egg allergy arises from the albumin fraction. Propofol contains no bacteriocidal or bacteriostatic agent, so it is strictly for single-patient use. It should be withdrawn from the ampule in an aseptic manner (10). Improper handling of propofol in a syringe or its use for multiple patients has led to severe infections in a few patients (11). A loading port to refill syringes in a pump has been described, but its use is questionable because of possible contamination of propofol in the stopcock (12).

The recommended anesthetic induction dose for healthy adults is 1.5 mg/kg to 2.0 mg/kg, followed by further increments of 20–30 mg, if necessary, to cause loss of consciousness. For elderly or more seriously ill patients, the dose should be reduced to 1–1.5 mg/kg. A single induction dose should be effective for 3 to 5 minutes. Although a longer duration of effect can be accomplished with intermittent doses of about 25% of the induction dose, a smoother anesthetic course is achieved when propofol is given by a continuous infusion. When given by a calculator pump, the infusion rates for maintenance of anesthesia are generally between 6 mg/kg and 12 mg/kg per hour (100–200 μg/kg/min).

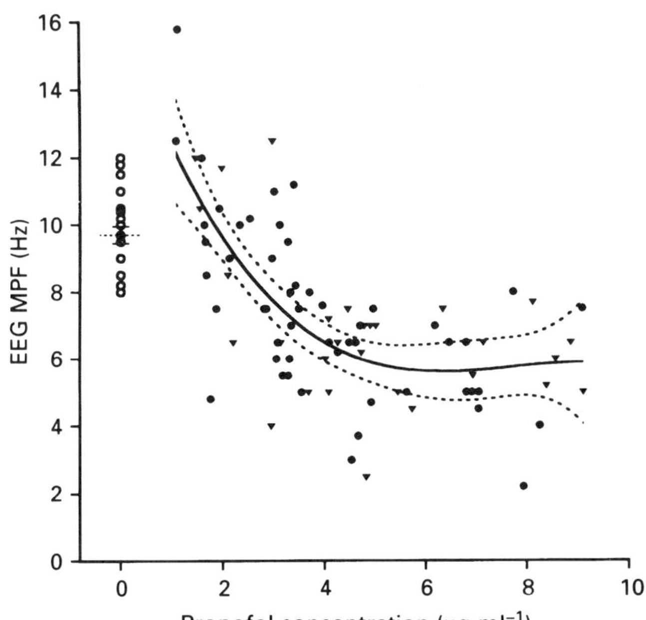

FIG. 5. Relationship between MPF (median power frequency) and whole blood propofol concentration. The values at a concentration 0 are baseline MPF values in fully awake patients before the start of infusion. ○ = mean baseline value (9.7 Hz); ● = 30 min, = 45 min after the start of infusion. - - - - = 95% confidence limits for mean MPF values. (From Forrest et al., ref. 14, with permission.)

TABLE 2. *Pharmacokinetic microconstants to program a computer program for computer-assisted continuous infusions of propofol for pediatric and adult patients.*

Microconstant		Pediatric	Adult
Vc	ml/kg	343	228
K_{10}	min	0.1	0.119
K_{12}	min	0.0855	0.112
K_{13}	min	0.021	0.0419
K_{21}	min	0.033	0.055
K_{31}	min	0.0033	0.0033

Propofol can be given by a computer-driven pump based on an algorithm derived from its pharmacokinetics. Instead of bolus doses and infusion rates, a target plasma concentration can be chosen and the computer will determine the infusion rates over time. Theoretically, it is possible to correlate target concentrations and depth of anesthesia by correlating the target concentrations with blood propofol concentrations or with a derivative of the EEG. Marsh et al. (13), in patients premedicated with benzodiazepines but receiving no opioids, determined that the target blood propofol concentration necessary to induce unconsciousness was 4–6 μg/ml in adults and 14 μg/ml in children. The infusion rates necessary to maintain unconsciousness were about 20% greater in pediatric patients than in adults. Forrest et al. (14) showed a good correlation between plasma concentration and the maintenance infusion rate (Fig 4). They also showed that patients were unconscious when the median frequency of the EEG was less than 6.8 Hz and the target plasma concentration was 4–6 μg/ml (Fig. 5). The EEG, however, may not be a good predictor of whether patients will move after a skin incision because it was shown in animals that immobility in response to skin incision may be caused by depressed spinal motor neurons, thus a spinal cord function rather than a cerebral cortical effect (15). For those interested in establishing a pharmacokinetic model-driven infusion of propofol, the data set in Table 2 is recommended.

Side effects are dose related in incidence and severity and are related to the speed of injection except in young healthy adults. The incidence of pain on injection is about 40% when propofol is injected into veins in the back of the hand or wrist and about 10% when injected into larger veins. In one study, the incidence of this side effect decreased from 73% to 32% by injection of 2 ml of 1% or 2% lidocaine (16) or decreased from 84% to 36% by injection of an opioid such as 1 mg of alfentanil in the same vein before injecting propofol (17). The severity of the pain also decreased.

Effects on Body Systems

Before using propofol for neurosurgical anesthesia, one must understand its EEG, evoked potential, and intracranial effects. When given in doses sufficient to cause drowsiness in patients who can be awakened, 1 mg/kg followed by less than 100 ug/kg/min, propofol can change the awake alpha rhythm of the EEG to a predominantly beta rhythm. When this sedative infusion is stopped, the EEG reverts to control rhythm in about 30 minutes (18). When there is increased beta activity, especially in the anterior leads of the EEG, partial amnesia may exist (19). This was achieved in one study with a bolus propofol dose of 0.5 mg/kg followed by an infusion rate of 75 μg/kg/min. The mean blood propofol concentration produced by this regimen was 0.86 ± 0.14 μg/ml. This change to beta rhythm can be used to guide dosing of midazolam to sedative-amnestic levels as well (20). When larger doses of propofol are given to induce and maintain unconsciousness, the EEG power is decreased to slower frequencies in a dose-related manner until burst suppression occurs. At burst suppression, there is about a 20% decrease in heart rate, mean arterial pressure, cardiac index, and left ventricular stroke work index in relatively healthy hydrated patients (21). Increasing the propofol dose also decreases the amplitude and increases the latency in some segments of auditory evoked potentials (22) and somatosensory evoked potentials (SSEP) (23). However, propofol infusions given simultaneously with opiate infusions can be used successfully for neurosurgical patients during monitoring of evoked potentials. During TIVA, evoked potential signals are usually of better quality than during inhalation anesthesia.

If electrocorticography will be used to optimize regional brain resection, it would be best to avoid propofol infusions for sedation until the recordings are completed because propofol can depress the EEG (24). Propofol has been used at an infusion rate of 600 mg/hr to control otherwise resistant seizure activity that had been unsuccessfully treated with diazepam and phenytoin (25).

The bispectral analysis of the EEG shows relatively good correlation with movement to skin incision during propofol-N_2O anesthesia (Fig 6). Bispectral analysis

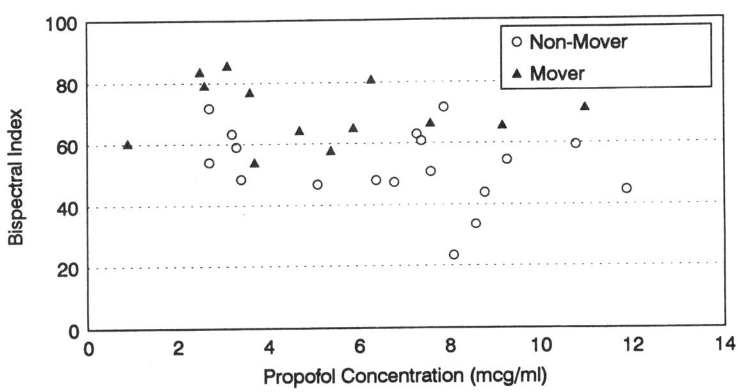

FIG. 6. Plasma propofol concentrations determined from blood samples drawn within 2 min of skin incision in movers and nonmovers compared with the bispectral index values immediately before that incision. (From Kearse et al., ref. 26, with permission.)

quantifies nonlinear phase locking and quadratic energy coupling within various frequencies of the EEG. It is not a "depth of anesthesia" monitor, but it may predict when anesthesia is insufficient to prevent movement to a painful stimulus. The bispectral index is a better movement predictor than propofol blood concentrations or other EEG measurements such as the spectral edge or median frequency (26).

Propofol decreases cerebrospinal fluid pressure and increases cerebral vascular resistance in patients undergoing craniotomy whether or not they show preexisting rises in intracranial pressure (ICP) (27–29). Because thiopental causes less decrease in systemic blood pressure than propofol does, some may prefer it to propofol because cerebral perfusion pressure may be better maintained. Cerebral perfusion pressure (CPP) is intracranial pressure minus mean arterial pressure, and a safe CPP is above 50 mmHg. However, propofol may be useful for neurosurgical anesthesia when a quicker recovery after the IV hypnotic infusion is desirable. Particular attention must be paid to the propofol dose and arterial pressure support. Propofol has advantages over the volatile anesthetics that cause cerebral vasodilation and increased ICP. If N_2O is given with propofol, it does not affect the cerebral vasoconstrictive properties of propofol and reactivity to carbon dioxide (CO_2) is preserved (Fig. 7) (30).

Propofol also reduces intraocular pressure, a benefit in ophthalmological procedures. Mirakhur et al. (31) prevented a rise in intraocular pressure above postin-

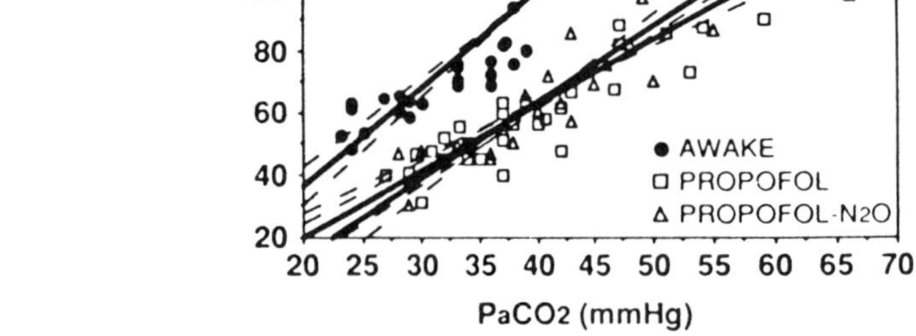

FIG. 7. A composite diagram plotting the relative middle cerebral artery flow velocity (V_{mca}) against corresponding $PaCO_2$ for all patients studied. Relative V_{mca} are calculated by expressing all flow velocity values as a percentage of awake V_{mca} at $PaCO_2$ of 40 mmHg. The respective linear regression and 95% confidence intervals for all experimental conditions are shown. Propofol and propofol-N_2O significantly reduced flow velocity at all levels of $PaCO_2$ with no differences among them. Although the CO_2 reactivity slope was reduced equally by both anesthetic conditions, the vasoconstrictive response to reduction in $PaCO_2$ was clearly preserved. (From Eng et al., ref. 30, with permission.)

duction values after tracheal intubation by giving a second dose of propofol, but not of thiopental, just before succinylcholine and tracheal intubation.

Propofol is a central respiratory depressant, depressing both the rate and depth of breathing. Short periods of apnea commonly occur after an induction dose is injected. Apnea occurs more frequently and lasts longer when patients breathe 100% oxygen rather than air (32) or when they are hyperventilated (33). If a patient receives a 6 mg/kg/hr infusion of propofol during spontaneous breathing, tidal volume decreases about 30% and respiratory rate increases to the same degree (32).

When drugs that depress the respiratory rate (opiates) are combined with propofol, the combination causes greater respiratory depression than does either drug alone. Even during sedative infusions of propofol, the tidal volume and minute ventilation were decreased, as was the slope of the ventilatory response curve to hypoxia in isohypercapnic patients (34). Propofol causes neither bronchoconstriction nor bronchodilation. However, it depresses airway reactivity to a greater extent than does an equivalent dose of thiopental (35). This makes instrumentation of the airway, insertion of artificial airways or insertion of a laryngeal mask airway, easier after propofol induction but could lead to a greater incidence of aspiration in cases with a high risk of vomiting (36). The Sellick maneuver can overcome this disadvantage. Hypoxic pulmonary vasoconstriction is preserved when a propofol infusion is given during one-lung ventilation; in this respect, it acts like other IV anesthetics but differs from volatile anesthetic agents (37).

Propofol causes cardiovascular depression—its major drawback. It causes arterial hypotension without the compensatory increase in heart rate common after IV barbiturates. The baroreflex is reset to allow a lower heart rate for a given blood pressure, but its reactivity remains intact (38).

Because of its vagotonicity, propofol can result in marked bradycardia when combined with other vagotonic drugs such as opiates and succinylcholine (39,40). Glycopyrrolate may be a better anticholinergic drug than atropine when given before propofol, especially when propofol will be combined with an opiate (41). However, pretreatment with glycopyrrolate did not influence the degree of hypotension (42). No other cardiac arrythmias have been reported after propofol injection.

There is evidence that propofol causes a dose-related degree of hypotension by both a negative ionotropic action and decreased tone in both arterioles and veins (43). Propofol, 1.5–2.5 mg/kg, caused a more pronounced and longer-lasting hypotension than did 4.0–6.5 mg/kg of thiopental (44). Recovery of depressed contractility occurs after blood concentrations decrease (45). Despite the negative inotropic effect, left ventricular performance was preserved after propofol but not after methohexital (46). Greater venodilation was demonstrated by occlusive phlethysmography during a propofol infusion at a rate of 200 μg/kg/min than at lower rates of infusion of 50 or 100 μg/kg/min (47). A decrease in systemic vascular resistance (SVR) without a change in cardiac output (CO) occurred in the following patient groups after receiving propofol and fentanyl: Those with coronary artery disease (CAD) who were taking their cardiac medications but were not premedicated and not hydrated before anesthetic induction (48), those with CAD but good left ventricular function (49), and spontaneously breathing elderly patients (aged 63 yrs ± 8 yrs) premedicated with lorazepam and given a propofol infusion of 6 mg/kg/hr after a 2 mg/kg anesthetic induction dose of propofol (50). This contrasts with studies that show direct myocardial depression and a decrease in CO and SVR (51,52).

In dogs, collateral-dependent myocardium tolerated adverse hemodynamic effects after propofol, whereas ischemic myocardium had impaired function (53). There is no good reason to use propofol in patients with poor ventricular function or in those for whom decreases in blood pressure, SVR, or myocardial contractility would be detrimental. It is important to avoid administering propofol to hypovolemic patients. A fluid load of 300 ml to 500 ml is recommended before anesthetic induction in patients who receive nothing by mouth for 6 hours or more before elective surgery.

Propofol has a direct antiemetic effect (54). The incidence of nausea and vomiting is lower after propofol than after other IV sedative-hypnotic drugs. This distinct benefit can be put to practical advantage, especially for procedures associated with a high incidence of these symptoms. Children undergoing strabismus surgery have less emetic symptoms and a faster recovery when propofol by bolus and infusion is the sole maintenance anesthetic. However, the incidence of oculocardiac reflex is greater than when inhalation anesthetic agents are used (55–57). Adult patients have significantly less emetic symptoms when propofol rather than methohexital is the anesthetic induction agent (Table 3) (58,59). When another group of outpatients received a propofol infusion and N_2O, they had significantly less nausea and vomiting than did patients whose N_2O was supplemented with either isoflurane or enflurane (60). The administration of propofol alone causes fewer emetic episodes that its administration with either N_2O or N_2O plus enflurane (61).

No other effects of propofol on the body are known. Cirrhotic patients have a slower recovery from a given dose of propofol than do normal patients, even though the pharmacokinetics are the same (62). Propofol can be used to induce and maintain anesthesia in patients with a history of acute intermittent porphyria (63) or malignant hyperpyrexia (64).

TABLE 3. *Antiemetic effects of propofol*

	Incidence of emetic symptoms			
	0–1 hr postoperatively		1–6 hr postoperatively	
Premedication	Methohexital	Propofol	Methohexital	Propofol
Morphine	8	0	13	5
Meperidine	4	2	5	1
Total	12	2*	18	6*

From McCallum et al., ref. 58, with permission.
*$p < 0.05$.

During recovery, patients describe a sense of well-being and have less impairment of mood state after propofol compared with thiopental when either drug is used to induce anesthesia for outpatients (65). Recovery is usually rapid after a propofol infusion is stopped; the recovery time is directly related to the dose administered (how much the effect site concentration of propofol is above the recovery concentration) (66). Pain on injection of propofol is not associated with postoperative thrombophlebitis, and intraarterial injection results in pain on injection but no permanent sequelae (67). When propofol rather than midazolam is used to sedate colonoscopy patients, the swallowing reflex returns sooner (68). Thus, oral intake can begin safely at an earlier time.

Propofol has no important interactions with the commonly used nondepolarizing muscle relaxants or succinylcholine. Finally, measurements of immunoglobulin, complement (C3), or histamine show no change after propofol administration (69), but anaphylactoid reactions have been reported (70). Their incidence, however, is probably lower than 1:250,000.

Uses and Infusion Techniques

Propofol infusions are used as the hypnotic component of a "balanced anesthetic technique," usually with N_2O and sometimes with the addition of an opiate, to cause light sleep in patients under local or regional anesthesia and cause light sleep (sedation) in patients either undergoing diagnostic procedures or being ventilated in ICUs.

Most infusions for propofol are based on the BET infusion scheme, which is designed to provide a bolus dose to fill the central volume of distribution, a maintenance infusion rate to compensate for elimination, and an exponentially decreasing infusion rate to compensate for transfer from the central to the peripheral compartments. This scheme is ideal but requires a computer-run infusion pump. A more practical method uses intermediate infusion rates between the bolus and final infusion rate. Because infusion rates are based on pharmacokinetic values derived from a small group of healthy patients, blood concentrations that result from these infusions are apt to vary from predicted concentrations. The variability after propofol may be less than the usual four- to fivefold variations seen with most drugs. Furthermore, blood concentrations and clinical effects are poorly correlated for a given patient. Population pharmacokinetics helps to define effective blood concentrations for a large group of people, but it has not been determined for propofol or other IV hypnotics. Therefore, suggested dose regimens are designed to achieve blood (or better, effect site) concentrations that are close to the therapeutic range and that must be individually adjusted according to a patient's needs at a particular moment.

The results of many studies show successful dose regimens of propofol-N_2O anesthesia with various premedicants or adjuncts. A 2.5 mg/kg induction dose of propofol followed by a three-stage maintenance propofol infusion, decreasing from 12 mg/kg/hr to 9 mg/kg/hr to 6 mg/kg/hr over 40–60 minutes, results in faster discharge than does a comparative volatile anesthetic (71–74). When compared with the shorter-acting volatile anesthetic desflurane, recovery times after a propofol technique are similar (75).

Although initial recovery was similar when either propofol or methohexital was given with N_2O for brief gynecological surgery, orientation to time and place was faster and ambulation was possible 14 minutes sooner after propofol (58) (Table 3). In this study and most other studies, the propofol infusion was stopped about 5 minutes before the end of surgery.

In techniques where propofol will be given with a computer-controlled infusion pump, target plasma concentrations rather than bolus doses and infusion rates will be selected. When target concentrations were used for anesthetic induction, 40% of patients lost consciousness at a target concentration of 3 µg/ml; 75%, at 4 µg/ml; and 90%, at 5 µg/ml (76). Thus, for patients premedicated with a benzodiazepine, a good starting target concentration would be 5 µg/ml, followed by an increase in the concentration for those who fail to lose consciousness in a short time. These are slightly higher figures than those determined by Vuyk et al. (77).

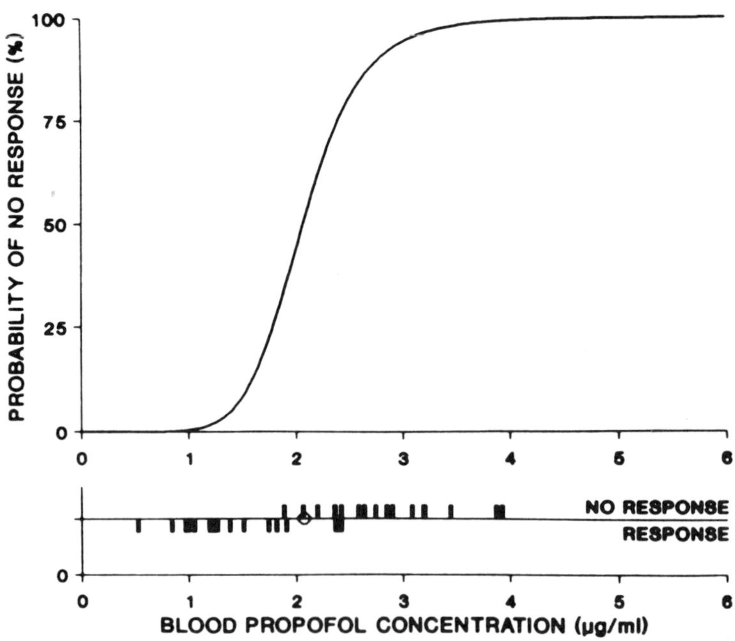

FIG. 8. The concentration-effect relationship for loss of eyelash reflex in patients who received a propofol infusion with either the Titration of Intravenous Agents by Computer (TIAC, Janssen Scientific Instruments, Janssen Pharmaceutica, Beerse, Belgium) or an Ohmeda 9000 infusion pump controlled by an Atari Portfolio pocket computer. Beneath each curve, the response/no response data versus the blood propofol concentration and the EC_{50} (circle) are displayed. (From Vuyk et al., ref. 77, with permission.)

At a target blood propofol concentration of 1 μg/ml, female patients who were not premedicated were relaxed and comfortable, at 2–3 μg/ml they could be aroused and were talkative, and at more than 3 μg/ml many lost consciousness. Their ED_{90} for loss of eyelash reflex was 2.78 μg/ml and their ED_{90} for loss of consciousness was 4.34 μg/ml (Figs. 8 and 9) The recommended starting blood propofol concentration of 5 μg/ml is still appropriate, but 6 μg/ml might be better for adults who are not premedicated adults.

A morbidly obese patient can be dosed on the basis of corrected body weight, calculated as the ideal weight (0.4 x the excess weight). In a study of such patients who were premedicated with 10 mg of diazepam and 0.4 mg of atropine and were breathing N_2O, satisfactory anesthesia was produced with an initial propofol infusion rate of 21 mg/kg/hr for 5 minutes, 12 mg/kg/hr for 10 minutes, and then 6 mg/kg/hr until 5 minutes before the end of surgery (78). Morphine premedication reduces the ED_{90} maintenance infusion rate compared with that necessary after lorazepam premedication (79,80). An infusion scheme designed to achieve and maintain a plasma propofol concentration of 3 μg/ml within 2 minutes of the start of propofol injection used an initial dose of 1 mg/kg, an initial

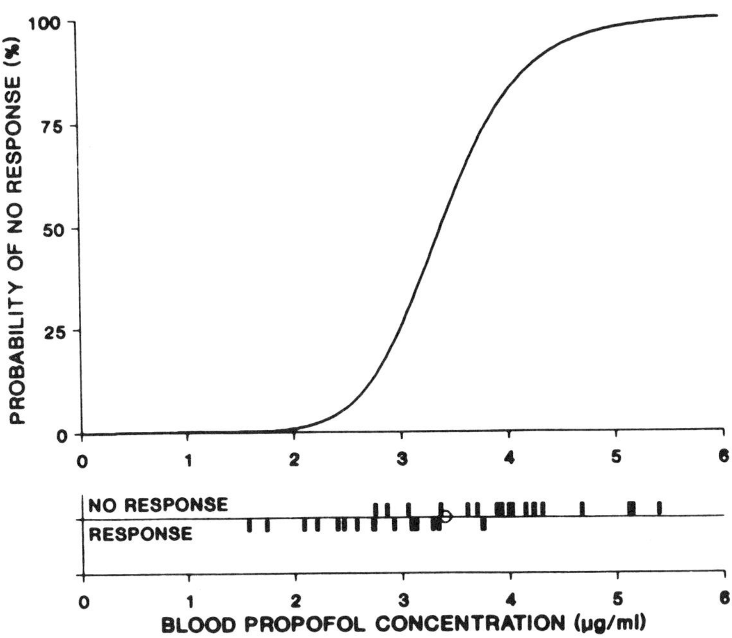

FIG. 9. The concentration-effect relationship for loss of consciousness in patients who received a propofol infusion with either the Titration of Intravenous Agents by Computer (TIAC, Janssen Scientific Instruments, Janssen Pharmaceutica, Beerse, Belgium) or an Ohmeda 9000 infusion pump controlled by an Atari Portfolio pocket computer. Beneath each curve, the response/no response data versus the blood propofol concentration and the EC_{50} (circle) are displayed. (From Vuyk et al., ref. 77, with permission.)

infusion rate of 10 mg/kg/hr for 10 minutes, a second infusion rate of 8 mg/kg/hr, and a final infusion rate of 6 mg/kg/hr. This regimen was administered to premedicated patients breathing 67% N_2O and resulted in plasma concentrations of propofol that were slightly higher than predicted (81). Using a variable-rate infusion of propofol from 0–20 mg/min and intermittent bolus doses of 10–20 mg/min with N_2O and meperidine, Shafer et al. (82) found that the average required propofol blood concentration was 4 ± 1 μg/ml for major surgery and 3 ± 1 μg/ml for minor surgery. Their EC_{50} awake was 1.07 μg/ml, orientation was 0.95 μg/ml, and return of psychomotor performance to preanesthetic values was about 0.4 μg/ml (Fig. 10) Patients undergoing superficial surgery, premedicated with 150 μg/kg of morphine and breathing 67% N_2O, required a propofol infusion rate of 73.4 μg/kg/min (range, 38–155 μg/kg/min) after a 2.5 mg/kg induction dose when the anesthesiologist could adjust the rate according to patients' requirements (83).

All of these schemes for the infusion of propofol with N_2O and other adjuvant drugs during surgery are similar in design, and with any of them, recovery occurs a few minutes after the infusions are stopped. Because recovery occurs rapidly, the muscle relaxant must be pharmacologically reversed or its effects spontaneously worn off so patients will not be awake and paralyzed at the end of the surgical procedure. Adequate early analgesia after a painful surgical procedure also is important because the patient may be more alert sooner than is the case after other IV hypnotics.

Lower-dose infusions of propofol can be used for sedation (light sleep from which the patient is easily roused to an awake but tranquil state). When various

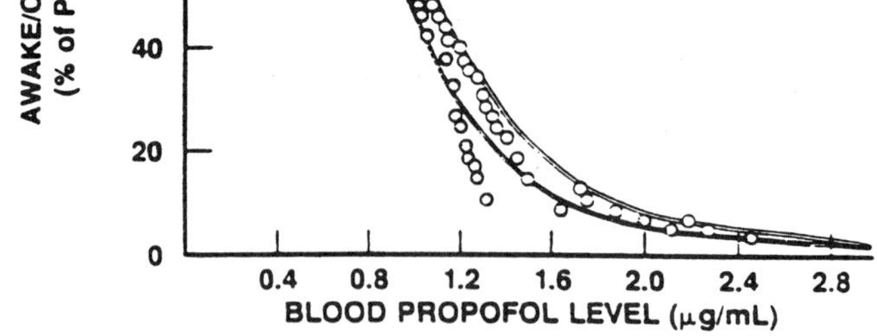

FIG. 10. Concentration-response curves for awakening and orientation as a function of blood propofol levels (μg/ml). The cumulative percentage of patients who awoke or were oriented at various blood propofol levels are shown. (From Shafer et al., ref. 82, with permission.)

sedative infusion rates of propofol up to 4 μg/kg/hr were given during regional block, the correlation between propofol blood concentrations and the degree of drowsiness was poor. Amnesia was not reliably produced by these infusion rates (84). In another study, propofol by infusion was a better sedative technique than midazolam was with or without pharmacological reversal with flumazenil (85). Mackenzie and Grant (86) determined that a rate of 4 mg/kg/hr (range, 2.6–5.6 mg/kg/hr) was required for patients younger than 65 years and a 3 mg/kg/hr dose (range, 2.3–3.5 mg/kg/hr) was necessary for those older than 65 years when propofol was used to sedate patients under regional anesthesia. This infusion rate kept patients in a state of light sleep, able to respond to verbal or tactile stimuli and with their eyelash reflex intact. An infusion rate of 6 mg/kg/hr produced light sleep without patient response (87).

When a surgical procedure outlasts the regional block, increasing the infusion rate to 10 mg/kg/hr while the patient breathes 67% N_2O will convert a regional anesthetic with sedation to a general anesthetic. The blood propofol concentrations produced by propofol infusion rates of 3, 6, and 9 mg/kg/hr and the decrease in concentrations when the infusions were stopped, shown in Figs. 11 and 12, allow one to predict times to unconsciousness and recovery (88).

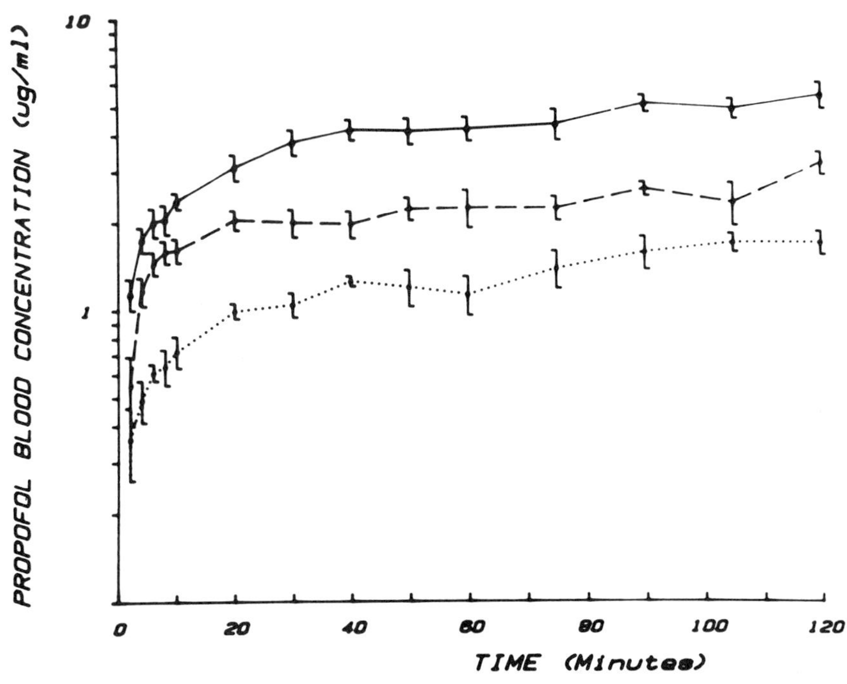

FIG. 11. Mean propofol blood concentrations ± SEM as a function of time during propofol infusions at 3 (. . .), 6 (- - -), or 9 (___) mg/kg/hr. (From Gepts et al., ref. 88, with permission.)

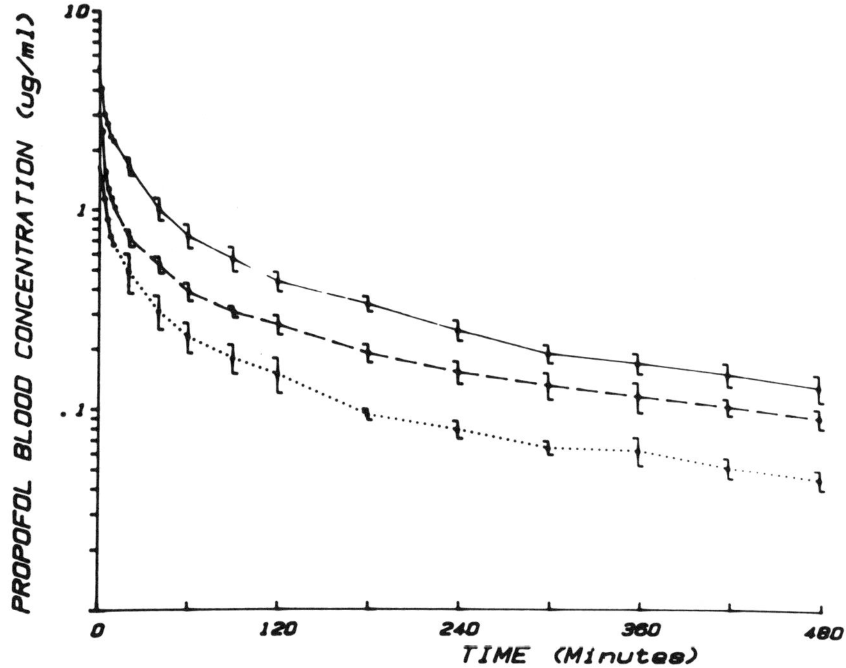

FIG. 12. Mean propofol blood concentrations ± SEM as a function of time after cessation of propofol infusions at 3 (...), 6 (- - -), or 9 (___) mg/kg/hr. For clarity, SEM of the first 10 min of data are omitted. (From Gepts et al., ref. 88, with permission.)

Propofol is an option for sedating patients undergoing diagnostic procedures without local anesthesia. Such procedures should be performed only in an operating room-like setting because a 6 mg/kg/hr infusion rate producing apnea and hypotension during colonoscopy has been reported (89). However, a technique in which propofol was given by a computer-controlled infusion pump at an initial blood target concentration of 1.5 μg/ml, which could be increased by increments of 0.25 μg/ml, provided quicker recovery than did IV midazolam given by bolus and infusion for outpatient bronchoscopy. Midazolam produced a longer amnestic period and greater motor dysfunction (90). In addition to clinical signs, the P_{300} of the auditory evoked response can be used to quantify the degree of propofol's effect because it is depressed in a concentration-dependent manner when sedative doses of the drug are administered (91). Blood pressure, heart rate, and pulse oximetry should be monitored by properly trained professionals when propofol is used for sedation.

In the ICU, the dose of propofol necessary to sedate patients maintained on mechanical ventilation depends on the residual anesthetic effects plus the particular opioid drug and the dose co-administered. Relatively low doses of 13–32 μg/kg/min can cause hypotension and are expensive when used over a long period (92,93).

However, rapid recovery after the infusion is stopped may outweigh these disadvantages because there are many ways to support blood pressure in the ICU. In one study, a 57% decrease in the blood concentration of propofol occurred 10 minutes after a mean infusion of propofol of 86 hours even though the terminal elimination half-life increased to as much as 1,411 minutes (94).

MIDAZOLAM

Midazolam is a water-soluble imidazobenzodiazepine that has multiple uses in the practice of anesthesiology (95). It can be used for intramuscular or IV premedication, IV sedation, and induction and maintenance of unconsciousness as a component of balanced or total IV anesthesia. It is formulated as 1 mg/ml, 2 mg/ml, and 5 mg/ml concentrations in a buffered aqueous solution. The steep dose-response curve of midazolam relative to other benzodiazepines (96) (Fig. 13) and its pharmacokinetics suggest that the drug would be a reasonable one to use by infusion: better than other benzodiazepines, but not as good as propofol. Recovery is slower after midazolam infusions without pharmacological reversal than after propofol. Midazolam infusions have been used appropriately for relatively long surgical procedures when rapid recovery is unimportant.

The availability of flumazenil, a specific benzodiazepine-competitive antagonist at the $GABA_A$ receptor (97), now makes it possible to awaken patients receiving a midazolam infusion. Flumazenil reverses all the effects of the benzodiazepines: sedation, amnesia, hypnosis, and respiratory depression. However, the drug's short elimination half-life of about 1 hour compared with 3–4 hours for midazolam (98) presents a problem. Therefore, the recommended method of titrating flumazenil in increments of 0.2 mg to a total dose of 1 mg can result in manifest residual drowsiness and recurrence of amnesia after the initial awakening.

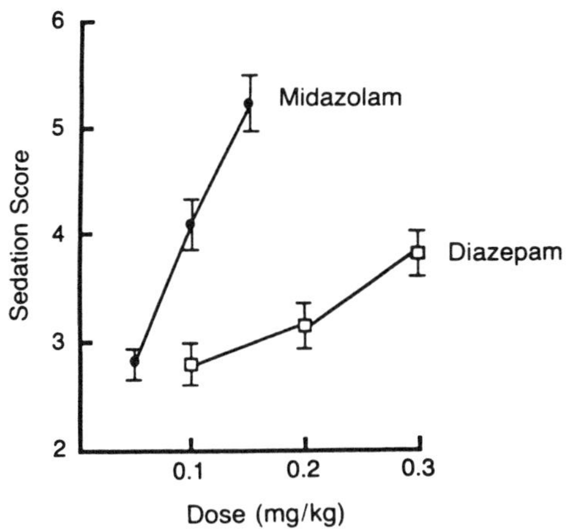

FIG. 13. Relationship between the sedation (drowsiness) score and the initial IV dose of midazolam and diazepam (mg/kg). Sedation scores of 2 (awake/relaxed) to 6 (asleep/not arousable). (From White, ref. 96, with permission.)

The degree to which this occurs depends on the total dose of midazolam, the dose of flumazenil, and the time interval between administration of the two drugs. After an infusion of midazolam, a 10-mg dose of flumazenil kept patients awake for more than 2 hours (99). Prolonged reversal is possible with additional doses of flumazenil when patients appear to be drowsy. In outpatients, 1 mg of flumazenil given after a midazolam infusion caused recovery equivalent to that seen after a propofol infusion for 1 hour, but mild residual drowsiness appeared thereafter (100). This is the typical time course of events when flumazenil is used to antagonize the effects of a midazolam infusion. Titrated use of flumazenil has no adverse effects of its own (101). If given too rapidly or in a high enough dose, it can precipitate excitement reactions. Chronic benzodiazepine users should not be given flumazenil. Flumazenil can also reverse the occasional excitement reaction seen after injection of a benzodiazepine agonist.

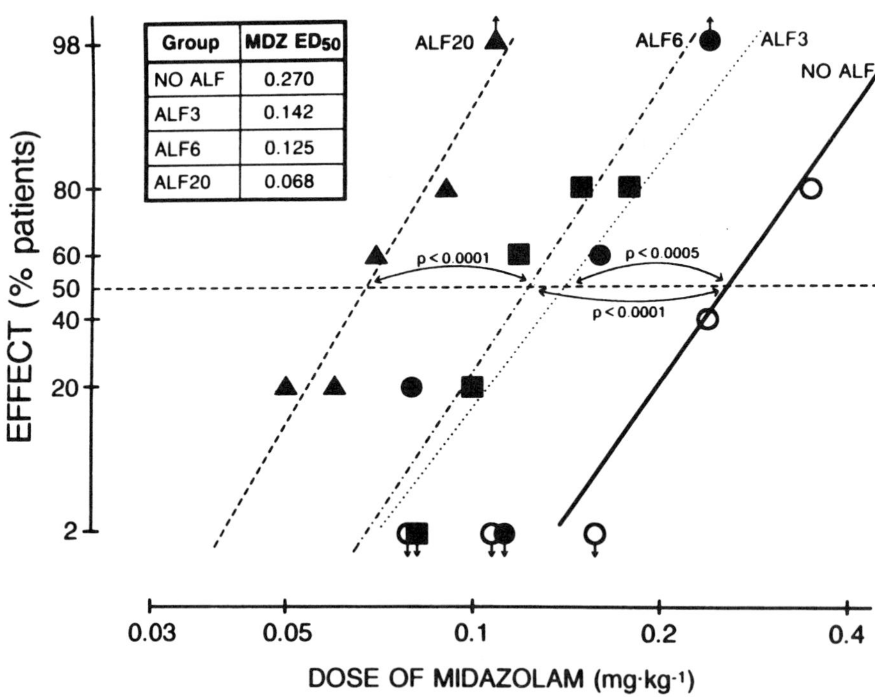

FIG. 14. Effect of alfentanil on the midazolam dose-response curves for induction of anesthesia. NO ALF (open circles)—the midazolam dose-response curve without the addition of alfentanil (saline only). ALF 3 (filled circles), ALF 6 (squares), and ALF 20 (triangles)—the midazolam dose-response curves with the addition of alfentanil in the doses 3, 6, and 20 µg/kg, respectively. Each circle, square, or triangle represents the effect in a subgroup of five patients at the indicated dosage. Arrow superimposed on symbols indicates that their actual locations are higher or lower (restriction caused by probit scale of the figure). The inset represents midazolam ED_{50} values for the four dose-response curves. (From Kissin et al., ref. 104, with permission.)

The ED_{95} for producing amnesia with midazolam is 50 μg/kg, although the slope of the amnesia dose-response curve is flat, indicating individual variability. Amnesia usually occurs when the concentration of midazolam in plasma is 100 ng/ml and when the $beta_1$/alpha ratio of the EEG is 1 (an increase of 20% in the beta power of the EEG). An EC_{50} of midazolam for amnesia in most studies is reported to be 64–81 ng/ml (102). The addition of 6 μg/kg of alfentanil increases the amnestic effect by more than 50% (103). Alfentanil also can potentiate the hypnotic effect of midazolam. Alfentanil decreased the ED_{50} of midazolam to produce unconsciousness from 270 μg/kg to as low as 68 μg/kg, depending on the alfentanil dose given (104) (Fig. 14) The anesthetic induction dose of midazolam, 0.2 mg/kg, does not reliably cause unconsciousness in all patients despite its steeper dose-response curve compared with other benzodiazepines (Fig. 12). Rather than administer larger doses of midazolam, a small dose of a more potent hypnotic (e.g., 30–50 mg of propofol or 50–100 mg of thiopental) will usually complete the induction of anesthesia. Both thiopental (105) and propofol (106) act synergistically with midazolam. Midazolam, 2 mg IV, increases drowsiness, anxiolysis, and amnesia without prolonging recovery time when given before a sedative propofol infusion versus a propofol infusion alone (107).

Effects on Body Systems

Except for cardiorespiratory depression, midazolam causes essentially no side effects of induction or recovery except that recovery can be prolonged and amnesia can persist after patients appear to be awake. Impairment of psychomotor performance after midazolam is dose related; greater impairment is seen after a 150 μg/kg dose than after a 50 μg/kg or 100 μg/kg dose. However, 300 μg/kg of diazepam causes less psychomotor impairment than 100 μg/kg of midazolam does, but its duration is much longer (108). Midazolam, 70 μg/kg, given by a 10-minute infusion, causes changes in the auditory event-related potential that is present for 50 minutes after the infusion is stopped. Despite a normal clinical picture during this time, there is the potential for drug interactions, especially with opiates that may be given in the recovery room (109).

After midazolam doses of 50–150 μg/kg, the tidal volume decreases and the respiratory rate increases to about the same extent, resulting in only a 10% rise in expired CO_2 (110). The addition of an opiate blunts the compensatory increase in respiratory rate. A slower injection time does not alter the respiratory depression (111).

The dose-related cardiovascular effects usually result in mild hypotension with little change in heart rate. However, cardiovascular depression is greater in patients who are hypovolemic rather than normovolemic, are on beta-adrenergic blocking drugs, or have myocardial dysfunction; therefore, caution should be used if midazolam is given to such patients. Midazolam does not cause arrythmias and has no adverse effects on other organs. It is associated with a low incidence of postoperative nausea and vomiting and does not cause thrombophlebitis (95).

Uses and Infusion Techniques

After the initial induction dose, midazolam infusions of about 5 mg/hr can maintain amnesia, if not unconsciousness. This infusion rate was used with 67% N_2O, fentanyl, and vecuronium after induction with 0.25 mg/kg of midazolam for patients undergoing maxillofacial surgery (112). It was also used to maintain postoperative sedation for tracheal intubation. The postoperative plasma concentrations of 133 ng/ml to 163 ng/ml were less than the concentrations of 300 ng/ml to 500 ng/ml considered necessary for a profound hypnotic effect during surgery. Although recovery is fairly rapid after midazolam infusions are discontinued, infusion rates should be individually adjusted to the minimum necessary for the desired level of sedation. Midazolam infusions should be discontinued at least 20 minutes, or possibly 40 minutes, before the end of a long period of anesthesia unless pharmacological reversal is anticipated.

Midazolam infusions can be used to sedate patients during regional anesthesia. This was accomplished in one study by giving an initial infusion rate of 36 ml/hr with a solution of 0.67 mg/ml until the desired effect was reached (10–12 min), then decreasing it to 9 ml/hr. A methohexital infusion of 8.33 mg/ml or an etomidate infusion of 2.0 mg/ml can be infused at the same rate to provide equivalent sedation. Adjustments should be made when necessary to maintain the desired effect (113). To infuse midazolam in a volumetric pump, prepare a solution of 20 μg/ml by adding 5 mg of midazolam to 250 ml of solution. A pump setting of 50 mg/hr will equal 1 mg/hr of midazolam. If the midazolam concentration is doubled, the 50 ml/hr will infuse a dose of 2 mg/hr. One can adjust these numbers easily to derive the appropriate dose in a volume suitable for the patient. A dose of 3–5 mg/hr is usually needed for sedation with regional anesthesia. Midazolam will have a greater effect if given in the presence of erythromycin, which appears to inhibit the metabolizing enzymes of the drug (114).

ETOMIDATE

Etomidate is a carboxylated imidazole prepared as a stable 2%, 20-ml solution dissolved in 35% propylene glycol. A new solvent proposed for etomidate, 2-hydroxypropyl-b-cyclodextrin (HCPD), results in less pain on injection, less thrombophlebitis, and no hemolysis compared with the current propylene glycol formulation and with no important alterations in its pharmacology (115). Etomidate is widely distributed throughout the body and rapidly cleared by the liver, where it is metabolized to inactive metabolites that are excreted mainly by the kidney. Elimination clearance approaches liver blood flow and the elimination half-life of a single dose is 2.9 ± 1.1 hr (116) (see Table 1). The pharmacokinetics of etomidate were determined during and after a 2-day infusion used to sedate healthy patients in an ICU after maxillofacial surgery. The elimination half-life was 5.5 hours (117). These patients took about 40 minutes to recover: four times longer than after infusions of about an hour (116). Etomidate acts in one arm-brain circulation time when an induction dose of 200–300 μg/kg is given intravenously. The side effects of pain on injection and myoclonus can be reduced in incidence and severity by slowing the rate of injection into the tubing of a rapidly running IV infusion and by preceding etomidate with a small dose of an IV opiate (e.g., 100 μg of fentanyl or 500 μg of alfentanil). Myoclonus is probably caused by a disinhibiting effect at the level of the spinal cord. Unconsciousness can be maintained with intermittent doses of 25% to 50% of the induction dose or by a continuous infusion.

Effects on Body Systems

Etomidate decreases ICP, cerebral blood flow, cerebral metabolic rate for oxygen, and intraocular pressure (118–120). Cerebral vascular resistance increases. The signal amplitude of SSEPs will be enhanced, which can make etomidate preferable to other hypnotic infusions for use during neurosurgery in patients with low amplitude signals (121).

Respiratory depression is short-lived and less than that observed after equivalent doses of thiopental or propofol. Respiratory upset rarely occurs and bronchomotor tone is unaffected. Hemodynamic stability is maintained after etomidate administration probably by preserving sympathetic outflow and autonomic reflexes (122). In contrast, propofol inhibits the sympathetic nervous system and impairs the baroreflex (122). Unlike other IV hypnotics, etomidate causes coronary blood flow to increase without a corresponding increase in myocardial metabolism (123). This suggests that etomidate may have a nitroglycerin-like effect and would be a preferred IV hypnotic for patients with coronary artery disease, those who are debilitated, and possibly for those undergoing neurosurgery. It can be administered to patients with a history of acute intermittent porphyria (124).

Recovery after etomidate infusion is fairly rapid, depending on the total dose administered and length of the infusion, but it is slower than after either propofol or methohexital infusions. Restlessness may occur from the time of initial recovery until patients are completely awake (116). Nausea and vomiting frequently occur after etomidate administration. Venous complications also are fairly common, the incidence of thrombophlebitis being higher than that after other IV hypnotics (125).

Etomidate should not be used for long-term infusions in an ICU because it led to increased mortality among multiple trauma patients who received a combination of an etomidate infusion and morphine (126). Subsequent studies revealed that etomidate causes adrenocortical suppression, the duration of which is dose related (127,128). Despite the inability to prove increased morbidity or mortality in patients who received etomidate for anesthesia, its use by continuous infusion is not approved in the United States and its use is infrequent in other countries.

Uses and Infusion Techniques

The pharmacokinetics of etomidate favor its use by continuous infusion. An infusion scheme beginning with a loading dose of 100 μg/kg/min for 3 minutes, followed by 20 μg/kg/min for 27 minutes, and then 10 μg/kg/min for the rest of the infusion allows recovery about 10 minutes after the infusion ceases for most patients (116). A simpler infusion scheme, 100 μg/kg/min for 10 minutes and a terminal infusion of 10 μg/kg/min for the remainder of the procedure, produces similar recovery times (129).

Apparently, most patients who receive etomidate infusions for maintenance of anesthesia with N_2O or with opiates require 400–500 ng/ml blood concentrations, which can be achieved by the infusion rates described. Awakening usually occurs when the blood etomidate concentration decreases below 300 ng/ml.

KETAMINE

Ketamine is a phencyclidine derivative prepared as a racemic mixture in a stable aqueous solution in concentrations of 10 mg/ml, 50 mg/ml, and 100 mg/ml. It can be dissolved in normal saline to make a 0.1% or 0.2% solution for IV infusion. It is the only drug described in this chapter that has analgesic as well as hypnotic properties. It is effective against somatic but not visceral pain.

Effects on Body Systems

The initial dose of ketamine should be administered over a minute and be preceded by a hypnotic drug (a barbiturate, propofol, or a benzodiazepine) to reduce both sympathetic stimulation and the incidence and severity of postoperative psychotomimetic reactions (130).

Ketamine is a poor choice for either neurosurgical or ophthalmologic procedures because it does not decrease intracranial or intraocular pressure (131). It may stimulate respiration and cause bronchodilation, making it advantageous in the asthmatic patient (130). When administered alone, ketamine stimulates the central sympathetic nervous system, resulting in tachycardia and hypertension (131). It may increase demand for myocardial oxygen. The vasodilating properties of ketamine are offset by sympathetic stimulation. In chronically ill patients, catacholamines may be depleted, leading to cardiovascular depression rather than stimulation (132). The baroreceptor mechanism remains intact. Ketamine is safe to use for patients with porphyria and malignant hyperpyrexia. It is most commonly indicated for anesthetic induction in adults with hypovolemia, pericardial effusion, pericarditis, or bronchoconstrictive disease.

Uses and Infusion Techniques

A ketamine infusion technique that results in hemodynamic stability and reasonably rapid, smooth emergence can be used for general anesthesia for major surgery (133). After premedication with 10 mg of diazepam by mouth and 0.4 mg of atropine IV, an induction dose of 1.5 mg/kg of ketamine is administered over 3 minutes; 5 mg of diazepam is given after each minute for a total of 15 mg. Muscle relaxation is achieved with a nondepolarizing muscle relaxant during the second minute. Two minutes later, the larynx is sprayed with lidocaine, and the trachea is intubated a minute later. To accompany 67% N_2O by inhalation, ketamine is infused at a rate of 0.2 mg/kg/hr for the first hour and 5 mg of diazepam is given IV every 30 minutes. The rest of the anesthetic consists of 0.1 mg/kg/hr of ketamine, 2.5 mg of diazepam every 30 minutes, and muscle relaxant to maintain surgical relaxation. Other ketamine techniques of equal or greater advantage are now possible by using midazolam instead of diazepam and shorter-acting nondepolarizing relaxants for quicker recovery.

A different dosage scheme is used for ketamine infusions in outpatients. After thiopental induction, and with N_2O by inhalation, a variable-rate ketamine infusion produces adequate anesthesia, faster recovery, and fewer side effects than does an intermittent bolus technique using the same agents (134).

METHOHEXITAL

Methohexital, constituted as a 1% solution, is recommended for anesthetic induction in a dose of 1.5 mg/kg. It is a methylated oxybarbiturate, introduced as a barbiturate with a shorter elimination half-life (about one-third shorter than that of thiopental) and more rapid metabolism (135). When methohexital rather than thiopental is used for anesthetic induction, recovery is only slightly faster because redistribution is the main factor terminating clinical effects. When patients are given a continuous infusion to maintain anesthesia, recovery is faster after methohexital than after thiopental (135). The context-sensitive half-time increases rapidly as the duration of the infusion becomes longer, but not to the same extent as occurs after thiopental (see Fig. 1). The pharmacokinetics of methohexital are similar in younger and older adults (136).

Effects on Body Systems

Methohexital causes some pain on injection and muscle movement, coughing, and hiccups. These symptoms are usually mild in severity and incidence when patients are premedicated with an opiate. Methohexital depresses both the respiratory and cardiovascular systems. It depresses myocardial contractility, dilates capacitance vessels, and may affect SVR. The resultant hypotension is partially offset by tachycardia (137). The drug has no particular advantages over thiopental for neurosurgical procedures.

Uses and Infusion Techniques

After anesthesia is induced with methohexital, the drug can be administered by infusion as part of a "balanced" anesthetic technique with N_2O, an opiate, and a muscle relaxant, if indicated. One regimen used a maintenance infusion rate of 3 mg/kg/hr, adjusted according to a patient's requirements (138). Another dose scheme is a maintenance dose similar to that recommended for propofol after the usual methohexital induction dose (58).

Methohexital infusions also have been titrated to produce light sleep during local or regional anesthesia (139). The recommended loading dose is 0.5–2.0 mg/kg of a 0.1% to 0.2% solution, followed by an infusion rate of 0.15 mg/kg/min, with adjustments as necessary. A similar technique for thiopental uses an infusion rate of 0.3 mg/kg/min after a 1–4 mg/kg loading dose. Emergence from these dose schemes is usually smooth but not as rapid as after propofol infusions.

THIOPENTAL

Thiopental, considered the gold standard of IV anesthetics, is the least desirable of the agents discussed in this chapter for use by continuous infusion. It has a rapid equilibration time, but the context-sensitive half-time increases quickly. Thiopental is metabolized in the liver, and the hepatic extraction ratio is low compared with the other drugs.

A study of the effect of different rates of thiopental infusion on the dose to produce unconsciousness and EEG burst suppression resulted in an equilibration time of 0.29 minutes, a median effect site concentration for loss of consciousness of 11.3 mg/ml, and a concentration of 33.9 μg/ml for EEG burst suppression (140). Patient factors that influence the dose that will produce unconsciousness (syringe drop) are age, weight, and sex, whereas cardiac output, but not sex, also influences the dose that will cause EEG burst suppression (141).

Clinically, the adult induction dose of thiopental of 3–5 mg/kg causes unconsciousness in one arm-brain circulation time. The 2.5% solution can be given by 50–100 mg increments to maintain unconsciousness, or it can be given by continuous infusion. Chronic alcohol intake does not appear to change thiopental anesthetic requirements (142). Thiopental will form a precipitate if injected into IV tubing with most other anesthetic drugs that are acidic. If recovery is to occur within a reasonable time, thiopental infusions should be stopped at least 30 minutes before the end of a long procedure.

Effects on Body Systems

Thiopental is useful for neurosurgery because it reduces cerebral blood flow, cerebral metabolic rate for oxygen, and ICP and causes cerebral vasoconstriction (143). Cerebral perfusion pressure usually remains adequate. Because thiopental decreases intraocular pressure, it also is useful for ophthalmologic surgery (31).

Dose-related cardiorespiratory depression is a common effect of thiopental. The drug depresses both the rate and depth of breathing to the point of causing a few minutes of apnea after an anesthetic induction dose. It directly depresses the myocardium, venodilates, and decreases central catacholamine outflow. Heart rate increases through the baroreflex (144), and the drug causes a parallel decrease in coronary blood flow and myocardial oxygen consumption (145).

Thiopental is irritating to tissues if extravasated or injected intraarterially because of its high pH, but it is associated with a low incidence of induction and recovery side effects. Although contraindicated in patients with acute intermittent porphyria, thiopental is safe to use in patients with a history of malignant hyperpyrexia.

Uses and Infusion Techniques

Thiopental can protect the brain when there is focal rather than global ischemia. Maximum depression of cerebral metabolism (a flat EEG) usually accompanies an infusion rate of 4 mg/kg/hr. A rate of 3.05 ± 0.37 mg/kg/hr produces a plasma thiopental concentration of 31.8 ± 10.7 μg/ml, and an infusion rate of 4.2 ± 0.3 mg/kg/hr produces a plasma concentration of 48.9 ± 14.6 μg/ml. When the plasma concentration at the end of the infusion is less than 32 μg/ml, recovery occurs in 6–24 hours; when it is more than 35 μg/ml, recovery takes 30–60 hours. Infusions for this purpose should be monitored with plasma thiopental concentrations or an EEG or both (146).

Crankshaw et al. (147), using a computer-controlled infusion pump that is capable of delivering an exponentially decreasing infusion to achieve target plasma concentrations, found that plasma concentrations of 15–20 μg/ml induces anesthesia and 10–20 μg/ml maintains unconsciousness when patients are ventilated with 67% N_2O. Awakening occurs at a plasma concentration of 5.9 ± 1.1 μg/ml, 111 ± 34 minutes after the infusion is stopped.

REFERENCES

1. Fragen RJ, Avram MJ. Nonopioid intravenous anesthetics. In: Barash P, Stoelting RK, Cullen B, eds. *Clinical anesthesia*. Vol 1. Philadelphia, PA: JB Lippincott; 1989:227–254.
2. Barash PG, Stoelting RK, Cullen B. *Clinical anesthesia*. 2nd ed. Philadelphia, PA: JB Lippincott; 1993.
3. Miller RD. *Anesthesia*. 4th ed. New York: Churchill Livingstone; 1994.

4. Dundee JW, Wyant GM. *Intravenous anaesthesia.* 2nd ed. New York: Churchill Livingstone; 1988.
5. Jacobs JR, Reves JG. Effect site equilibration time is a determinant of induction dose requirements. *Anesth Analg* 1993;76:1–6.
6. Stokes DN, Hutton P. Rate-dependent induction phenomena with propofol: implication for the relative potency of intravenous anesthetics. *Anesth Analg* 1991;72:578–583.
7. Hughes MA, Glass PSA, Jacobs JR. Context-sensitive half-time in multicompartment pharmacokinetic models for intravenous anesthetic drugs. *Anesthesiology* 1992;76:334–341.
8. Veroli P, O'Kelly B, Bertrand F, Trouvin JH, Farinotti R. Extrahepatic metabolism of propofol in man during the anhepatic phase of orthotopic liver transplantation. *Br J Anaesth* 1992;68:183–186.
9. Sebel PS, Lowdon JD. Propofol: a new intravenous anesthetic. *Anesthesiology* 1989;71:260–277.
10. Zacher AN, Zornow MH, Evans G. Drug contamination from opening glass ampules. *Anesthesiology* 1992;75:893–895.
11. Carr S, Waterman S, Rutherford G, et al. Postsurgical infections associated with an extrinsically contaminated intravenous anesthetic agent: California, Illinois, Maine, and Michigan. *MMWR* 1990;39: 426–427,433.
12. O'Flynn RP, Siler JN. A "loading port" for syringe infusion pumps. *Anesth Analg* 1991;72:407–408.
13. Marsh B, White M, Morton N, Kenny GNC. Pharmacokinetic model driven infusion of propofol in children. *Br J Anaesth* 1991;67:41–48.
14. Forrest FC, Tooley MA, Saunders PR, Prys-Roberts C. Propofol infusion and the suppression of consciousness: the EEG and dose requirements. *Br J Anaesth* 1994;72:35–41.
15. King BS, Rampil IJ. Anesthetic depression of spinal motor neurons may contribute to lack of movement in response to noxious stimuli. *Anesthesiology* 1994;81:1484–1492.
16. King SY, Davis FM, Wells JE, Murchison DJ, Pryor PJ. Lidocaine for the prevention of pain due to injection of propofol. *Anesth Analg* 1992;74:246–249.
17. Fletcher JE, Seavell CR, Bowen DJ. Pretreatment with alfentanil reduced pain caused by propofol. *Br J Anaesth* 1994;72:342–344.
18. Seifert HA, Blouin RT, Conrad PF, Gross JB. Sedative doses of propofol increase beta activity of the processed electroencephalogram. *Anesth Analg* 1993;76:976–978.
19. Veselis RA, Reinsel RA, Wronski M, Marino P, Tong WP, Bedford RF. EEG and memory effects of low-dose infusions of propofol. *Br J Anaesth* 1992;69:246–254.
20. Breimer LTM, Hennis PJ, Burn AGL, et al. Quantification of the EEG effect of midazolam by aperiodic analysis in volunteers. Pharmacokinetic/pharmacodynamic modeling. *Clin Pharmacokinet* 1990;18:245–253.
21. Illievich UM, Petricek W, Schramm W, Weindlmayer-Goettel M, Czech T, Spiss CK. Electroencephalographic burst suppression by propofol infusion in humans: hemodynamic consequences. *Anesth Analg* 1993;77:155–160.
22. Thornton C, Konieczko KM, Knight AB, et al. Effect of propofol on the auditory evoked response and oesophageal contractility. *Br J Anaesth* 1989;63:411–417.
23. Maurette P, Simeon F, Castagnera L, Esposito J, Maconillard G, Heraut LA. Propofol alters somatosensory evoked cortical potentials. *Anaesthesia* 1988;43(Suppl):44–45.
24. Rampil IJ, Lopez CE, Laxer KD, Barbaro NM. Propofol sedation may disrupt interictal epileptiform activity from a seizure focus. *Anesth Analg* 1993;77:1071–1073.
25. Pitt-Miller PL, Elcock BJ, Maharay M. The management of status epilepticus with a continuous propofol infusion. *Anesth Analg* 1994;78:1193–1194.
26. Kearse LA, Manberg P, Chamoun N, de Bros F, Zaslavsky A. Bispectral analysis of the electroencephalogram correlates with patient movement to skin incision during propofol/nitrous oxide anesthesia. *Anesthesiology* 1994;81:1365–1370.
27. Ravussin P, Berger-Bayer M, Nydegger M, Freeman J. Thiopentone-isoflurane vs propofol in neuroanesthesia for intracranial surgery. *Anesthesiology* 1988;96:A577 (abst).
28. Ravussin P, Guinard JP, Ralley F, Thorin D. Effect of propofol on cerebrospinal fluid pressure in patients undergoing craniotomy. *Anaesthesia* 1988;43(Suppl):23–24.
29. Herregods L, Verbeke J, Rolly G, Colardyn F. Effect of propofol on elevated intracranial pressure. Preliminary results. *Anaesthesia* 1988;43(Suppl):107–109.
30. Eng C, Lam AM, Mayberg TS, Lee C, Mathisen T. The influence of propofol with and without nitrous oxide on cerebral blood flow velocity and CO2 reactivity in humans. *Anesthesiology* 1992;77: 872–879.
31. Mirakhur RK, Shepherd WF I, Darrah WC. Propofol or thiopentone: effects on intraocular pressure associated with induction of anaesthesia and tracheal intubation (facilitated with suxamethonium). *Br J Anaesth* 1987;59:431–436.

32. Thompson KB, Payne JB. Effect of oxygen on arterial saturation during induction of anaesthesia with propofol. *Br J Anaesth* 1987;59:1318P.
33. Goodman NW, Carter JA, Black AMS. Some ventilatory effects of propofol ("Dripivan") as a sole anaesthetic agent: preliminary studies. *Postgrad Med J* 1985;61(Suppl):21–22.
34. Blouin RT, Seifert HA, Babencott D, Conrad PF, Gross JB. Propofol depresses the hypoxic ventilatory response during conscious sedation and isohypercapnia. *Anesthesiology* 1993;79:1177–1182.
35. Barker P, Langton JA, Wilson IG, Smith G. Movements of the vocal cords on induction of anaesthesia with thiopentone or propofol. *Br J Anaesth* 1992;69:23–25.
36. McKeating K, Bali IM, Dundee JW. The effects of thiopentone and propofol on upper airway integrity. *Anaesthesia* 1988;43:638–640.
37. Van Keer L, Van Aken H, Vandermeersch E, Vermaut G, Lerut T. Propofol does not inhibit hypoxic pulmonary vasoconstriction in humans. *J Clin Anesth* 1989;1:284–288.
38. Cullen PM, Turtle M, Prys-Roberts C, Way WL, Dye J. Effect of propofol on baroreflex activity in humans. *Anesth Analg* 1987;66:1115–1120.
39. Baraka A. Severe bradycardia following propofol-suxamethonium sequence. *Br J Anaesth* 1988;61: 482–483.
40. Ganansia M, Francois TP, Ormezzano X, Pinaud ML, Lepage J. Atrioventricular mobitz I block during propofol anesthesia for laproscopic tubal ligation. *Anesth Analg* 1989;69:524–525.
41. Skues MA, Richards MJ, Jarvis AP, Prys-Roberts C. Preinduction atropine or glycopyrrolate and hemodynamic changes associated with induction and maintenance of anesthesia with propofol and alfentanil. *Anesth Analg* 1989;69:386–390.
42. Sneyd JR, Berry A. Effect of preinduction glycopyrrolate on the hemodynamic response to anesthesia with propofol. *Anesth Analg* 1991;72:831–834.
43. Pagel PS, Warltier DC. Negative ionotropic effects of propofol as evaluated by the regional preload recruitable stroke work relationship in chronically instrumented dogs. *Anesthesiology* 1993;78: 100–108.
44. Mulier JP, Wouters PF, Van Aken H, Vermout G, Vandermeersch E. Cardiodynamic effects of propofol in comparison with thiopental: assessment with a transesophageal echocardiographic approach. *Anesth Analg* 1991;72:28–35.
45. Coetzee A, Fourie P, Coetzee J, et al. Effect of various propofol plasma concentrations on regional myocardial contractility and left ventricular afterload. *Anesth Analg* 1989;69:473–483.
46. Lepage J-YM, Pinaud ML, Helia JH, Cozian AY, LeNormand Y, Souron RJ. Left ventricular performance during propofol or methohexital anesthesia: isotopic and invasive cardiac monitoring. *Anesth Analg* 1991;73:3–9.
47. Muzi M, Berens RA, Kampine JP, Ebert TJ. Venodilation contributes to propofol-mediated hypotension in humans. *Anesth Analg* 1992;74:877–883.
48. Lepage J-YM, Pinaud ML, Helias JH, et al. Left ventricular function during propofol and fentanyl anesthesia in patients with coronary artery disease: assessment with a radionuclide approach. *Anesth Analg* 1988;67:949–995.
49. Vermeyen KM, Erpels FA, Janssen LA, Beckman CP, Hanegreefs GH. Propofol-fentanyl anaesthesia for coronary bypass surgery in patients with good left ventricular function. *Br J Anaesth* 1987;59: 1115–1120.
50. Claeys MA, Gepts E, Camu F. Haemodynamic changes during anaesthesia induced and maintained with propofol. *Br J Anaesth* 1988;60:3–9.
51. Coates DP, Monk CR, Prys-Roberts C, Turtle M. Hemodynamic effects of infusions of the emulsion formulation of propofol during nitrous oxide anesthesia in humans. *Anesth Analg* 1987;66:64–70.
52. Brussel T, Theissen JL, Vigfusson G, Lundenheimer PP, Van Aken H, Lawin P. Hemodynamic and cardiodynamic effects of propofol and etomidate: negative ionotropic properties of propofol. *Anesth Analg* 1989;69:35–40.
53. Mayer N, Legat K, Weinstabl C, Zimpfer M. Effects of propofol on the function of normal, collateral-dependent and ischemic myocardium. *Anesth Analg* 1993;76:33–39.
54. Borgeat A, Wilder-Smith HG, Saiah M, Rifat K. Subhypnotic doses of propofol possess direct antiemetic properties. *Anesth Analg* 1992;74:539–541.
55. Watcha MF, Simeon RM, White PF, Stevens JL. Effect of propofol on the incidence of postoperative vomiting after strabismus surgery in pediatric outpatients. *Anesthesiology* 1991;75:204–209.
56. Weir PM, Munro HM, Reynolds PI, Lewis IH, Wilton NCT. Propofol infusion and the incidence of emesis in pediatric outpatient strabismus cases. *Anesth Analg* 1993;76:760–764.
57. Snellen FT, Vanacker B, Van Aken H. Propofol-nitrous oxide versus thiopental sodium-isoflurane-nitrous oxide for strabismus surgery in children. *J Clin Anesth* 1993;5:37–41.

58. McCallum JSC, Milligan KR, Dundee JW. The antiemetic action of propofol. *Anesthesia* 1988;43: 239–240.
59. Doze VA, Westphal LM, White PF. Comparison of propofol with methohexital for outpatient anesthesia. *Anesth Analg* 1986;65:1189–1195.
60. Korttila K, Faure E, Aplfelbaum J, Ostman P, Roizen M. Less nausea and vomiting after propofol than after enflurane or isoflurane anesthesia. *Anesthesiology* 1988;69:A578 (abst).
61. Gunawardene RD, White DC. Propofol and emesis. *Anaesthesia* 1988;43(Suppl):65–67.
62. Servin F, Desmonts JM, Farinotti R, Haberer JP, Winckler C. Pharmacokinetics of propofol administered by continuous infusion in patients with cirrhosis. *Anaesthesia* 1988;43(Suppl):37–41.
63. Mitterschiffthaler G, Theiner A, Hetzel H, Fuith LC. Safe use of propofol in a patient with acute intermittent porphyria. *Br J Anaesth* 1989;60:109–111.
64. Krivosic-Horber R, Reyfort H, Becq MC, Adnet P. Effect of propofol on the malignant hyperthermia susceptible pig model. *Br J Anaesth* 1989;62:691–693.
65. McDonald NJ, Mannion D, Lee P, O'Toole DP, O'Boyle C, Keane PK. Mood evaluation and outpatient anaesthesia: a comparison between propofol and thiopentone. *Anaesthesia* 1988;43(Suppl):68–69.
66. Wright PJ, Clarke RSJ, Dundee JW, Briggs LP, Greenfield AA. Infusion rates for anaesthesia with propofol. *Br J Anaesth* 1984;56:613–616.
67. Chong M, Davis TP. Accidental intra-arterial injection of propofol. *Anaesthesia* 1987;42:781.
68. Rimaniol JM, D'Honneur G, Duvaldestin P. Recovery of the swallowing reflex after propofol anesthesia. *Anesth Analg* 1994;79:856–859.
69. Doenicke A, Lorenz W, Stanworth D, Duka TL. Effects of propofol ("Diprivan") on histamine release, immunoglobulin levels and activation of complement in healthy volunteers. *Postgrad Med J* 1985; 61(Suppl):15–20.
70. Laxenaire M-C, Mata-Bermejo E, Moneret-Vautrin DA, Gueant J-L. Life-threatening anaphylactoid reactions to propofol (Diprivan). *Anesthesiology* 1992;77:275–280.
71. Sear JW, Shaw I, Wolf A, Kay NH. Infusions of propofol to supplement nitrous oxide-oxygen for the maintenance of anaesthesia: a comparison with halothane. *Anaesthesia* 1988;43(Suppl):18–22.
72. Gold MI, Sacks DJ, Grosnoff DB, Herrington CA. Comparison of propofol with thiopental and isoflurane for induction and maintenance of general anesthesia. *J Clin Anesth* 1989;1:272–276.
73. Cork RC, Scipione P, Vonesk MJ, Magarelli JL, Pittman RG. Propofol infusion vs. thiopental/isoflurane for outpatient anesthesia. *Anesthesiology* 1988;69:A563 (abst).
74. Valane J. Recovery and discharge of patients after long propofol infusions vs isoflurane anaesthesia for ambulatory surgery. *Acta Anaesth Scand* 1992;36:530–533.
75. Rapp SE, Conahan TJ, Pavlin DJ, et al. Comparison of desflurane with propofol in outpatients undergoing peripheral orthopedic surgery. *Anesth Analg* 1992;75:572–579.
76. Chaudhri S, White M, Kenny GNC. Induction of anaesthesia with propofol using a target-controlled infusion system. *Anaesthesia* 1992;47:231–233.
77. Vuyk J, Engbers FHM, Lemmens HJM, et al. Pharmacodynamics of propofol in female patients. *Anesthesiology* 1992;77:3–9.
78. Servin F, Farinotti R, Haberer J-P, Desmonts J-M. Propofol infusions for maintenance of anesthesia in morbidly obese patients receiving nitrous oxide: a clinical and pharmacokinetic study. *Anesthesiology* 1993;78:657–665.
79. Spelina KR, Coates DP, Monk CR, Prys-Roberts C, Norley I, Turtle MJ. Dose requirements of propofol by infusion during nitrous oxide anaesthesia in man. *Br J Anaesth* 1987;58:1080–1084.
80. Turtle MJ, Cullen P, Prys-Roberts C, Coates DP, Monk CR, Faroqui MH. Dose requirements of propofol by infusion during nitrous oxide anaesthesia in man. *Br J Anaesth* 1987;59:283–287.
81. Roberts FL, Dixon J, Lewis GTR, Tackley RM, Prys-Roberts C. Induction and maintenance of propofol anaesthesia: a manual infusion scheme. *Anaesthesia* 1988;43(Suppl):14–17.
82. Shafer A, Doze VA, Shafer SI, White PF. Pharmacokinetics and pharmacodynamics of propofol infusions during general anesthesia. *Anesthesiology* 1988;69:348–356.
83. Kay NH, Uppington J, Sear JW, Allen WC. Use of an emulsion of ICI 35868 (propofol) for the induction and maintenance of anaesthesia. *Br J Anaesth* 1985;57:736–742.
84. Smith I, Monk TG, White PF, Ding Y. Propofol infusion during regional anesthesia: sedative, amnestic, and anxiolytic properties. *Anesth Analg* 1994;79:313–319.
85. Kestin IG, Harvey PB, Nixon C. Psychomotor recovery after three methods of sedation during spinal anaesthesia. *Br J Anaesth* 1990;64:675–681.
86. Mackenzie N, Grant IS. Propofol for intravenous sedation. *Anaesthesia* 1987;42:3–6.
87. Mackenzie N, Grant IS. Propofol infusion for sedation in the intensive care unit. *Br Med J* 1987;294:774.

88. Gepts E, Camu F, Cockshott ID, Douglas EJ. Disposition of propofol administration at a constant rate infusion in humans. *Anesth Analg* 1987;66:1256–1263.
89. Gepts E, Claeys MA, Camu F, Smekens L. Infusion of propofol ("Diprivan") as a sedative technique for colonoscopies. *Postgrad Med J* 1985;61(Suppl):120–126.
90. Crawford M, Pollack J, Anderson K, Glavin RJ, MacIntyre D, Vernon D. Comparison of midazolam with propofol for sedation in outpatient bronchoscopy. *Br J Anaesth* 1993;70:419–422.
91. Sneyd JR, Samra SK, Davidson B, Kishimoto T, Kadoya C, Domino EF. Electrophysiologic effects of propofol sedation. *Anesth Analg* 1994;79:1151–1158.
92. Newman LH, McDonald JC, Wallace FGM, Ledingham IMcA. Propofol infusion for sedation in the intensive care unit. *Br Med J* 1987;294:970.
93. Ground RM, Lalor JM, Lumley J, Royston D, Morgan M. Propofol infusion for sedation in the intensive care unit: preliminary report. *Br Med J* 1987;294:397–400.
94. Bailie GR, Cockshott ID, Douglas EJ, Bowles BJW. Pharmacokinetics of propofol during and after long term continuous infusion for maintenance of sedation in ICU patients. *Br Med J* 1992;68:486–491.
95. Reves JG, Fragen RJ, Vinik HR, Greenblatt DJ. Midazolam: pharmacology and uses. *Anesthesiology* 1985;62:310–324.
96. White PF. Use of midazolam infusion during regional blockade. In: Vinik HR, ed. *Midazolam infusion for anesthesia and intensive care*. Princeton, NJ: Excerpta Medica; 1989:21–25.
97. Polc R, Bonetti EP, Schaffner R, Haefely W. A three-state model of the benzodiazepine receptor explains the interaction between the benzodiazepine antagonist RO 15-1788, benzodiazepine tranquilizers, beta carbolines, and phenobarbitone. *Arch Pharmacol* 1982;321:260–264.
98. Klotz U, Ziegler G, Reimann IW. Pharmacokinetics of the selective benzodiazepine antagonist RO 15-1788 in man. *Eur J Pharmacol* 1984;27:115–117.
99. Lauven PM, Schwilder H, Stoeckel H, Greenblatt DJ. The effects of a benzodiazepine antagonist RO 15-1788 in the presence of stable concentrations of midazolam. *Anesthesiology* 1985;63:61–64.
100. Ghouri AF, Ramirez Ruiz MA, White PF. Effect of flumazenil or recovery after midazolam and propofol sedation. *Anesthesiology* 1994;81:333–339.
101. Fisher GC, Hutton P. Cardiovascular responses to flumazenil-induced arousal after arterial surgery. *Anaesthesia* 1989;44:104–106.
102. Veselis RA, Reinsel R, Alagesan R, Heino R, Beford RF. The EEG as a monitor of midazolam amnesia: changes in power and topography as a function of amnestic state. *Anesthesiology* 1991;74: 866–874.
103. Vinik HR, Bradley EL Jr, Kissin I, Mayeaux CA, Nielson VG, Waring PH. Midazolam induced amnesia: dose-response curve and potentiation by alfentanil. *Anesth Analg* 1990;70:S417.
104. Kissin I, Vinik HR, Castillo R, Bradley EL Jr. Alfentanil potentiates midazolam-induced unconsciousness in subanalgesic doses. *Anesth Analg* 1990;71:65–69.
105. Tverskoy M, Fleyshman G, Bradley EL Jr, Kissin I. Midazolam–thiopental anesthetic interaction in patients. *Anesth Analg* 1988;67:342–345.
106. Teh J, Short TG, Wang J, Tan P. Pharmacokinetic interactions between midazolam and propofol. *Br J Anaesth* 1993;72:62–65.
107. Taylor E, Ghouri AF, White PF. Midazolam in combination with propofol for sedation during local anesthesia. *J Clin Anesth* 1992;4:213–216.
108. Nuotto EJ, Korttila KT, Lichtor JL. Ostman PL, Rupani G. Sedation and recovery of psychomotor function after intravenous administration of various doses of midazolam and diazepam. *Anesth Analg* 1992;74:265–271.
109. Reinsel RA, Veselis RA, Heino R, Miodownik S, Alagesan R, Bedford RF. Effect of midazolam on the auditory event-related potential: measures of selective attention. *Anesth Analg* 1991;73: 612–618.
110. Forster A, Morel K, Bachmann M, Gemperle M. Respiratory depressant effects of different doses of midazolam and lack of reversal with naloxone—a double-blind randomized study. *Anesth Analg* 1983; 62:920–924.
111. Alexander CM, Teller LE, Gross JB. Slow injection does not prevent midazolam-induced ventilatory depression. *Anesth Analg* 1992;74:260-264.
112. Driessen JJ, Dirksen MSC, Rutten JMJ, Santman F, van Egmond J, Vree TB. Continuous infusion of midazolam during anaesthesia and postoperative sedation after maxillofacial surgery. *Acta Anaesth Scand* 1989;68:116–121.
113. Urquart ML, White PF. Comparison of sedative infusions during regional anesthesia—methohexital, etomidate, and midazolam. *Anesth Analg* 1989;68:249–254.

114. Hiller A, Olkkola KT, Ksohammi P, Saarnivaara L. Unconsciousness associated with midazolam and erythromycin. *Br J Anaesth* 1990;65:826–828.
115. Doenicke A, Roizen MF, Nebauer AE, Kugler A, Hoernecke R, Beger-Hintzin H. A comparison of two formulations for etomidate, 2-hydroxypropyl-b-cyclodextrin (HCPD) and propylene glycol. *Anesth Analg* 1994;79:933–939.
116. Fragen RJ, Avram MJ, Henthorn TK, Caldwell NJ. A pharmacokinetically designed etomidate infusion for hypnosis. *Anesth Analg* 1983;62:654–660.
117. Hebron BS, Edbrooke DL, Newby DM, Mather SJ. Pharmacokinetics of etomidate associated with prolonged I.V. infusion. *Br J Anaesth* 1983;55:281–287.
118. Moss E, Powell D, Gibson RM, McDowall DG. Effect of etomidate on intracranial pressure and cerebral perfusion pressure. *Br J Anaesth* 1979;51:347–352.
119. Renou AM, Vernheit J, Macrez P, et al. Cerebral blood fow and metabolism during etomidate anaesthesia in man. *Br J Anaesth* 1978;50:1047–1051.
120. Famewo CE, Adighesion CO, Ostuntakum OD. Effect of etomidate on intraocular pressure. *Can Anaesth Soc J* 1977;24:712–715.
121. Sloan TB, Ronai AK, Toleikis JR, Koht A. Improvement of intraoperative somatosensory evoked potentials by etomidate. *Anesth Analg* 1985;67:582–585.
122. Ebert J, Muzi M, Berens R, Goff D, Kampine JP. Sympathetic response to induction of anesthesia in humans with propofol or etomidate. *Anesthesiology* 1992;76:725–733.
123. Kettler D, Sonntag H, Wolfram-Donath U, Hoeft HJ, Regensburger D, Schenk HD. Haemodynamics, myocardial function, oxygen requirements and oxygen supply of the human heart after administration of etomidate. In: Doenicke AE, ed. *Etomidate—an intravenous hypnotic agent.* New York, Springer Publishing; 1977:81–94.
124. Blekkenhorst GA, Hansen GE, Cook ES, Eales L. Screening of certain anaesthetic agents for their ability to elicit acute porphyric phases in susceptible patients. *Br J Anaesth* 1980;52:759–762.
125. Korttila K, Aromaa U. Venous complications after intravenous injections of diazepam, flunitrazepam, thiopentone and etomidate. *Acta Anaesth Scand* 1980;24:227–230.
126. Ledingham IA, Watt I. Influence of sedation on mortality in critically ill multiple trauma patients. *Lancet* 1983;i:1270–1271.
127. Wagner RL, White PF. Etomidate inhibits adrenocortical function in surgical patients. *Anesthesiology* 1984;61:647–651.
128. Fragen RJ, Shanks CA, Molteni A, Avram MJ. Effects of etomidate on hormonal responses to surgical stress. *Anesthesiology* 1984;61:652–656.
129. Sear JW, Walters FJM, Wilkins DG, Willatts SM. Etomidate by infusion for neuroanaesthesia: kinetic and dynamic interactions with nitrous oxide. *Anaesthesia* 1984;39:12–18.
130. White PF, Way WL, Trevor AJ. Ketamine—its pharmacology and therapeutic uses. *Anesthesiology* 1982;56:119–136.
131. Silvay G. Ketamine. *Mt Sinai J Med* 1983;50:300.
132. Gooding JM, Darrich AR, Tovakoki M, Corssen G. A physiologic analysis of cardiopulmonary response to ketamine anesthesia in non-cardiac patients. *Anesth Analg* 1977;56:813–816.
133. Aldrete JA, McDonald JS. Low dose ketamine-diazepam prevents adverse reactions. In: Aldrete JA, Stanley TH, eds. *Trends in intravenous anesthesia.* Chicago: Year Book Medical Publishers, 1980; 813–816.
134. White PF. Use of continuous infusion versus intermittent bolus administration of fentanyl or ketamine during outpatient anesthesia. *Anesthesiology* 1983;59:294–300.
135. Hudson RJ, Stanski DR, Burch PG. Pharmacokinetics of methohexital and thiopental in surgical patients. *Anesthesiology* 1983;59:215–219.
136. Ghoneim MM, Chiang CK, Schoenwold RD, Lilburn JK, Dhanaraj J. The pharmacokinetics of methohexital in young and elderly subjects. *Acta Anaesth Scand* 1985;29:480–482.
137. Bernhoff A, Eklund B, Kaijser L. Cardiovascular effects of short-term anaesthesia with methohexitone and propanidid in normal subjects. *Br J Anaesth* 1972;44:2–6.
138. Breimer DD. Pharmacokinetics of methohexitone following intravenous infusion in humans. *Br J Anaesth* 1976;48:643–649.
139. Philip BK, Covino BG. Local and regional anesthesia. In: Wetchler BV, ed. *Anesthesia for ambulatory surgery.* Philadelphia, PA: JB Lippincott, 1985;233.
140. Gentry WB, Krecjie TC, Henthorn TK, et al. Effect of infusion rate on thiopental dose-response relationships. *Anesthesiology* 1994;81:316–324.
141. Avram MJ, Sanghvi R, Henthorn TK, et al. Determinants of thiopental induction dose requirements. *Anesth Analg* 1993;76:10–17.

142. Swerdlow BM, Holley FO, Maitre PO, Stanski DR. Chronic alcohol intake does not change thiopental anesthetic requirement, pharmacokinetics or pharmacodynamics. *Anesthesiology* 1990;72:455–461.
143. Samuels SI. Anesthesia for supratentorial tumors. In: Cottrell JE, Turndorf H, eds. *Anesthesia and neurosurgery* St. Louis: CV Mosby, 1980;150–167.
144. Reves JG, Flezzani P, Kissin I. Pharmacology of intravenous anesthetics. In: Kaplan J, ed. *Cardiac anesthesia*. New York; Grune & Stratton, 1983;125–150.
145. Reiz S, Balfors E, Friedman A, Haggmark S, Peter T. Effects of thiopentone on cardiac performance, coronary haemodynamics, and myocardial oxygen consumption in chronic ischaemic heart disease. *Acta Anaesth Scand* 1981;25:103–110.
146. Turcant A, Delhumeau A, Premel-Cabric A, et al. Thiopental pharmacokinetics under conditions of long-term infusions. *Anesthesiology* 1985;63:50–54.
147. Crankshaw DP, Edwards NE, Blackman GL, Boyd MD, Chan HNJ, Morgan DJ. Evaluation of infusion regimens for thiopentone as a primary anaesthetic agent. *Eur J Clin Pharmacol* 1985;28:543–552.

Drug Infusions in Anesthesiology, Second Edition,
edited by R. J. Fragen. Lippincott-Raven Publishers,
Philadelphia © 1996.

4

Opiate Infusions

Thomas K. Henthorn

Department of Anesthesia, Northwestern University Medical School, Chicago, Illinois 60611

Opiates have been used for surgical anesthesia or analgesia since Claude Bernard first used morphine as premedication in 1869. Morphine with scopolamine was used intraoperatively as a totally intravenous (IV) technique near the turn of the century (1).

Opiates are both important and popular as the analgesic component of IV anesthetic techniques because hypnotic drugs, with the exception of ketamine, have no appreciable analgesic effect and because of the relatively benign profile of side effects. The mood-altering effects of opiates are sometimes beneficial preoperatively, and their potent analgesic effects are useful pre-, intra-, and postoperatively. They have little, if any, adverse effect on cardiovascular stability or, if ventilation is adequately maintained, on cerebral blood flow. They do depress airway reflexes, which is also clinically important to the conduct of anesthesia.

This chapter brings the clinician up to date on the potential role of opiate infusions in anesthetic techniques and discusses the principles behind IV infusion protocols for these drugs. The partial agonists and agonist-antagonist opiates, such as nalbuphine and butorphanol, are not included because they possess insufficient analgesic efficacy to be primary agents for use during surgical anesthesia. Theoretically, they could be secondary or tertiary agents, but the dearth of information about their pharmacokinetics and pharmacodynamics for surgical anesthesia limits their use at this time.

Although many opioid analgesics are widely used as components of balanced anesthetic techniques, only a few are widely accepted for continuous infusion techniques. These are fentanyl, alfentanil, sufentanil, and meperidine. It appears that remifentanil will soon be added to this list. The discussion in this chapter will be limited to the fentanyl analogues. Their relatively rapid onset and, especially, offset of effect during the distribution phase gives these drugs advantages not enjoyed by morphine and methadone. Other factors such as specificity of effect without undesirable side effects also make these drugs preferred for infusions.

CLINICAL PHARMACOLOGY

Pharmacodynamics

Opiates produce their pharmacologic effects mainly through interaction with opioid receptors. At least nine separate classes of opioid receptors, scattered throughout the central nervous system (CNS) in both gray and white matter, have been identified (2). They are found in structures associated not only with pain transmission, but also with respiration, gastrointestinal function, cardiovascular regulation, motor control, and behavior (2). Multiple endogenous peptides that bind with these receptors have been identified. To date, no drug available has the capacity selectively to produce only a single effect (e.g., analgesia) by interacting with only a specific subset of opiate receptors; instead, all these systems are affected to varying degrees when opiates are administered.

Analgesia

Opiates are used clinically primarily for their analgesic effect resulting from their interaction with μ receptors. Opiates also interact with the κ opiate receptors to produce significant sedative effects. In selected patients who are undergoing certain operations, such as cardiac surgery, these drugs are used to produce both analgesia and unconsciousness (3). However, opiate/oxygen/muscle relaxant anesthesia generally results in an unacceptably high rate of awareness during most operations. Narcotic-based anesthesia is most often accompanied by additional centrally acting agents such as hypnotics, N_2O, benzodiazepines, or low-inspired concentrations of potent volatile anesthetics. Wong (4) stated in an editorial that narcotics should not be expected to produce unconsciousness.

The concept that opiates are incomplete anesthetics is probably best supported by studies that determine the degree to which various opiates reduce the minimum alveolar concentration (MAC) of volatile anesthetics in dogs. Fentanyl, sufentanil, and alfentanil can reduce the MAC of enflurane to a maximum of 66% (5–7). Therefore, opiate infusions should be designed to produce target blood concentrations that provide optimal analgesia for the various intensities of painful stimuli encountered intraoperatively but should not be expected to render a patient unconscious or amnesic.

Studies by Austin et al. (8) and Ausems et al. (9) demonstrated that the plasma concentration-response curve for the analgesic effect of opiates is rather steep. That is, plasma concentrations are inadequate for pain relief for a given stimulus, as evidenced by pain scores (8) or autonomic response (9), until a threshold concentration is reached. Plasma opiate concentrations that exceed this threshold by as little as 10% to 25% will rapidly produce maximal analgesia. Concentrations that are much higher than this threshold can provide no further therapeutic benefit and result in the loss of some of the advantages of using continuous infusion techniques, namely controllability and predictability.

Like other drugs with large therapeutic indexes (e.g., muscle relaxants), opiates are in no real danger of producing clinically significant side effects when excessive doses are administered to ventilated patients. However, the clinically important side effects of respiratory depression and sedation may have unpredictably long durations of action if excessive opiate plasma concentrations are produced.

This concept is key to understanding the benefits of continuous infusion of opiates. White (10) correctly argued that the practice of large "up front" doses of opiates at the beginning of operations (e.g., 50–150 μg/kg of fentanyl for cardiac surgery) is inefficient and against general principles. Administering 16.2 mg of pancuronium, calculated on the basis of pharmacokinetic/pharmacodynamic information appearing in Chapter 5 (half-life, 107 min), to produce a 75% neuromuscular blockade at the end of a 4-hour operation is analogous to giving a high dose of fentanyl "up front." Although some clinicians might give such a dose, how many would give the 76.7 mg "up front" calculated for an 8-hour case? In his review, White (10) cited several studies that demonstrated lower overall doses, improved postoperative analgesia, less postoperative respiratory depression, and less postoperative sedation when opiate infusions were compared with conventional repeated-bolus techniques. The underlying pharmacokinetic explanation for this is provided in Chapter 1.

Ventilation

All opioid agonists produce roughly equivalent plasma concentration-dependent respiratory depression (11). This depression of brainstem respiratory centers is typically expressed as a ventilatory response to a CO_2 challenge. Progressively higher opiate plasma concentrations tend to shift the $PaCO_2$ versus alveolar ventilation curve to the right. Thus, more $PaCO_2$ is required to stimulate a given level of alveolar ventilation. The slope of the curve is preserved until unconsciousness occurs, at which time the slope becomes depressed.

Although the effect of opiates on hypoxic respiratory drive is controversial, it is apparent that an intact hypoxic respiratory drive may be important in maintaining ventilation after opiate administration and that the effects of volatile anesthetics on this drive may be detrimental (12). Other drugs that depress the CNS will exacerbate opiate respiratory depression. Painful stimulation can counteract these effects. The decline in stimulation during the first one or two postoperative hours, along with the onset of sleep, may be an important factor in recurrent, clinically significant respiratory depression. This so-called biphasic response is occasionally seen postoperatively despite falling plasma opiate concentrations.

Cardiovascular Effects

Although most opiates, even in high doses, do not adversely affect myocardial function, they have pronounced effects on the cardiovascular system. Opiates produce a dose-dependent bradycardia, possibly by stimulating the medullary vagal nucleus (13). This vagal response is easily counteracted by atropine or pancuronium (14). Meperidine differs from morphine and the fentanyl congeners in that it is a direct myocardial depressant at clinical dosage levels, which limits its clinical usefulness for continuous infusion during surgery (15).

Hypotension, which occasionally is clinically significant, may accompany the administration of any opiate. The opioid agonists, especially morphine, increase venous capacitance, apparently by increasing the tone of postcapacitance resistance vessels, particularly in the splanchnic bed (16). At the same time, morphine appears to have the opposite effect on arteriolar resistance vessels, producing vasodilatation. This latter effect may be mediated via histamine release, an action not shared by meperidine and the fentanyl analogues (17,18). Alfentanil, given rapidly as a loading dose, produces transient hypotension (19,20). Prior induction of anesthesia with propofol may enhance the hypotensive effects of alfentanil (21) or fentanyl (22). Speiss et al. (23) reported four cases of precipitous hypotension when sufentanil was administered after IV lorazepam. Although the mechanism is unknown, it may be related to diminished central sympathetic tone (24).

Gastrointestinal and Hepatic Effects

Opiates cause an increase in smooth muscle tone at the sphincter of Oddi (25). This may cause problems for anesthesiologists and their patients for two reasons. First, spasm may cause biliary colic in patients premedicated with opiates, particularly morphine. The resulting epigastric distress may mimic angina pectoris. Its relief by naloxone would point toward opiate-induced biliary colic and therefore help in the differential diagnosis; the presence of changes in the electrocardiogram (ECG) would indicate a cardiac origin. Nitroglycerine may complicate the picture because it can relieve angina as well as spasm of the sphincter of Oddi. Second, spasm caused by preoperative or intraoperative opiates can interfere with intraoperative cholangiography. Reversal with naloxone is an unsatisfactory solution because it would play havoc with a narcotic-based anesthetic technique. In most cases, it is probably best to avoid anesthetic techniques based on narcotic infusions in patients in whom cholangiography is anticipated.

Opiates increase the resting tone of the gastrointestinal tract by both centrally mediated effects and interaction with opiate receptors in the gut itself (26). The resultant decrease in gastric motility and increase in antral tone slows gastric emptying, which delays systemic absorption of oral medication given preoperatively and increases the likelihood of pulmonary aspiration of gastric contents in patients medicated or fed after receiving a dose of narcotic. These drugs also cause constipation.

Miscellaneous Effects

Opiates commonly produce nausea and vomiting by their direct action at emetic chemoreceptors in the medulla (26). Patients receiving opiates are more sensitive to vestibular stimulation. This effect may become apparent or aggravated with postoperative movement or ambulation. Although opiate antagonists reverse nausea and vomiting, administration of an antiemetic drug such as droperidol is preferable because the opiate analgesic effect remains.

Urethral and detrusor muscle tone is increased with opiate administration. The resulting postoperative urinary retention can be antagonized by nalbuphine or naloxone, although catheterization may be required.

Morphine, meperidine, and the fentanyl congeners readily cross the placenta. Although they are considered to be nonteratogenic and can be used in early pregnancy, they should be used with caution for labor or cesarean section before delivery of the fetus because opiate effects can be seen in the newborn.

When opiates are used with the benzodiazepines, there may be a synergistic effect. Persson et al. (27) showed that alfentanil added to a midazolam infusion regimen caused increased and prolonged (more than additive) sedative and respiratory depressant effects postoperatively. Tverskoy et al.'s report (28) that the sedative interaction between morphine and midazolam was only additive indicates that the nature of this interaction has not been resolved.

Opiates inhibit the secretion of hypothalamic-releasing factors, resulting in decreased circulating levels of luteinizing hormone, follicle-stimulating hormone, adrenocorticotropic hormone, beta-endorphin, testosterone, and cortisol. These actions are in direct opposition to the effects of surgical trauma. The fentanyl analogues in particular have been used to reduce the metabolic stress response to surgical trauma to produce so-called "stress-free anesthesia." Opiates may or may not block antidiuretic hormone released by surgical stimulation (26).

Skeletal muscle rigidity is a significant effect seen with all opioid agonists (29) and with the fentanyl congeners in particular (30). An animal model has demonstrated that this action arises in the brainstem at the nucleus raphe pontis (31); opiates have no effect at the neuromuscular junction. Perhaps because this region of the brain is a major source of ascending and descending serotonergic projections, Weinger et al. (32) were able to reverse this rigidity by pretreating rats with the serotonin antagonist ketanserin.

Skeletal muscle rigidity may be related to a mammalian behavior of "freezing" just before explosive attempts to flee when attacked by predators (T.A. Blasco, *personal communication*). Regardless of the teleological underpinnings, virtually all skeletal muscle exhibits increased tone when this effect occurs. The muscles that affect the airway (e.g., massaters, neck, glottis) and respiration (e.g. thoracic, abdominals) are the most obvious to anesthesiologists attempting to maintain ventilation (30). The onset of rigidity may also be accompanied by significant increases in intracranial pressure (33). Rigidity appears to occur most frequently with loss of consciousness and accordingly occurs virtually 100% of the time when alfentanil is given as a bolus injection at a dose of 175 μg/kg (30), although an 8% incidence has been reported with IV fentanyl doses of only 80–200 μg (34).

Attenuating this effect is important because such rigidity is likely to occur during infusion of the loading doses proposed in this chapter. Pretreatment with small doses of neuromuscular blocking agents (e.g., 1 mg of vecuronium) was used to decrease the incidence or severity of rigidity (34). Larger doses were used to attenuate occurrences of rigidity. Pretreating patients with centrally acting GABAergic agents such as thiopental or diazepam resulted in limited success (35). Future work with serotonin antagonists may eventually lead to more effective pretreatments to prevent this effect.

Alternatively, one can simply induce unconsciousness with a hypnotic agent (e.g., thiopental, propofol, midazolam) and then administer a partial or full paralyzing dose of a neuromuscular blocking agent before administering the loading dose of an opiate. This seems to be the most logical approach because some degree of muscle relaxation is usually advised (see Chapter 5) for most IV infusion anesthesia techniques.

Clinical Requirements

Opiates serve two clinical purposes during the conduct of anesthesia; they provide analgesia and they reduce the requirement for other anesthetic drugs [the so-called MAC-sparing effect (5–7)], perhaps by virtue of the former effect. The painful or noxious stimuli for which analgesia is required begins with laryngoscopy and tracheal intubation, continues through surgical incisions and manipulations, and concludes with postoperative pain resulting from the surgical trauma. As practitioners of anesthesia know, these stimuli vary greatly in their intensity. The anesthetic drug levels required to suppress the perception of pain, or the reflex autonomic response to the pain in the unconscious patient, vary in parallel.

Three options are available to the clinician attempting to maintain adequate analgesia with an opiate infusion during the course of surgery. First, one could select a target plasma concentration that lies two or three standard deviations above the estimated EC_{50} anticipated to be necessary for maximum stimulation. Although this may provide adequate analgesia in the vast majority of cases, opiate side effects such as sedation and respiratory depression may last an undesirably long time postoperatively. Respiratory depression may not be a problem when postoperative ventilation is part of the clinical plan.

Second, one could target a concentration near the EC_{50} and add another anesthetic agent, such as a potent volatile anesthetic, should analgesia prove to be inadequate. Third, one could plan to titrate the opiate infusion to analgesic effect. The infusion rate could be diminished if the patient showed no signs of inadequate analgesia or if the estimated concentration could be raised in anticipation of an increased level of surgical stimulation or in response to movement or autonomic reflex activity indicating that analgesia is inadequate.

In the unconscious patient, there is no reliable measure of opiate effect. Roizen et al. (36) advocated the concept of minimum analgesic concentration to maintain baseline autonomic response (MAC-BAR). Others, concerned that autonomic response cannot be depended on to reveal inadequate analgesia, particularly in patients with cardiovascular disease or on drugs that moderate cardiovascular tone, have sought an electroencephalogram (EEG) measure of opiate effect. Although opiates can produce characteristic graded changes in the EEG, these changes are as yet unrelated to clinical response or the potential for awareness. At present, although using movement and autonomic response to judge the adequacy of analgesia, or even anesthesia, seems imprecise at best, the method appears to work reasonably well.

Ausems et al. (9) used a variable-rate alfentanil infusion along with 67% inspired N_2O in O_2 during superficial and intra-abdominal operations as part of a study in which plasma samples were collected periodically to measure plasma alfentanil concentrations. Criteria for bolus and upward adjustments in infusion rate were established on the basis of changes from baseline systolic blood pressure or heart rate, movement (patients were kept only partially paralyzed), or other autonomic responses such as tearing. Infusion rates were decreased if all signs remained at or below baseline for 15 minutes. The investigators collected blood samples periodically during operation and whenever signs of inadequate analgesia were observed. The collected data were used to generate concentration-response curves (see Fig. 1) based on a logistic regression for individuals or for the various surgical stimuli for their entire patient sample. These data form the basis of

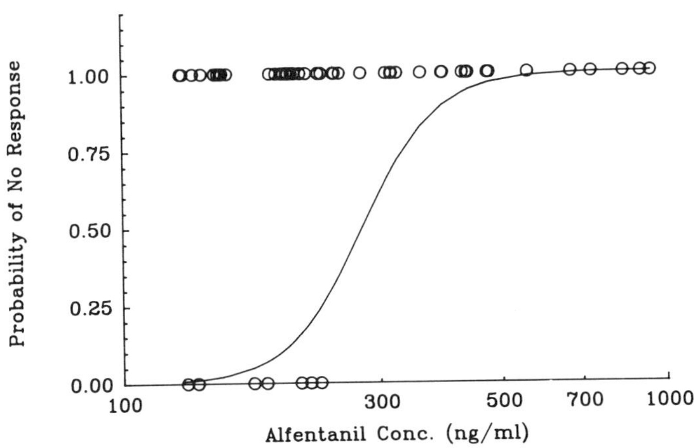

FIG. 1. Alfentanil plasma concentration data from a surgical patient. Open circles represent measured concentrations and are plotted either at 0.0 (patient responding to surgical stimulus) or 1.0 (patient not currently responding). Solid line is fit of these data to a probability model (9). Note that the Cp_{50} for this patient (alfentanil plasma concentration at which the patient has a 50:50 chance of response) is approximately 275 ng/ml. (Prepared according to Ausems et al., ref. 9.)

TABLE 1. *Opioid target plasma concentrations to be used for continuous infusions in adult patients expressed in ng/ml*

	Meperidine (10) ng/ml	Fentanyl (41) ng/ml	Sufentanil (41) ng/ml	Alfentanil (9) ng/ml
During surgery with N_2O/O_2	300–2000	2.5–10	0.25–1.0	200–800
During surgery with O_2 alone		15–60	2–8	1000–4000
Adequate postoperative ventilation	150 (?)	1.5	0.25	125

the detailed information concerning alfentanil target concentrations in Table 1. This approach, in which infusion rates are adjusted in accordance with clinical response or anticipated clinical need, appears to be the most sound; in fact, it mirrors the technique of adjusting inspired volatile anesthesia concentrations with which practitioners of anesthesia are already familiar.

Pharmacokinetics

Before discussing pharmacokinetic variables, some basic concepts will be reviewed. To establish a clear picture of the pharmacokinetic differences among the various opiates, one must understand the kinetic biophase. The biophase, or effect compartment, is a compartment (with imaginary drug concentrations) in which the time course of drug concentrations, or the kinetic profile, actually reflects concentrations at the active site. The kinetics of this biophase are determined by the time course of the measured drug effect (or pharmacodynamics) and an assumed (or otherwise determined) concentration-effect model. An example of such a model is the sigmoid E_{max} or Hill model that is used extensively when examining the pharmacokinetic-pharmacodynamic relationship of neuromuscular blocking agents (Eq. 1, Chapter 5).

Quantifying such relationships requires a graded measure of drug effect, which coincides with the desired clinical effect. One could argue that there is a continuum in the ability to assess these relationships. The precise, continuously scaled, second-to-second measured, directly clinically relevant determination of muscle relaxant effect represents one extreme. The difficult to quantitate, often nominally or quantally scaled, slowly acquired observation of centrally acting drugs such as analgesics or hypnotics represents the other. Ironically, the centrally acting drugs often have the more evanescent effects and possess the more important secondary effects, making the elucidation of a full pharmacokinetic-pharmacodynamic model more important.

The group at Stanford led by Drs. Stanski and Shafer (37,38) attempted to bring objective pharmacodynamic measures, much like those available for neuromuscular blockade, to bear on the study of centrally acting hypnotic drugs by using the processed EEG to measure the CNS effects of opiates as well as hypnotics.

This method affords the second-to-second acquisition of continuously scaled effect data that are necessary to estimate pharmacokinetic-pharmacodynamic models accurately for rapidly acting drugs such as the fentanyl analogues.

This approach suffers on such theoretical grounds as the lack of correspondence of the 95% spectral edge of the processed EEG with any clinically important opiate effect. Often, no maximal EEG effect is attained or a plateau approached even though a sigmoid E_{max} concentration-effect model is used. However, these EEG effects presumably model the same biophase as the effect of interest (i.e., analgesia) and are useful in characterizing the kinetics of the plasma concentration-effect relationship.

Recently, the Stanford group (39) used the EEG as a surrogate opioid effect marker to evolve an ambitious blueprint for Phase I drug investigations. This approach involves comparing the pharmacokinetics and EEG pharmacodynamics of a new drug under study with a well-studied opioid currently in widespread clinical use (e.g., fentanyl). If the new drug is mechanistically similar to older drugs in its therapeutic class (e.g., μ-receptor agonist), it is likely that valid clinical dose-response relationships can be estimated from a study with a small number of subjects, thus fingerprinting the new drug relative to its pharmacologic peers. This scheme also permits the clinician to couple these potency comparisons made on the basis of EEG studies with pharmacokinetic data to devise rational dosing regimens.

After the introduction of a pulse dose to the central compartment of a mammillary multicompartmental model, peripheral compartment concentrations (including the effect compartment) will rise toward those of the central driving compartment. This occurs at a rate determined by the ratio of the rate constants defining the peripheral compartment until a pseudoequilibrium is reached. The concentrations will subsequently remain higher than and fall roughly parallel to those of the central compartment. A study by Scott et al. (38) showed that alfentanil equilibrates between blood and the CNS biophase approximately five times more rapidly than does fentanyl. Such a model can define more clearly the already clinically appreciated differences in time to maximum effect observed following IV administration of these drugs. The model also sheds light on previously difficult to interpret observations such as the seemingly incongruous data on potency ratios between these drugs. Fentanyl is only 4 times as potent as alfentanil when given as a bolus (40) but is 60 times as potent when steady-state plasma concentrations are compared (Table 1). This is because a drug such as alfentanil, which equilibrates rapidly with its biophase, will have early, relatively more intense effects than will a drug such as fentanyl, which equilibrates more slowly. The example in Fig. 2 shows two drugs that produce similar plasma concentration-versus-effect profiles, allowing normalization of concentrations to equivalent doses. Once normalized, lipid-soluble drugs will have nearly superimposable pharmacokinetic curves for about the first half-hour after bolus injection in an adult. Therefore, for purposes of demonstration (Fig. 2), the pharmacokinetic profiles of the two drugs are represented by a single curve.

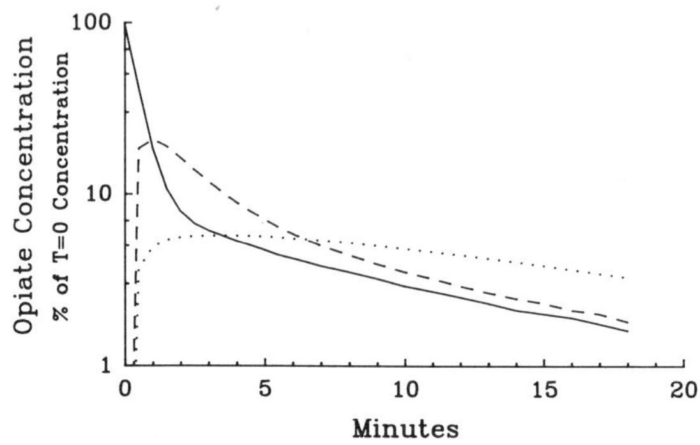

FIG. 2. Simulation of plasma and effect site concentrations for two putative fentanyl analogues. Plasma concentrations (solid line) are normalized for two drugs. Effect site concentrations rise toward the plasma concentrations at different rates; drug A (dashed line), which has a rapid *t*1/2 k_{eo} (like alfentanil), equilibrates more quickly than drug B (dotted line), which has a slower *t*1/2 k_{eo} (like fentanyl). This allows drug A to reach approximately four times greater relative effect site concentrations at peak.

Note that after pseudoequilibration of drug B, the one with a longer $t1/2_{Keo}$, the drug concentrations in the biophase have a similar time course except that those for drug B remain approximately two times greater. However, drug A equilibrates sooner at a much higher concentration (approximately four times greater).

This principle explains more than half of the apparent 15-fold difference in potency ratio between the bolus IV doses of the drugs and their plasma concentrations at steady state. The remaining disparity may relate to the accuracy of the determination of the original 4:1 potency ratio and actual differences in early pharmacokinetic profiles for the two drugs; this simulation assumed them to be identical.

These kinetic factors are of primary importance when considering the use of opiates by continuous infusion during anesthesia, particularly because they tend to fly in the face of common clinical impressions about these drugs. First, the ability of relatively small doses of alfentanil (in relation to its recommended infusion rate) to "pack more of a punch" when given as a bolus has nothing to do with a potency or efficacy advantage over other opiates. Believing otherwise may lead one to administer too small a loading dose when a step change in alfentanil infusion rate is deemed necessary.

Second, 5–10 minutes after a bolus dose or short infusion, alfentanil biophase concentrations fall at a rate similar to those of fentanyl and sufentanil until the terminal or elimination portion of the curve is reached about an hour or two later. Therefore, the extremely rapid falloff of effect seen after small IV injections of alfentanil will not be experienced when large doses are given or after relatively prolonged infusions—situations in which the effects of rapid equilibration of the biophase are lost.

To reiterate, the extremely rapid dissipation of effect seen after impulse IV doses of alfentanil are not a result of its plasma pharmacokinetics but rather the kinetics of its pharmacodynamics. Alfentanil does have a shorter $t_{1/2\beta}$ than any other narcotic (approximately 100 min), but this is not sufficiently brief to influence falloff of effect after infusion for surgical procedures of 1 hour to 4 hours in duration. Shafer and Varvel (41) published an article in which the implications of these principles are graphically demonstrated with the extensive use of pharmacokinetic simulations of fentanyl analogue infusions.

Another underappreciated pharmacokinetic principle of importance to the clinical use of opiate infusions concerns time to reach steady-state concentrations. It is generally taught that at 3.3 half-lives, 90% of steady-state concentration is reached. This is true and is a useful rule for single-compartment or monoexponential models used to explain, say, digoxin or theophylline kinetics; however, it is not accurate or particularly useful for situations encountered in anesthetic practice in which multicompartmental considerations are very important.

No easy formula is available to explain the rise to steady-state during constant infusion for a multicompartmental model. Roughly speaking, however, the rate of rise toward steady state is governed by the half-lives of the distributional and elimination phases in proportion to the contribution of each exponential phase to the overall area under the concentration-time curve after an impulse dose. What this means in practical terms is that these opiates have "sizable" distributional phases, so one can expect to reach the eventual steady-state level much more rapidly than would be predicted by single-compartment approximations.

Figure 3 illustrates the difference in predicted rise of sufentanil plasma concentrations using a single- versus a three-compartmental model. Unfortunately,

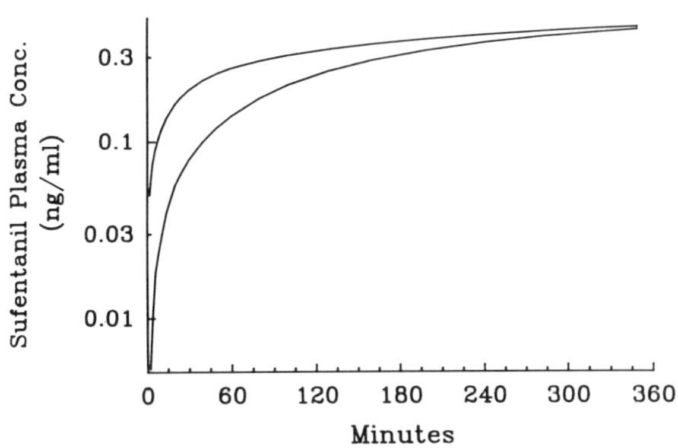

FIG. 3. Simulations of sufentanil plasma concentration versus time curves during steady, constant-rate infusions for one-compartment (lower curve) versus three-compartment (upper curve) models, assuming similar volumes and identical elimination clearances for both models. Note that although both rise to the same eventual steady-state concentration, only the three-compartment plot accurately depicts the early rapid rise to near plateau concentrations.

short of complex calculations or simulations, there is no easy way to represent meaningfully the relative rates of rise toward target concentrations for these opiates. Table 2 includes columns giving the times to reach 50%, 75%, and 90% of steady-state concentrations assuming constant infusion without a loading dose into the appropriate multicompartmental system. Obviously, loading doses and certain computer-controlled infusion pumps (42,43) designed to circumvent the slow concentration rise of constant infusion will essentially render these figures useless.

Practitioners of anesthesiology should be cognizant of the importance of multicompartmental considerations as they pertain to the use of opiate infusions. Unfortunately, most equipment now available to administer these drugs works as if the drugs obeyed single-compartment rules. One purpose of this chapter is to explain how to use this equipment to administer opiate infusions optimally and to demonstrate the multicompartmental result.

Technological advances have been made that allow drug infusion equipment to make ongoing calculations based on the multicompartmental behavior of drugs in patients. Infusion devices capable of accepting serial input from a PC computer can be controlled to allow infusion rates to be altered continuously to hold plasma- or effect-compartment concentrations steady (42,43). These devices greatly simplify the rational administration of opiates during anesthesia but are not yet commercially available.

Simulation algorithms for hand-held calculators (44) and programs for microcomputers (45) that can calculate estimates of current (or forecasted) plasma concentrations are already available. Such calculations are useful for at least two reasons. By associating concentration estimates with actual clinical effect seen, one can improve control of the concentration in relation to desired effect by changing the infusion rate, which results in proportional changes in concentration. Also, the ability to predict when concentrations associated with minimal respiratory depression will occur after discontinuation of infusions of whatever length will increase the likelihood that such concentrations will be realized when the patient arrives in the recovery room. To this end, Maitre and Stanski (46) studied the use of Bayesian statistical techniques and their ability to refine greatly the estimates

TABLE 2. *Pharmacokinetics of the opioids commonly used for continuous infusion for adult patients*

Opioid	Vd_{ss} (L/kg)	Cl_E(ml/min)	$t1/2_\beta$ (hr)	$t_{50\%}$ (hr)[a]	$t_{75\%}$ (hr)	$t_{90\%}$ (hr)	References
Fentanyl	2–4	850	3–5	1.0	4.8	9.8	50–53,56–59
Sufentanil	2–4	850	3–5	0.9	3.3	6.8	48,53,54,59
Alfentanil	0.2–0.5	275	1–3	1.7	3.75	6.5	45,47,51,57
Meperidine[b]	2–4	850	3–5				49,55

[a]Time for a constant rate infusion to reach stated percentage of the steady-state level.
[b]Full three-compartmental kinetics not available.

of individual pharmacokinetic variables when intraoperative opiate concentrations are known. However, rapid and inexpensive techniques of opiate assay, although feasible, appear to be somewhere in the future.

Because a patient may have either an unexpectedly increased or a decreased demand for these drugs, one should anticipate the need to adjust the infusion rate during the course of anesthesia from that initially predicted. As previously mentioned, this need may result from the significant interindividual differences in the pharmacokinetics of these drugs that may translate into variable dose-response relationships among patients. Equally variable concentration-response relationships may compound or amplify the need to change infusion rates upward or downward.

Selected pharmacokinetic variables for the commonly used opiates are shown in Table 2. In general, the pharmacokinetics of fentanyl and sufentanil are similar. Alfentanil differs from the other opiates by virtue of its lower Vd and Cl_E. The lower hepatic clearance of alfentanil means that it is influenced less by changes in hepatic blood flow, as indicated by the lack of a correlation between alfentanil and indocyanine green clearances (47).

Fentanyl, sufentanil, and meperidine have large steady-state distribution volumes (approx. 2–4 L/kg), perhaps reflecting their high lipid solubility. They are metabolized in the liver by oxidative pathways and have high hepatic extraction ratios (near 0.7). This means that elimination clearance is approximately 70% of liver blood flow and is sensitive to factors affecting hepatic blood flow. Thus, the poor oral bioavailability of these drugs is due to extensive first pass metabolism.

The metabolites of these drugs are thought to be inactive, although the N-demethylated metabolite of meperidine (normeperidine) has CNS excitatory effects that may lead to seizures. Normeperidine pharmacokinetics indicates that concentrations will reach problematic levels only during chronic parenteral administration, but similar concentrations will result from prolonged oral administration because of increased normeperidine creation with first pass metabolism.

INFUSION SCHEMES

As was detailed in Chapter 2, the primary determinants of an infusion regimen are pharmacodynamic data, or target plasma concentrations, and pharmacokinetic variables. Table 1 provides reasonable estimates for concentrations associated with good clinical response during general anesthesia in which the opiate is given with either N_2O/O_2 or O_2 alone. Some data suggest that requirements for opiates given in conjunction with infusions of hypnotic agents such as propofol, etomidate, or midazolam as part of a totally IV anesthetic technique are roughly equivalent to values given for N_2O/O_2. This may be because the pharmacodynamic data of the opiates given at lower doses with adjunct anesthetic drugs such as N_2O reflect more purely the analgesic efficacy of opiates rather than their secondary effects of sedation when given at high doses alone.

Because opiate drugs have relatively high margins of safety a bolus plus infusion regimen along the lines of that proposed by Mitenko and Ogilvie (48) is generally sufficient. The bolus dose and infusion rate are selected on the basis of the following:

Bolus dose = target concentration – distribution volume [1]

Infusion rate = target concentration – elimination clearance, [2]

where the target concentration is selected on the basis of the expected level of surgical stimuli and the use of adjunct anesthetic drugs. High plasma concentrations seen during the distribution phase, when the bolus dose is based on total distribution volume rather than an initial distribution volume, should not produce significant adverse effects.

Often, significant hypotension is seen after loading doses of opiates, especially alfentanil (30). This may occur particularly when the opiate is administered just after induction of anesthesia with a hypnotic drug, especially propofol (21). To avoid unnecessarily high plasma opiate concentrations, one can give the bolus dose divided into roughly four equal parts over approximately 45 minutes.

To understand the effect of the drug in patients, it is necessary to simulate the multicompartmental pharmacokinetic behavior of dosing regimens designed on

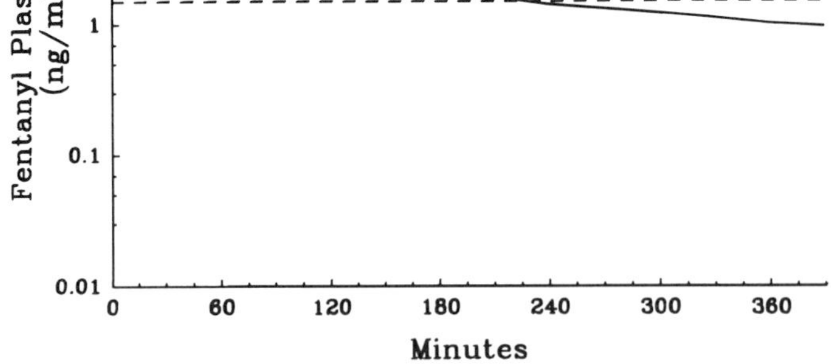

FIG. 4. Simulation of three-compartmental "behavior" of fentanyl plasma concentrations after a loading dose and infusion scheme based on one-compartment pharmacokinetic estimates from Table 1 and target concentrations from Table 2. The loading dose, determined by multiplying the volume of distribution and the target concentration (upper dashed line), was given as four separate boluses 10 min apart. The infusion, calculated by multiplying clearance and the target concentration, was terminated at 120 min. Note that the time to reach fentanyl plasma concentrations consistent with normal ventilation is approximately 100 min after termination of the infusion.

the basis of single-compartmental concepts. The simulations in Figs. 4 through 6 demonstrate that opiate concentrations remain near the target concentration using the technique of four divided loading doses. One might consider giving the second bolus before intubation and the fourth before the start of surgery to correlate high biophase concentrations more closely with painful stimuli. If the duration of surgery is less than 1 hour, these stimulations indicate that only two or three of the quartered loading doses may be required to maintain analgesic plasma concentrations.

Because of previously mentioned interindividual variability in pharmacokinetics and pharmacodynamics of the opiates and the occurrence of repeated and varied painful surgical stimuli during the course of an operation, one should expect to titrate opiate infusions much as one would a volatile anesthetic. The scheme proposed by Ausems et al. (9) is generally sound. After the loading dose designed to establish a target concentration, one gives an additional bolus to raise plasma concentrations immediately and increases the infusion rate by increments equal to 50% of the initially predicted rate when movement or autonomic response results from surgical stimuli. Correspondingly, one decreases the infusion rate by increments

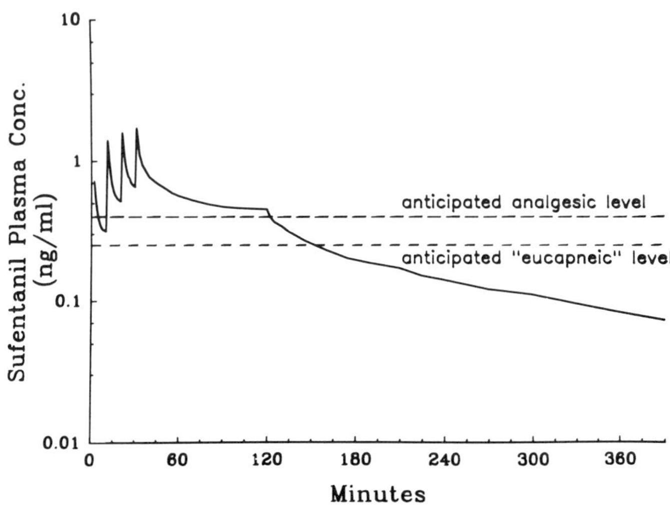

FIG. 5. Simulation of three-compartmental "behavior" of sufentanil plasma concentrations after a loading dose and infusion scheme based on one-compartment pharmacokinetic estimates from Table 1 and target concentrations from Table 2. The loading dose, determined by multiplying the volume of distribution and the target concentration (upper dashed line), was given as four separate boluses 10 min apart. The infusion, calculated by multiplying clearance and the target concentration, was terminated at 120 min. Note that the time to reach sufentanil plasma concentrations consistent with normal ventilation is approximately 30 min after termination of the infusion. This rapid dissipation of effect is partly the result of its distribution kinetics, which differ from the other two fentanyl analogues, and a reported (and yet unconfirmed) smaller relative difference between surgical analgesic and normal ventilatory plasma concentrations.

equal to 25% of the initial rate when 15 minutes or 20 minutes elapse, during which painful surgical stimuli have not elicited any response from the patient. This titration procedure greatly improves the likelihood that respiratory depressant effects will be sufficiently low to render the patient eucapnic postoperatively.

Fragen et al. (21) used this approach with alfentanil along with either N_2O/O_2 or propofol given by continuous infusion. In their study, the alfentanil infusion scheme of Ausems et al. (9) was modified so that the additional boluses of alfentanil were intended to attain analgesic levels immediately and to serve as adequate loading doses for the rapid attainment of the higher plasma concentration resulting from the increased rate of infusion.

Whereas Ausems et al.'s intraoperative boluses of 7 μg/kg were sufficient to attenuate the patient's response to pain, they did not constitute a sufficient loading dose based on the principles in Eqs. 1 and 2. One would predict that 25 μg/kg would be the proper loading dose. The tendency to give inadequate loading doses for intraoperative step changes in plasma concentration arises as a result of the large but short-lived effect that a smaller impulse dose of alfentanil produces. Instead, Fragen et al. gave 25% of an approximate initial loading dose for a small adult (1 mg) in response to appropriate clinical signs. A need for this bolus to be repeated within 15 minutes (after the dissipation of alfentanil's additional "punch"; see Fig. 1) indicated that a higher target concentration was needed and served as

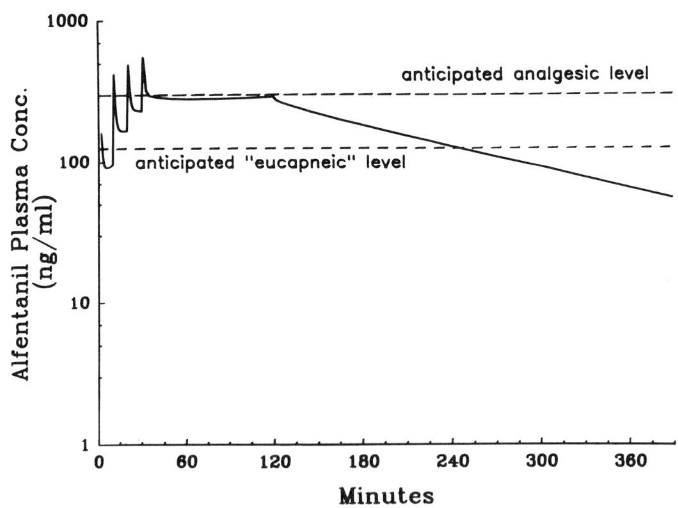

FIG. 6. Simulation of three-compartmental "behavior" of alfentanil plasma concentrations after a loading dose and infusion scheme based on one-compartment pharmacokinetic estimates from Table 1 and target concentrations from Table 2. The loading dose, determined by multiplying the volume of distribution and the target concentration (upper dashed line), was given as four separate boluses 10 min apart. The infusion, calculated by multiplying clearance and the target concentration, was terminated at 120 min. Note that the time to reach alfentanil plasma concentrations consistent with normal ventilation is approximately 110 min after termination of the infusion.

a sufficient load to allow more rapid achievement of the new target concentration that an increase equal to 50% of the initial infusion rate should eventually reach. Figure 7 shows both the bolus/infusion scheme and the resulting plasma alfentanil concentrations.

The rate at which opiate concentrations fall after termination of an infusion depends on the pharmacokinetics of the particular drug and the length of the infusion (see Chapter 1). Typically, the longer an infusion runs, the closer one comes to true steady-state conditions. At steady state, a minimum rate of decline in plasma drug concentrations is seen when the infusion is stopped. However, even at steady state, the time for the initial 50% decrease in plasma concentration is less than the terminal elimination half-life. Conversely, with shorter infusions, the distribution phases continue to manifest greater influences on the rate at which drug concentration declines at the end of infusion.

Fortunately, most surgical procedures are brief enough (less than about 6 hrs) to allow distributional processes to contribute to lowering plasma opiate concentrations after termination of the infusion, at least for fentanyl and sufentanil. This means that one should expect a 50% decrement in plasma concentration in 25–40 minutes after a 2-hour infusion of either fentanyl or sufentanil (see Figs. 4 and 5) rather than that predicted by the t1/2 in Table 2. On the other hand, it takes alfen-

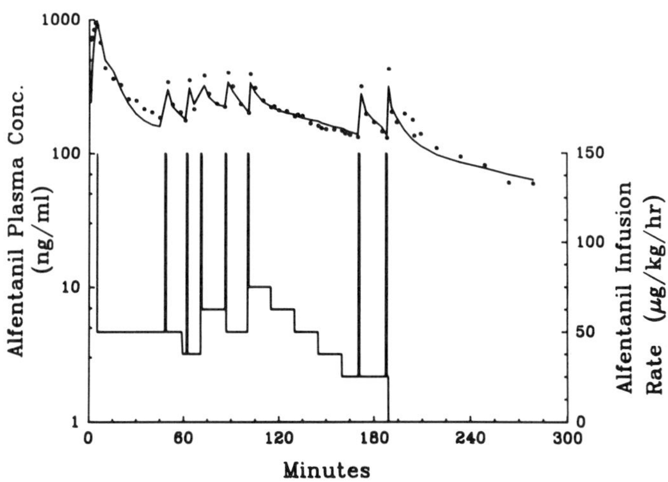

FIG. 7. Alfentanil plasma concentration versus time profile during continuous infusion in which the infusion rate was adjusted according to the patient's needs. The lower curve with the right vertical axis represents the alfentanil infusion rate. The infusion was begun by giving the loading dose of 150 µg/kg over 5 min. The maintenance infusion was started at a rate of 50 µg/kg/hr. If the patient responded to stimuli, a 1.0 mg alfentanil bolus was given (vertical spikes). Two such bolus doses in any 15-min period prompted the infusion rate to be increased by 25 µg/kg/hr. With the absence of patient response in any 15-min period after surgery began, the infusion was decreased by 12.5 µg/kg/hr. Note that the infusion rate was mistakenly turned down rather than up after the bolus at approximately 80 min. The solid circles represent the actual arterial plasma alfentanil concentrations, and the solid line is the fit by least-squares nonlinear regression.

tanil plasma concentrations nearly a full half-life (99 min in the example in Fig. 6) to fall 50% after a similar infusion.

Because levels adequate for analgesia during surgical anesthesia are generally twice those that allow for adequate ventilation, one should attempt to discontinue opiate infusions at a time that would allow the concentrations to fall by one-half on the patient's anticipated arrival in the recovery room. A comparison of Figs. 4 through 6 suggests that the fractional difference between analgesic levels and levels associated with adequate ventilation is less for sufentanil than for either fentanyl or alfentanil. Other recent evidence seems to support this earlier observation (49). If this is true, then the time required for plasma sufentanil concentrations to fall from levels sufficient for surgical analgesia to those allowing adequate ventilation might be significantly shorter.

Generally, surgical manipulations associated with operative closure are less stimulating and are compatible with the reduced opiate levels seen in the minutes after cessation of the infusion. Again, the rate of opiate level falloff after termination of infusion is a complex issue with no easy rules of thumb. It is analogous

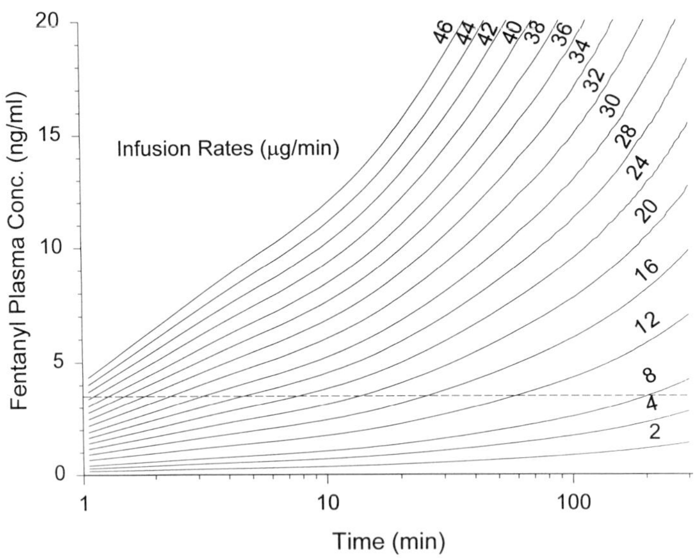

FIG. 8. Isoconcentration nomogram for fentanyl in a healthy adult. To maintain a plasma fentanyl concentration of at least 3.5 ng/ml, start with an infusion rate of 38 µg/min. Then from the horizontal line drawn at 3.5 µg/ml, change to the next infusion rate (36 µg/min) at the time its concentration versus time curve intersects the horizontal (approximately 1.5 min). Alternatively, one could elect to be less fussy and allow the plasma fentanyl concentration to rise higher above the target until, for example, it reached 6 ng/ml, at which time (approximately 3.5 min) the infusion would be changed to 28 µg/min. For this example, the new infusion rates in micrograms per minute at time (in minutes) are 24 at 7, 20 at 13, 16 at 22, 12 at 55, 8 at 190. (Prepared according to Shafer, ref. 50.)

to the time necessary to reach 90% of steady state discussed above and depends on the duration of continuous infusion and the kinetics of the opiate. Shafer and Varvel's report (41) devoted an extensive discussion to this issue and the further issue of continued decreases in opiate levels that would allow a patient to be discharged from the hospital.

Another practical way of "controlling" a "dumb" infusion pump is the use of the isoconcentration nomogram developed by Steven L. Shafer (50) (Figs. 8–10). These are constructed by superimposing simulations of constant-rate infusions, such as the one shown in Fig. 3, at incremental rates. One can use them by placing a horizontal line at the desired target plasma concentration. The active infusion rate is the one with the simulated concentration versus time profile that is most recently intersected by the horizontal line. One manually switches to the next infusion rate at the times corresponding to the points of intersection. Target concentrations can be redrawn according to clinical demand.

Remifentanil is a new μ-agonist opioid that was in Phase III trials as of this writing. Although it shares almost identically the pharmacodynamic profile of the

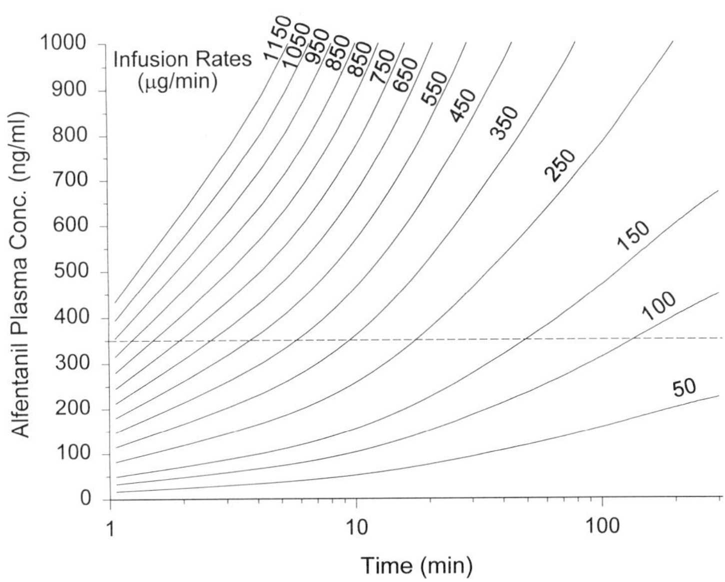

FIG. 9. Isoconcentration nomogram for alfentanil in a healthy adult. To maintain a plasma alfentanil concentration of at least 350 ng/ml, begin with an infusion rate of 950 μg/min. Then, from the horizontal line drawn at 350 ng/ml, change to the next infusion rate (850 μg/min) at the time its concentration versus time curve intersects the horizontal (approximately 1.5 min). Alternatively, one could elect to be less fussy and allow the plasma alfentanil concentration to rise higher above the target until, for example, it reached 600 ng/ml, at which time (approximately 4 min) the infusion would be changed to 550 μg/min. For this example, the new infusion rates in micrograms per minute at time (in minutes) are 450 at 5, 350 at 8, 250 at 12, 150 at 42, 100 at 120. (Prepared according to Shafer, ref. 50.)

other opioids discussed in this chapter, it is remarkably different in its pharmacokinetics because it is eliminated extremely rapidly by tissue-nonspecific esterases (51,52). The elimination clearance is a remarkable 3–4 1/min in adults. In vitro tests indicate that remifentanil is not a good substrate for pseudocholinesterase. Pharmacokinetic studies of remifentanil show that the time for a 50% decrease in plasma concentration asymtotically approaches 3 minutes with increasing duration of infusion and that this holds across various patient populations.

Carl Rosow (53) editorialized that the general problem of interindividual variability in pharmacokinetics and pharmacodynamics can be addressed in two ways: (1) develop a reliable opioid-effect monitor against which the clinician can titrate the drug or (2) develop an opioid that confers a greater margin of error in our currently crude titration methods. It appears that remifentanil offers the second solution. It should be useful in any situation where rapid termination of opioid effect is desirable. Intraoperative use will certainly require a constant infusion. Glaxo has provided guidelines for its use (Table 3), nevertheless, the company recommends checking the package insert before these recommendations are followed.

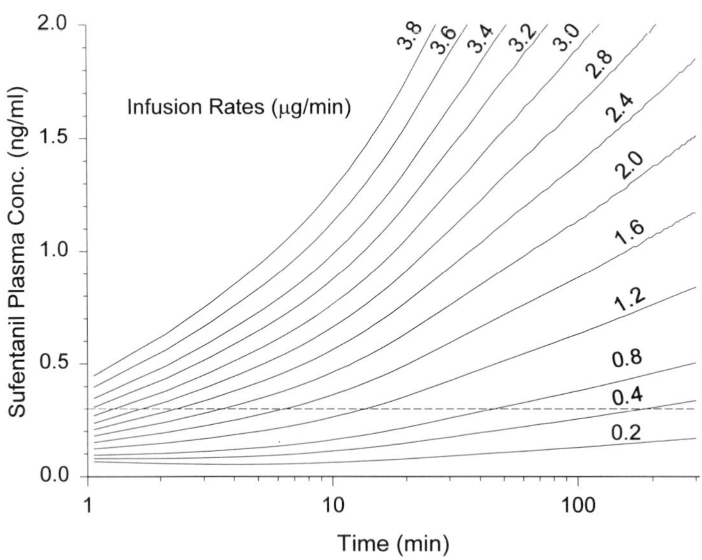

FIG. 10. Isoconcentration nomogram for sufentanil in a healthy adult. To maintain a plasma sufentanil concentration of at least 3.0 ng/ml, begin with an infusion rate of 3.0 μg/min. Then, from the horizontal line drawn at 3.0 ng/ml, change to the next infusion rate (2.8 μg/min) at the time its concentration versus time curve intersects the horizontal (approximately 1.8 min). Alternatively, one could elect to be less fussy and allow the plasma sufentanil concentration to rise higher above the target until, for example, it reached 0.5 ng/ml, at which time (approximately 3.5 min) the infusion would be changed to 2.0 μg/min. For this example, the new infusion rates in micrograms per minute at time (in min) are 1.6 at 6, 1.2 at 12, 0.8 at 42, 0.4 at 180. (Prepared according to Shafer, ref. 50.)

TABLE 3. *Projected doses for remifentanil*[a]

Use	Bolus (μg/kg)	Infusion (μg/kg/min)
Induction	0.5–2	1
Maintenance with 0.67 N_2O	1–2	0.5
Maintenance with propofol	1–2	0.25–0.5
Monitored anesthesia care	1–2	0.05–0.2
Post-operative pain relief	—	0.025–0.2

[a] From Glaxo, with permission.

Armed with a thorough knowledge of the clinical pharmacology of the opioid analgesics, the clinician should be able to manage a continuous infusion of these synthetic opiates in a rational, if not deft, manner. The current state of the art has not progressed much beyond simple infusion pumps and clinical observation for endpoints of pharmacologic effects. Progress is being made on both fronts with current developments on computer-driven infusion pumps for administering the drugs with greater ease and accuracy as well as on electrophysiologic monitors for quantitating their effects. Although infusion-pump technology is progressing at a rapid rate and soon will be commonly available, the appearance of an "analgesometer" does not seem imminent. The skilled clinician will still have to understand and use basic pharmacokinetic and pharmacodynamic principles in using these pumps to provide optimal anesthetic conditions, but infusions offer enough advantages to make such efforts worthwhile.

REFERENCES

1. Smith RR. Scopolamine-morphine anaesthesia, with report of two hundred and twenty nine cases. *Surg Gynecol Obstet* 1908;7:414–420.
2. Olley JE. Opiate receptors: ligands and methods of study. *Clin Exp Pharmacol Physiol* 1989;16: 535–538.
3. de Lange S, Boscoe M, Stanley TH, Pace N. Comparison of sufentanil-O_2 and fentanyl-O_2 for coronary artery surgery. *Anesthesiology* 1982;56:112–118.
4. Wong KC. Narcotics are not expected to produce unconsciousness and amnesia. *Anesth Analg* 1983; 62:625–626 (editorial).
5. Hall RI, Szlam F, Hug CC Jr. The enflurane-sparing effect of alfentanil in dogs. *Anesth Analg* 1987; 66:1287–1291.
6. Hall RI, Murphy MR, Hug Jr CC. The enflurane-sparing effect of sufentanil in dogs. *Anesthesiology* 1987;67:518–525.
7. Murphy MR, Hug CC Jr. The anesthetic potency of fentanyl in terms of its reduction of enflurane MAC. *Anesthesiology* 1982;57:485–488.
8. Austin KL, Stapleton JV, Mather LE. Relationship between blood meperidine concentrations and analgesic response: a preliminary report. *Anesthesiology* 1980;53:460–466.
9. Ausems ME, Hug CC Jr, Stanski DR, Burm AG. Plasma concentrations of alfentanil required to supplement nitrous oxide anesthesia for general surgery. *Anesthesiology* 1986;65:362–373.
10. White PF. Clinical uses of intravenous anesthetic and analgesic infusions. *Anesth Analg* 1989;68: 161–171.
11. Hickey RF, Severinghaus JW. Regulation of breathing: drug effects and disease. In: Hornbein TF, ed. *Regulation of breathing*. Vol. 17, Part II. New York: Marcel Decker; 1981:1251–1298.

12. Abdul-Rasool IH, Ward DS. Ventilatory and cardiovascular responses to sufentanil infusion in dogs anesthetized with isoflurane. *Anesth Analg* 1989;69:300–306.
13. Laubie M, Scmitt H. Sites of the vagally mediated bradycardia induced by morphine-like agents and opioid peptides. In: Buckley JP, Ferrario CM, eds. *Central nervous system mechanisms in hypertension.* New York: Raven Press; 1981:235–247.
14. Hill DC, Chelly JE, Dlewati A, Abernethy DR, Doursout MF, Merin RG. Cardiovascular effects of and interaction between calcium blocking drugs and anesthetics in chronically instrumented dogs. VI. Verapamil and fentanyl-pancuronium. *Anesthesiology* 1988;68:874–879.
15. Strauer BE. Contractile responses to morphine, piritramide, meperidine and fentanyl: a comparative study of effects on the isolated ventricular myocardium. *Anesthesiology* 1972;31:304–311.
16. Green JF, Jackman AP, Parsons G. The effects of morphine on the mechanical properties of the systemic circulation in the dog. *Circ Res* 1978;42:474–478.
17. Rosow CE, Moss J, Philbin DM, Savarese JJ. Histamine release during morphine and fentanyl anesthesia. *Anesthesiology* 1982;56:93–96.
18. Rosow CE, Philbin DM, Keegan CR, Nfoss J. Hemodynamics and histamine release during induction with sufentanil and fentanyl. *Anesthesiology* 1984;60:489–491.
19. Morton NS, Hamilton WF. Alfentanil in an anesthetic technique for penetrating eye injuries. *Anaesthesia* 1986;41:1148–1151.
20. Crawford DC, Fell D, Achola KJ, Smith G. Effects of alfentanil on the pressor and catecholamine responses to tracheal intubation. *Br J Anaesth* 1987;59:707–712.
21. Fragen RJ, Avram MJ, Henthorn TK, Asada A, Pemberton D, Correll T. Total intravenous anesthesia with propofol, alfentanil, and vecuronium for superficial surgery. *Anesth Analg* 1990;70:S112.
22. Van Aken H, Meinshausen E, Prien T, Brussel T, Heinecke A, Lawin P. The influence of fentanyl and tracheal intubation on the hemodynamic effects of anesthesia induction with propofol/N_2O in humans. *Anesthesiology* 1988;68:157–163.
23. Speiss BD, Satoff RH, El-Ganzouri ARS, Ivankovich AD. High-dose sufentanil: four cases of sudden hypotension on induction. *Anesth Analg* 1986;65:703–705.
24. Kien ND, Reitan JA, White DA, Wu CH, Eisele Jr JH. Hemodynamic responses to alfentanil in halothane-anesthetized dogs. *Anesth Analg* 1986;65:765–770.
25. Radnay PA, Duncalf D, Novakovic NI, Lesser ML. Common bile duct pressure changes after fentanyl, morphine, meperidine, butorphanol, and naloxone. *Anesth Anaig* 1984;63:441–444.
26. Jaffe JH, Martin WR. Opioid analgesics and antagonists. In: Gilman AG, Goodman LS, Rall TW, Niles AS, Taylor P, eds. *The pharmacologic basis of therapeutics.* 8th ed. New York: Macmillan; 1990:485–521.
27. Persson MP, Nilsson A, Hartvig P. Relation of sedation and amnesia to plasma concentrations of midazolam in surgical patients. *Clin Pharmacol Ther* 1988;43:324–331.
28. Tverskoy NF, Fleyshman G, Ezry J, Bradley L Jr, Kissin I. Midazolam-morphine sedative interaction in patients. *Anesth Analg* 1989;68:282–285.
29. Wand P, Kuschinskv K, Sontag KH. Morphine-induced muscular rigidity in rats. *Eur J Pharmacol* 1973;24:189–193.
30. Benthuysen JL, Smith NT, Sanford TJ, Head N, Dec-Silver H. Physiology of alfentanil-induced rigidity. *Anesthesiology* 1986;64:440–446.
31. Blasco TA, Lee DE, Amalric M, Swerdlow NR, Smith NT, Koob GR. The role of the nucleus raphe pontis and the caudate nucleus in alfentanil rigidity in the rat. *Brain Res* 1986;386:280–286.
32. Weinger MB, Cline EJ, Smith NT, Koch GF. Ketanserin pretreatment reverses alfentanil-induced muscle rigidity. *Anesthesiology* 1987;67:348–354.
33. Benthuysen JL, Kien ND, Quam DD. Intracranial pressure increases during alfentanil induced rigidity. *Anesthesiology* 1988;68:438–440.
34. Moldenhauer CC, Hug CC Jr. Use of narcotic analgesics as anaesthetics. *Clin Anaesth* 1984;2(1): .
35. Blasco TA, Smith NT, Sanford TJ, Benthuysen J, Dec-Silver H, Head N. A clinical study of the effects of various pretreatment agents on alfentanil-induced rigidity: EMG data. *Anesthesiology* 1985; 63:A380(abst).
36. Roizen MF, Horrigan RW, Frazer BM. Anesthetic doses blocking adrenergic (stress) and cardiovascular responses to incision-MAC BAR. *Anesthesiology* 1981;54:390–398.
37. Homer TD, Stanski DR. The effect of increasing age on thiopental disposition and anesthetic requirement. *Anesthesiology* 1985;62:714–724.
38. Scott JC, Ponganis KV, Stanski DR. EEG quantitation of narcotic effect: the comparative pharmacodynamics of fentanyl and alfentanil. *Anesthesiology* 1985;62:234–241.

39. Egan TD, Lemmens HJM, Fiset P, Hermann DJ, Muir KT, Stanski DR, Shafer SL. The pharmcokinetics of the new short-acting opioid remifentanil (GI87084B) in healthy adult male volunteers. *Anesthesiology* 1993;79:881–892.
40. Stanski DR, Hug CC Jr. Alfentanil—a kinetically predictable narcotic analgesic. *Anesthesiology* 1982; 57:435–438(editorial).
41. Shafer SL, Varvel JR. Pharmacokinetics, pharmacodynamics, and rational opioid selection. *Anesthesiology* 1991;74:53–63.
42. Shafer SL, Siegel LC, Cooke JE, Scott JC. Testing computer-controlled infusion pumps by simulation. *Anesthesiology* 1988;68:261–266.
43. Alvis JM, Reves JG, Govier AV, et al. Computer-assisted continuous infusions of fentanyl during cardiac anesthesia: comparison with a manual method. *Anesthesiology* 1985;63:41–49.
44. Maitre PO, Shafer SL. A simple pocket calculator approach to predict anesthetic drug concentrations from pharmacokinetic data. *Anesthesiology* 1990;73:332–336.
45. Schüttler J, Kloos S. IVA-SIM: A program to stimulate intravenous anaesthesia. Bonn: Institut für Anästhesiologie; 1989.
46. Maitre PO, Stanski DR. Bayesian forecasting improves the prediction of intraoperative plasma concentrations of alfentanil. *Anesthesiology* 1988;69:652–659.
47. Henthorn TK, Avram MJ, Krejcie TC. Alfentanil clearance is independent of the polymorphic debrisoquin hydroxylase. *Anesthesiology* 1989;71:635–639.
48. Mitenko PA, Olgilvie RI. Rapidly achieved plasma concentration plateaus, with observations on theophylline kinetics. *Clin Pharmacol Ther* 1972;13:329–335.
49. Bailey PL, Streisand JB, East KA, et al. Differences in magnitude and duration of opioid-induced respiratory depression and analgesia with fentanyl and sufentanil. *Anesth Analg* 1990;70:8–15.
50. Shafer SL. Towards optimal intravenous dosing strategies. *Semin Anesth* 1993;42:222–230.
51. Lemmens HJM, Dyck JB, Shafer SL, Stanski DR. Pharmacokinetic-pharmacodynamic modeling in drug development: application to the investigational opioid trefentanil. *Clin Pharmacol Ther* 1994; 56:261–271.
52. Westmoreland CL, Hoke JF, Sebel PS, Hug CC, Muir KT. Pharmacokinetics of remifentanil (GI87084B) and its major metabolite (GI90291) in patients undergoing elective inpatient surgery. *Anesthesiology* 1993;79:893–902.
53. Rosow C. Remifentanil: a unique opioid analgesic. *Anesthesiology* 1993;79:875–876.
54. Bovill JG, Sebel PS, Blackburn CL, Heykants JJ. The pharmacokinetics of sufentanil in surgical patients. *Anesthesiology* 1984;61:502–506.
55. Mather LE, Tucker GT, Pflug AE, Lindop MJ, Wilkerson C. Meperidine kinetics in man: intravenous injection in surgical patients and volunteers. *Clin Pharmacol Ther* 1975;17:21–30.
56. McClain DA, Hug CC Jr. Intravenous fentanyl kinetics. *Clin Pharmacol Ther* 1980;28:106–114.
57. Scott JC, Stanski DR. Decreased fentanyl and alfentanil dose requirements with age: a simultaneous pharmacokinetic and pharmacodynamic evaluation. *J Pharmacol Exp Ther* 1987;240:159–166.
58. Singleton MA, Rosen JI, Fisher DM. Pharmacokinetics of fentanyl in the elderly. *Br J Anaesth* 1988; 60:619–622.
59. Stanski DR. Narcotic pharmacokinetics and dynamics: the basis of infusion applications. *Anaesth Intens Care* 1987;15:23–26.

Drug Infusions in Anesthesiology, Second Edition,
edited by R. J. Fragen. Lippincott-Raven Publishers,
Philadelphia © 1996.

5

Infusions of Muscle Relaxants

Colin A. Shanks

Department of Anesthesia, Northwestern University Medical School, Chicago, Illinois 60611

Some anesthesiologists restrict continuous infusion of neuromuscular blocking agents (NMBAs) to the depolarizing relaxant, succinylcholine. They use it for the ability to change the intensity of blockade rapidly, despite its potential to cause tachyphylaxis and Phase II block. The intermediate-duration nondepolarizing relaxants, such as atracurium, vecuronium, and rocuronium, come closer to the ideal of rapid control than the traditional long-acting NMBAs do, and their residual effects can be reversed more easily. The introduction of shorter-acting nondepolarizing agents such as mivacurium allows the anesthesiologist to respond quickly to altered surgical needs for muscle relaxation and for the swift return of muscle power postoperatively. The nondepolarizing NMBAs permit the anesthesiologist to use train-of-four stimulation to monitor the adequacy of surgical relaxation merely by counting the number of responses. This chapter provides guidelines for continuous infusion of NMBAs in the care of patients whose surgery requires neuromuscular blockade.

The initial reason to use NMBAs is to facilitate tracheal intubation. Unlike many other drugs administered during anesthesia, the NMBAs can be administered to the ventilated patient in doses considerably greater than those required for tracheal intubation. The intubating dose of succinylcholine represents an overdose, but usually the enzymatic degradation of the drug metabolizes this overdose rapidly. Rarely, prolonged neuromuscular block occurs with succinylcholine because the activity of pseudocholinesterase is reduced and cannot metabolize the drug quickly.

The urgent need for additional drug to increase the intensity of neuromuscular blockade during surgery can be unmistakable, yet administration of too large a bolus dose of a nondepolarizing agent can result in prolonged paralysis. During the infusion of NMBAs, neuromuscular monitoring facilitates achievement of optimal relaxation, varying the dosage according to the patient's responses to train-of-four stimulation. Some anesthesiologists apply stimulator electrodes at induction of anesthesia to determine when sufficient relaxation is obtained for tracheal intubation. The shorter-acting NMBAs enable rapid recovery from blockade, an advantage when the "wake-up test" is used to assess motor function during major spinal surgery (1). At the completion of surgery, rapid return of full motor power enhances the patient's ability to protect the airway and to ventilate satisfactorily.

NEUROMUSCULAR BLOCKING AGENTS

Pharmacodynamics

The effects of NMBAs can be graded from 0% to 100% for each individual. This contrasts with the problems of all-or-none quantitative responses such as awake/asleep, in which dosage can be characterized only in terms of a patient group. Ninety-five percent depression of the single twitch response (ED_{95}) is sufficient to facilitate tracheal intubation, although most clinicians reduce the time of onset with a larger dose.

Intraoperative Monitoring of Neuromuscular Responses

The intensity of neuromuscular blockade is best monitored intraoperatively by observing the muscle response to stimulation of a motor nerve. Because NMBAs act at neuromuscular junctions, the muscle can still respond if stimulated directly. Inappropriate responses are seen when electrodes to stimulate the facial nerve are placed too near the eye, over the orbicularis oculi muscle.

Most nerve stimulators now in clinical practice are constant current devices, which automatically adjust to a supramaximal stimulus intensity. Units that measure the mechanical or electrical muscle responses to nerve stimulation remain expensive and are seldom available. Most clinicians attach the stimulator after the administration of the NMBA because they do not have access to equipment that quantifies muscle responses. Train-of-four stimulation (four stimuli in 2 sec, repeated at 12 sec intervals) does not require control values. The adequacy of paralysis is assessed by counting the number of responses (2). The palpation or visualization of four responses indicates a need for further NMBA, whereas fewer than three responses are usually associated with good surgical relaxation (3–6). If a more profound blockade is desired, the drug effect can be monitored by counting the number of posttetanic twitch responses to stimuli delivered at 1-second intervals (7).

It should be emphasized that most investigators report the intensity of paralysis for the adductor pollicis muscle. In humans, this muscle is more sensitive to the effects of NMBAs than the diaphragm, which is blocked earlier and less completely and recovers more quickly than the thumb muscle (8,9). Orbicularis oculi showed a pattern of paralysis dissimilar to that of adductor pollicis (10); its time course more closely resembles that of the laryngeal muscles.

Postoperative Reversal and Residual Blockade

If the responses to nerve stimulation are quantified by a machine, a 70% train-of-four ratio can indicate adequate reversal of blockade (11). If the train-of-four ratio is not measured objectively, even experts are unable to assess it by tactilely or visually (12). The best indicator of adequate reversal is the patient's ability to sustain a head lift for 5 seconds (13). If the patient is unable to perform this maneuver, the nerve stimulator should be switched to 100 Hz tetanus and the response to a 5-second burst should be observed in the hope of obtaining a sustained response without fade. To avoid the effects of posttetanic potentiation, tetanic stimuli should not be reapplied within the next 2 minutes.

Classification

The traditional curariform agents have a relatively slow onset of action (4–10 min) and an expected duration of action of 45–70 minutes. The classification of Savarese and Kitz (14) was modified by the editor (RJF) to include both ultrashort and short-duration categories to the now standard intermediate and long-acting groupings of NMBAs (Table 1). The results of human studies with ORG 9487, a new rapid-onset, short-acting, nondepolarizing NMBA (15) are awaited with interest.

The duration of blockade is reported differently by various authors. Many report the time interval between administration of a single intravenous (IV) dose and spontaneous recovery of the twitch response to 25% of its control height (i.e., 75% twitch depression), a value thought to reflect the duration of useful surgical relaxation. This interval is dose dependent, but not necessarily in a linear fashion: the long-acting agents can show marked prolongation of surgical paralysis at an increased dose, an effect attributable to the shape of the concentration-time curve in the therapeutic concentration range. When the concentration-time curve in this range is steep, spontaneous recovery is rapid. The more

TABLE 1. *A modified classification of the NMBAs, based on the average time course of paralysis induced by a clinically useful bolus dose*

	Time intervals and percent twitch depression			
Class	Onset time (min) to 95%	Useful duration (min) to 75%	Recovery index, 75–25% (min)	Min to 5%
Ultrashort	1–1.5	5–8	4–8	10–15
Short	1–2.5	15–20	6–7	25–35
Intermediate	2–3	20–30	10–15	40–60
Long-acting	4–6	45–60	20–60	90–3 hr

Based on Savarese and Kitz, ref. 14.

rapid and complete the return of muscle tone, the less likely are problems caused by continuing postoperative paralysis. When spontaneous recovery following an intravenously injected (bolus) dose is extremely rapid, the unsuspecting anesthesiologist may find that only a few minutes separate good from inadequate surgical relaxation.

Table 1 classifies NMBAs according to the time course of neuromuscular blockade when they are administered in an "intubating dose": i.e., at about 1.5 to 2 times the ED_{95}. It is possible to intubate the trachea with an ED_{95} dose of an NMBA, but adequate relaxation takes longer to develop than with a larger dose.

Pharmacokinetics

Concepts

Spontaneous recovery from blockade is related to NMBA plasma concentrations that may decrease to nontherapeutic levels as a result of redistribution, clearance, or both. A large initial dose both hastens the onset of blockade and increases its duration. With the long-acting NMBAs, this increase in duration may be greater than proportional to the increase in dose. Although the effects of the smaller dose dissipate during redistribution, drug concentrations from larger doses can still be in the effective range during the elimination phase. Redistribution seems to be a major factor with spontaneous recovery from the newer steroidal NMBAs, whereas a rapid clearance underlies the short duration of action with mivacurium, atracurium, and its isomer, cis-atracurium (51W89). All agents are cleared via the liver and kidneys, but drugs that rely wholly on organ function for elimination are likely to show prolonged action in the presence of hepatic or renal pathophysiology. Enzymatic degradation by pseudocholinesterase occurs with several of the isoquinoline derivatives, particularly mivacurium. Atracurium is degraded by carboxylases and Hoffmann elimination; the cis-isomer should resemble the parent mixture.

A true steady state is achieved when the amount of drug infused is equal to that being cleared by the body. With complex, often computer-adjusted, dosing patterns, it is possible to achieve a plateau in plasma concentrations almost immediately. Both the steady state and the plateau are associated with a constant intensity of blockade, but any plateau will require further adjustment in the dosage pattern for this to continue. When a drug is infused at a fixed rate, it takes more than four half-lives to reach steady state. As a corollary, adjustments in the infusion rate are effective more rapidly for drugs having a shorter half-life.

If an appropriate bolus dose is injected when the infusion is started, the increase in plasma concentrations resulting from the infusion are matched by the decreasing values from the bolus, which produces an early, but not immediate, plateau. An ED_{95} dose produces high plasma concentrations, which quickly introduce relaxant into the "effect compartment"; the infusion maintains these. The longer the interval between administering the bolus dose and starting the infusion, the greater the additional dose of relaxant necessary to "catch up." This bolus-plus-infusion technique enables both rapid onset of blockade from the bolus and control of its intensity with the infusion. Monitoring-evoked twitch responses allows the anesthesiologist to change the infusion rate to maintain adequate surgical relaxation and to discontinue the infusion as surgery nears completion.

The pharmacokinetics of the relaxants have been studied extensively for patients under many conditions; those for normal patients are shown in Table 2. Single-dose studies with plasma concentration-time data show curves that contain either two or three exponents. When compartmental modeling is used, most are two- or three-compartment open mammillary models, with elimination from the central compartment.

Non-Organ Clearance

Atracurium is metabolized by carboxylases throughout the body and spontaneously undergoes Hoffmann elimination (16). As drug is cleared from both central and peripheral compartments, most investigators report only the distribution volume, Vd (area), for atracurium (Table 2). Kitts et al. (17) modeled atracurium pharmacokinetics by deriving an in vitro metabolic-rate constant from blood drawn before drug administration. Assuming this in vitro value to be true for non-organ elimination from all compartments, Kitts et al. then estimated organ elimination

TABLE 2. *Pharmacokinetics of the neuromuscular blocking agents (NMBAs), quoting the largest series of normal adult subjects*

NMBA	Steady-state distribution volume (l/kg)	Total body clearance (ml/kg/min)	Elimination half-life (min)[a]	Number of subjects (refs)
Long-acting				
Alcuronium	0.32	1.3	200	19 (110)
Doxacurium	0.21	1.7	136	10 (111)
Gallamine	0.24	1.3	142	31 (112)
Metocurine	0.51	1.1	345	14 (113)
Pancuronium	0.19	1.8	107	18 (114)
Pipecuronium	0.31	2.4	137	20 (115)
Tubocurarine	0.52	1.8	274	20 (116)
Intermediate-acting				
Atracurium	< 0.15[b]	5.1	20	19 (35)
	0.09	4.8	16	5 (18)
Vecuronium	0.25	4.3	58	14 (30)
Short-acting				
Mivacurium	0.20	54.5	17	5 (22)

[a] Calculated as 0.693/Beta.
[b] *Vd* (area), calculated as clearance/Beta.

of atracurium from the central compartment and derived a steady-state distribution volume (Table 2).

The pharmacokinetics of atracurium are unchanged by either renal or hepatic failure, even in combination (18). Concerns about atracurium arise because one of its major breakdown products—laudanosine, a tertiary amine capable of producing convulsions—is thought to be excreted by the kidney. In patients with acute renal failure, renal excretion of laudanosine is relatively unimportant, and it seems unlikely that toxic levels would be reached (19). The laudanosine levels were not particularly high during liver transplantation (20).

Mivacurium is catabolized by the plasma cholinesterase at approximately 88% of the rate of succinylcholine hydrolysis. No correlation exists between the activity of plasma cholinesterase and the duration of blockade, which suggests additional routes of elimination (21). The pharmacokinetic values of the pooled isomers of mivacurium shown in Table 2 are from a study containing many assumptions (22). These assumptions have been questioned (23), and have yet to be confirmed by other published studies. The least potent cis-cis isomers differ markedly in their pharmacokinetics from the cis-trans and trans-trans isomers (24); the authors believed that the cis-cis isomer was unimportant clinically. The cis-cis isomer does not accumulate in patients with low plasma cholinesterase activity (25) or during prolonged infusions during surgery (26).

Succinylcholine is the NMBA for which there is a direct relationship between duration of action and cholinesterase activity (27). Studies in humans that determined its pharmacokinetics were not based on assays of succinylcholine concentrations but on the assumptions of a one-compartment model combined with the time-course of blockade (28).

Organ Clearance

Most NMBAs are excreted in urine and bile. The many studies that examined patients with renal or hepatic dysfunction are reviewed elsewhere (29,30). Decreased clearance is likely to be associated with an increased duration of effect when large or repeated doses are administered. In most cases, a kinetic-dynamic model indicates that renal or hepatic diseases are not associated with altered sensitivity of the neuromuscular junctions.

There is extensive uptake of vecuronium by the liver. Human liver biopsies indicate that more than half the dose of vecuronium remains in the liver at 30 minutes (31). These results are unconfirmed by the low hepatic extraction of vecuronium in humans, accounting only for 18% to 35% of its total clearance (32). In patients with hepatic cirrhosis, vecuronium pharmacokinetics are either unchanged (33) or show a decrease in clearance together with prolonged neuromuscular blockade (34). The volume of distribution and elimination half-life of vecuronium is increased in patients who receive vecuronium for several days (35).

DOSE-RESPONSE RELATIONSHIPS

Kinetic-Dynamic Basis

The major value of clinical pharmacokinetics for the NMBAs derives from their applicability to predicting the time-course of paralysis obtained with various patient groups (29,30,36–38). Because the intensity of blockade is a graded response, the relationships among dose, concentration at site of action, and effect can be examined: simultaneous measurements of twitch responses and plasma NMBA concentrations allow the pharmacokinetics and the pharmacodynamics to be characterized for each subject and for the patient group. The elegant kinetic-dynamic model developed by Sheiner et al. (38) used tubocurarine data as its example. The model can use either bolus or infusion kinetic equations and will be illustrated below with data for atracurium (39), pancuronium, and vecuronium (40). "Effect compartment" pharmacokinetic equations require an additional rate constant (k_{eo}; these equations combine with a sigmoid curve equation to depict the effect-time relationships. The sigmoid E_{max} equation relates concentration (Conc) and effect (percentage paralysis), characterized by its midpoint (EC_{50}), and an exponent ($_s$) for slope:

$$\text{Percentage paralysis} = \frac{100\% \cdot \text{Conc}^s}{EC_{50}{}^s + \text{Conc}^s} \qquad [1]$$

Single Dose

Early pharmacokinetic-pharmacodynamic models examined the spontaneous recovery from blockade induced by a single dose, predicting the rate of decline of paralysis from a plasma concentration-time curve that included the range of effective concentrations of the NMBA (36). Assuming that the useful period of surgical relaxation is associated with blockade intensities in excess of 75% depression, then the duration of NMBA effect is related to time interval required for plasma concentrations to decay to the concomitant effective concentration, the EC_{75} (Fig. 1). If plasma concentrations following a small dose intersect with this concentration during the steeper "redistribution" phase, while those with twice the dose intersect during the terminal phase, then the larger dose will result in more than twice the duration of the smaller dose.

When the apparent rate of decline through the (log) EC_{75}–EC_{25} range of plasma concentrations is linear, as with atracurium (Fig. 1), then recovery between 25% and 75% twitch depression is also linear, reflecting the shape of the concentration-response curve between the EC_{25} and the EC_{75}. Recovery is least rapid when plasma concentrations decline through this range during the minimal slope of the concentration-time curve, during its terminal "elimination" phase (36), which makes atracurium modeling much simpler (41).

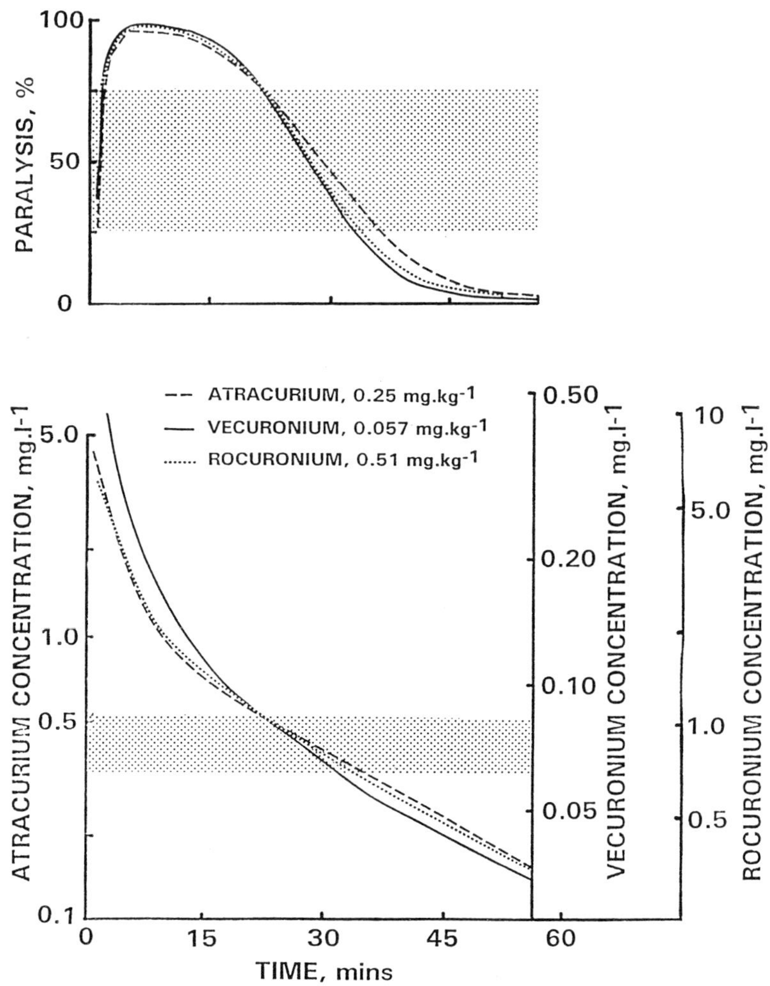

FIG. 1. Top: Simulations of the time-course of paralysis following atracurium, 0.25 mg/kg (dashed line); rocuronium, 0.51 mg/kg (dotted line); and vecuronium, 0.057 mg/kg (solid line). (Based on data from Weatherley et al., ref. 39; Sohn et al., ref. 40; and Shanks et al., ref. 147, respectively.) **Bottom:** Simultaneous plasma concentration-time curves, normalized for the 25%–75% effect concentration ranges of atracurium and vecuronium. These doses are equipotent for duration of blockade to 75% twitch depression. The recovery from vecuronium-induced blockade occurs during its redistributive phases.

Similar patterns of recovery from neuromuscular blockade are induced by single doses of either atracurium or vecuronium; yet Table 2 indicates that their pharmacokinetics are considerably different. This is explicable if the EC_{75}–EC_{25} plasma concentrations are superimposed (Fig. 1). The curve for atracurium is almost monoexponential, giving proportionality to the dose-duration relationships and a constant value for the recovery index. As recovery always occurred during the elimination phase, an increase in the atracurium dose did not alter the value of the recovery index (42). As is shown in Fig. 1, the duration of surgical relaxation and the recovery index seen with vecuronium remained comparable with atracurium because the curve for vecuronium redistribution approximates that for elimination of atracurium. The terminal (elimination phase) slope of the triexponential curve for vecuronium began late in the first hour, after the effects of the bolus dose dissipated. With a larger dose, the plasma concentration-time curve intersected the EC_{75}–EC_{25} range during the elimination phase (42): the recovery index modeled in Fig. 1 was 18 minutes, whereas a dose four times greater gave a recovery index of 37 minutes. The duration of surgical relaxation with vecuronium (0.057 mg/kg; above the stippled area in the figure) was 23 minutes. Modeling for two-to-four times this bolus dose gives roughly proportional durations of effect: 51 minutes, 70 minutes, and 87 minutes between administration and 75% twitch depression: times that agree with clinical findings (43).

Spontaneous recovery from continuous infusion of mivacurium occurs at a rate similar to that observed following various single bolus doses (21), suggesting that mivacurium cumulates minimally. The authors proposed the term "pharmacodynamic cumulation" to describe the relationship of rate of recovery from neuromuscular blockade (such as the 25%–75% recovery index) to the dose and duration of drug administration. Under this definition, cumulation is inversely related to any dose-dependent or time-dependent increase in the recovery index (21). As Fig. 1 suggests, a relaxant can lack "pharmacodynamic cumulation" only if its plasma concentration-time curve always declines through the range of effective concentrations during the elimination phase.

Multiple Doses

Pharmacokinetically, "cumulation" is traditionally described for fixed-dose, fixed-time interval dosing, which leads to a plateau in total body levels. Studies with the NMBAs use can also be designed for an initial dose, followed by increments given at a constant response intensity: e.g. whenever recovery reaches 75% depression. Cumulation is then defined as an increase in the time intervals between doses. Pancuronium was the example often quoted in an article in which four repeated doses were graphed to show an almost linear increase in blockade duration (44). Computer simulations confirmed these results, but they also indicated that the observations with pancuronium depend on the size of the

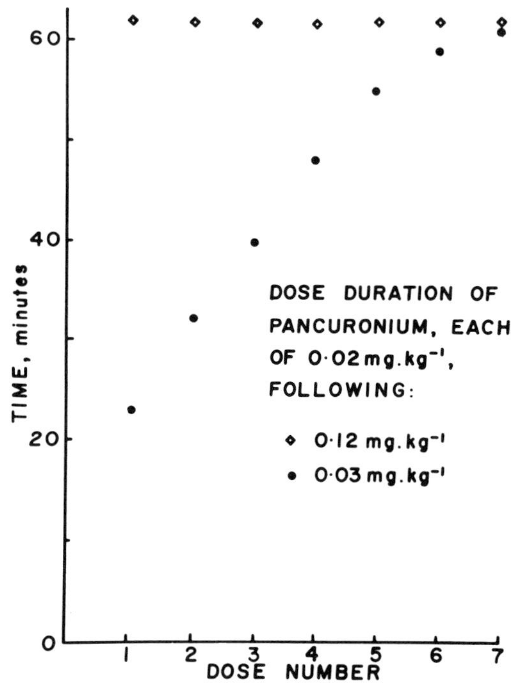

FIG. 2. Dose duration, with increments of pancuronium of 0.02 mg/kg repeated at spontaneous recovery to 75% twitch depression. These intervals do not change following an initial dose of 0.12 mg/kg (diamonds), but they show cumulation when the initial dose is 0.03 mg/kg (circles).

initial dose, or on the number of doses administered after a small initial dose (42,45) (Fig. 2).

Bolus and Infusion Regimens

The majority of the pharmacokinetic studies that have used a predetermined dosage regimen are based on the equations proposed by Mitenko and Ogilvie (46):

$$\text{Bolus dose} = \text{desired concentration} \cdot \text{distribution volume} \qquad [2]$$

$$\text{Infusion rate} = \text{desired concentration} \cdot \text{total clearance}, \qquad [3]$$

where the desired concentration might be that associated with 95% twitch depression, the EC_{95}. Any desired concentration can be calculated from the data in Table 3, using Equation 1. If the EC_{95} for atracurium is 1.3 mg/l and its clearance is 5.5 ml/kg/min (39), then the infusion rate becomes 7 μg/kg/min (Fig. 3). The dosage regimens predicted by this method for both an initial bolus and con-

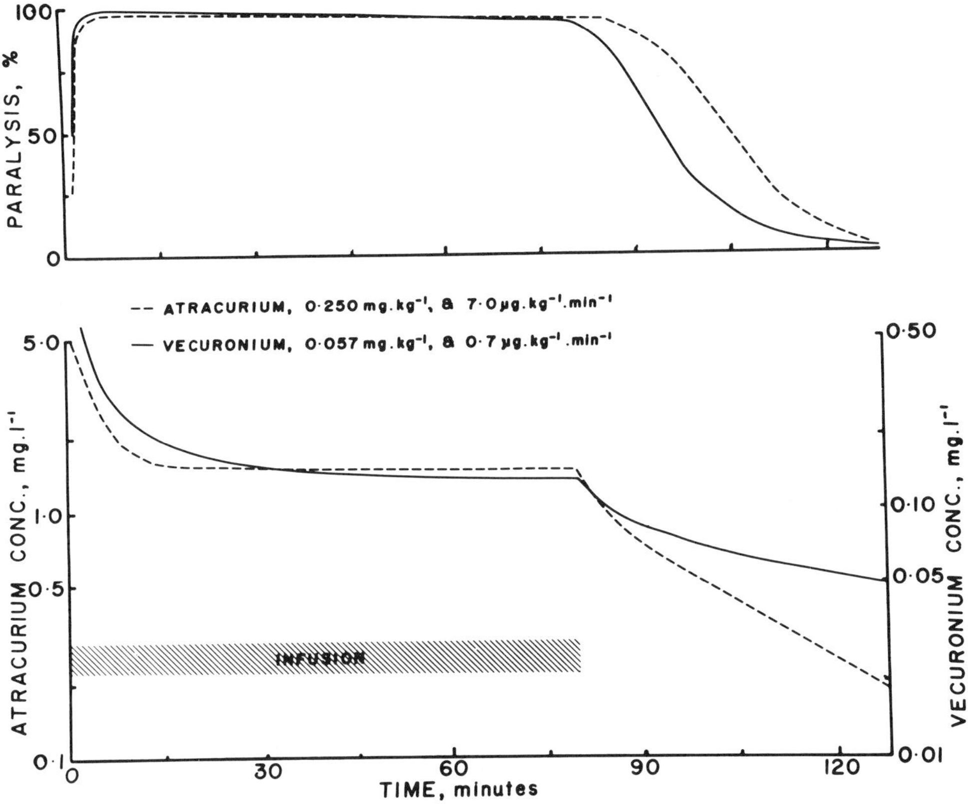

FIG. 3. Top: The time-course of paralysis associated with a bolus combined with an infusion for 80 min (diagonal lines). The recovery index for atracurium is unchanged, but that for vecuronium is less. The bolus doses are the same as those in Fig. 1; with these bolus doses, plasma concentrations always exceed those required to produce good surgical relaxation. **Bottom:** The scales of plasma concentrations are a decade apart, reflecting the proportionality of the infusion rates. Unlike those in Fig. 1, the y axes were not normalized for the concentration-effect relationships, making it difficult to predict the differing paralysis-time curves from the respective plasma concentration-time curves.

tinuous infusion are in agreement with those derived from dose-response studies (30).

Provided that patients remain well ventilated and normotensive, there are no restrictions on the size of the bolus dose, and a value in excess of the steady-state distribution volume can be used in calculation of the bolus dose using Equation 2. If the infusion is begun concomitantly, there is an early plateau in the plasma concentrations. With a large bolus dose, plasma concentrations always exceed the EC_{95} (Fig. 3). The duration of the fixed-rate atracurium infusion in this figure represents four half-lives and produces a pharmocokinetic steady state. Continuation

TABLE 3. *Pharmacodynamic values for the sigmoid curve equation, EC_{50} and exponent in Equation 1, and "effect compartment" rate constant, k_{eo}*[a]

NMBA	EC_{50} (mg/l^{-1})	Exponent	k_{eo} (min^{-1})	Number of subjects (ref)
Long-acting				
Alcuronium	0.50	5.4	0.24	12 (117)
Gallamine	5.40	4.8	0.16	10 (118)
Pancuronium	0.21	5.4	0.48	10 (119)
Tubocurarine	0.54	4.5	0.16	10 (118)
Intermediate-acting				
Atracurium	0.65	4.3	0.10	19 (35)
Vecuronium	0.20	5.5	0.10	10 (82)

[a] From Lebrault et al., ref. 34.

of the infusion will maintain the same blockade intensity. If the vecuronium infusion were to continue, its plasma concentrations would increase by 22% at its steady state several hours later. Because this increase is at the upper end of the sigmoid concentration-effect curve, only a 3% increase in the 94% twitch depression would occur. Calculation of clearance from Equation 3 assumes steady state, causing studies that maintain blockade at a constant intensity of approximately 95% to derive inaccurate estimates of clearance when single plasma samples are drawn before the true steady state.

PHARMACODYNAMICS OF INFUSION

Table 4 shows the average infusion rates that are associated with 90% twitch depression. A majority of studies that developed these data did not use the kinetic-dynamic approach outlined above but reported the mean infusion rates administered to maintain a 90% neuromuscular blockade during "balanced" anesthesia. Potentiation of competitive blockade by the potent inhalation anesthetic agents reduces their dose requirements.

TABLE 4. *Average relaxant requirements when administered by infusion*

NMBA	Dose (μg/kg/min)	Recovery index (min 75–25%)	Suggested dilution (μg/l)[a]
Succinylcholine	60–120	4–11	4000
Mivacurium	6.0–8.3	5–7	400
Atracurium	4.3–8.4	4–11	400
Vecuronium	1.0–1.7	13–16	60
Pancuronium	0.4–0.6	29–62	30

[a] This concentration can be infused with body weight in kg entered as ml/hr.

Individual Agents

Succinylcholine

Low cost and long familiarity make succinylcholine infusion a favorite choice of many clinicians. Prolonged surgery is a relative contraindication, which precludes its use in many teaching hospitals. Its dose averages 60–120 μg/kg/min (47,48), with considerable intra- and interindividual variability, especially in infants and children (49,50). Succinylcholine-induced neuromuscular blockade can be divided into two phases using the train-of-four ratio. The initial depolarizing block is usually accompanied by tachyphylaxis, but with minimal effect on the ratio. The second phase is characterized by a low ratio; Phase II block may have a rather abrupt onset (51) and an earlier development in the presence of isoflurane, halothane, or enflurane (48,52,53). Phase II block is usually, but not invariably, reversible with neostigmine (48).

Mivacurium

Mivacurium has a short duration of action, although longer than that of succinylcholine. Its margin of safety is similar to that of atracurium (21). Doses in excess of 0.2 mg/kg abolish the twitch responses in 2–3 minutes and are followed by 15–20 minutes of surgical relaxation; even at these doses, spontaneous recovery was almost complete in 30 minutes (21,54). Such doses produce brief decreases in arterial blood pressure that are associated with elevations of plasma histamine levels. Doses greater than 0.15 mg/kg allow good to excellent intubating conditions within 60 seconds.

A continuous infusion of mivacurium averaging 5–8 μg/kg/min during balanced anesthesia produces almost total depression of the twitch response (47,55–59). Postinfusion recovery data are shown in Table 4; recovery from mivacurium-induced blockade is more rapid than from the NMBAs of the intermediate-duration group. Requirements in children average 9–16 μg/kg/min (60,61). The mivacurium infusion rate is significantly less in the presence of isoflurane (57). With an infusion of mivacurium to maintain 90% twitch depression, reversal of blockade by neostigmine or edrophonium shorten recovery by 8–10 minutes (62).

Atracurium

Atracurium has been administered by continuous infusion during many types of prolonged surgery in both adults (5,6,21,56,63–82) and children (63,69,83,84). For infusion, atracurium is diluted best in normal saline because spontaneous degradation occurs rapidly in lactated Ringer's solution (85). During balanced anesthesia, 90–99% twitch depression is maintained by rates that average 4–9 μg/kg/min (see Table 4). The dosage is similar when atracurium is used for total

IV anesthesia with midazolam and alfentanil or with fentanyl and nitrous oxide (77). Prolonged administration does not alter the intraoperative requirements (78). The potent inhalational anesthetic agents reduced the dosage requirements (63,64,69), but there is considerable overlap. The interaction between enflurane and atracurium is time dependent (70). Dosage requirements are unaffected by age (65). Atracurium infusion requirements decrease during the anhepatic phase of liver transplantation (86) and hypothermic cardiopulmonary bypass (87,88).

cis-Atracurium

The cis-isomer of atracurium (51W89), administered in a dose of 0.1 mg/kg, appears to have neuromuscular effects similar to those of 0.5 mg/kg of atracurium. However, the cis-isomer lacks the cardiovascular effects (89).

Rocuronium

Rocuronium infusion requirements average 9.8–11.2 μg/kg/min (90,91). These are reduced in the presence of a volatile anesthetic agent. When 60 patients were randomly assigned to one of six sequences in which anesthesia was maintained with various agents, the interactions could be assessed as the infusion requirements. The mean values, calculated per lean body mass, were 0.64, 0.60, 0.61, 0.67, 0.63, and 0.39 mg/kg/hr in the etomidate, fentanyl, midazolam, propofol, thiopental, and isoflurane groups, respectively (91).

Vecuronium

Vecuronium infusion requirements average 1.0–1.5 μg/kg/min (5,56,68,92–99); they are unaffected by previous succinylcholine (94), but should be reduced for elderly patients (100) and during hypothermic cardiopulmonary bypass (87,88). Prolonged administration alters the intraoperative requirements, diminishing by 50% in the second to fourth hours (78). Dose requirements are reduced by halothane (101), enflurane, isoflurane, and sevoflurane (64). The suggestion that halothane increases neuromuscular sensitivity to vecuronium-induced blockade is unconfirmed (98). Children aged 3 years to 10 years may show increased dose requirements (102–104), whereas neonates may not.

Some patients receiving vecuronium infusions in the intensive care unit (ICU) show considerable variation in dose requirements, some of which are related to drug interaction (105); other patients may require significant increases in dosage over time to maintain adequate relaxation (106). The use of train-of-four monitoring appears to be associated with infusion requirements similar to those found intraoperatively (107).

Long-Acting Agents

This section mentions only pancuronium, although several of the long-acting agents have been given in infusion studies; these are reviewed elsewhere (30). Pancuronium infusion requirements average approximately 0.5 μg/kg/min (73,108,109). The advantages of a pancuronium infusion for prolonged surgery lie not only in its economics but also in neuromuscular monitoring to facilitate both maintenance of a precise intensity of blockade and an impression of the patient's clearance. A relatively low infusion requirement would prompt earlier than usual discontinuation of the pancuronium infusion.

Disadvantages

The major disadvantages of NMBA infusions are the time required to prepare the solution to be infused and to set up the equipment necessary for dependable drug delivery. Most hospitals have infusion pumps or other devices that can be adjusted to deliver solutions in milliliters per hour. If a solution is made up in a concentration indicated in Table 4, then the infusion rate can be set initially at the value of the patient's weight in kilograms, dialed as the delivery rate for milliliter per hour. For example, a 70 kg patient scheduled for a 3-hour procedure might have tracheal intubation facilitated by bolus administration of 5 mg of vecuronium. Another 15 mg is added to a 250-ml container, the contents of which are infused at a rate of 1 μg/kg/min—that is, a solution of 60 μg/ml given at a rate of 70 ml/hr. Those who have access to a programmed syringe pump such as the Bard Infusion Pump can make a solution of 0.5 mg/ml of vecuronium and use the same settings that are given for alfentanil. Use with 2 mg/ml of atracurium or mivacurium is facilitated by the application of a specific template for either drug. During prolonged surgery, it is only a minor task to assess tactile evaluation of the evoked thumb twitch, then adjust the individual infusion to maintain two palpable responses to train-of-four stimulation (3,5).

Several groups of workers developed closed-loop systems for automatic control of neuromuscular blockade, with feedback between either an evoked electromyogram or force transducer and the infusion pump (73,76,80,99,108,110–113). Programs for such devices incorporate a delay function to prevent their overreaction when the system must allow time for the delivered drug to have its effect.

REVERSAL OF BLOCKADE

The patient scheduled for major elective surgery requires prolonged paralysis. To avoid postoperative mechanical ventilation, the NMBA dosage must be tailored precisely to that patient's requirements. At present, the choice of NMBA is among atracurium, vecuronium, or a long-acting nondepolarizing NMBA such as pancuronium. Procedures in excess of 2 hours are likely to have Phase II block problems with succinylcholine infusion. Although a long-acting agent is more convenient during surgery, it is also more likely to cause residual paralysis postoperatively (114–116). This is reflected in an important outcome: a higher incidence of pulmonary complications after pancuronium than after atracurium blockade (117). Yet even 90 minutes after reversal of atracurium or vecuronium, diminution in peak expiratory flow is still detectable (118).

Whether neuromuscular blockade should be routinely reversed at the end of a surgical procedure is a subject of debate, with the conservatives advocating universal administration of an anticholinesterase. To make it routine is unacceptable to others, who usually add the caveat that the fractional train-of-four response should exceed 75% with mechonomyography. This caveat is based on studies with tubocurarine (11), although a similar adequacy of ventilatory reserves was confirmed for vecuronium in seven subjects (119). Some confusion also arises from the 75% value: this represents 25% depression of the height of the fourth response and differs from the 75% twitch depression desired during surgery. It is insufficient merely to observe four responses at the end of surgery; even expert observers are unable to estimate adequate spontaneous recovery of the train-of-four by palpation (12). The gold standard is the ability to sustain a head lift for 5 seconds.

For many years, edrophonium was considered to have too short a duration of action to be useful in reversing NMBA-induced paralysis; most clinicians used neostigmine or, occasionally, pyridostigmine. The onset of 0.5–1.0 mg/kg of edrophonium is faster than that of 0.03 to 0.06 mg/kg of neostigmine, but the intensity of effect is less. The relative efficacy depends on the extent to which neuromuscular blockade regressed spontaneously (120). Shortly after a large dose of NMBA, administration of neostigmine cannot reverse blockade (121). When blockade is profound but not total, neostigmine is slower but eventually more effective (122–126). If the evoked responses are in excess of 10% of their control values, both edrophonium and neostigmine are effective (63,126,127). The time required for reversal of intense blockade achieved with atracurium infusion similarly depends upon the degree of blockade at the time of reversal (128). Total recovery time is not shortened by an early injection of neostigmine.

PROLONGED USE IN INTENSIVE CARE

Neuromuscular blocking agents are used in intensive care to facilitate mechanical ventilation and reduce the metabolic rate. A national survey of the use of muscle relaxants by intensivists was published in 1992; the popular choices were vecuronium (52%), pancuronium (28%), metubine (5%), and atracurium (3%) (129). In the same year, the first major report of prolonged paralysis implicating vecuronium was published; 16 critically ill adults developed prolonged neuromuscular blockade (130). However, whether this is agent-specific is unclear. Some hypothesize that prolonged use of a nondepolarizing agent might enable penetration of the drug across cell membranes or cause up-regulation of receptors or that there is interaction with antibiotics and corticosteroids. Others point to the lack of neuromuscular monitoring in dose adjustment and state that such patients develop neuropathies or myopathies even in the absence of relaxants. A recent review (131) concluded that prolonged neuromuscular blockade can be divided into two types. One is pharmacokinetically based, caused by alterations in clearance and metabolite formation. The second occurs in patients without an etiology for drug clearance problems. Functional neuromuscular junction defects are the problem and may be the result of the underlying disease state in addition to, or regardless of, the use of neuromuscular blocking agents.

The use of atracurium has its strong advocates. Patients in renal failure reversed rapidly with the cessation of the atracurium infusion (71). Atracurium infusion can be used in the intensive care unit, although dose requirements are often greater than those shown in Table 4. Pediatric patients have increased dose requirements (132). The usual rate of recovery followed prolonged relaxation with atracurium, despite circulatory, renal, or hepatic dysfunction (71,133,134). Two of these studies included two patients with renal failure and seizure activity, possibly implicating accumulation of the metabolite laudanosine. In one case, trauma was followed by extensive intracerebral pathology. In the other, the patient developed generalized twitching; 2 hours after the last dose of atracurium was given, the plasma laudanosine level was 0.74 μg/ml—less than half the concentration associated with convulsions in dogs. Laudanosine is unlikely to be a clinical concern either during operative surgery (67) or in the ICU (19).

REFERENCES

1. Chamberlain ME, Bradshaw EG. The "wake-up test": a new approach using drug infusions. *Anaesthesia* 1985;40:780–782.
2. Lee CM. Train-of-4 quantitation of competitive neuromuscular block. *Anesth Analg* 1975;54:649–653.
3. Haraldsted VY, Nielsen JW, Joensen F, Dilling-Hansen B, Hasselstrom L. Infusion of vecuronium assessed by tactile evaluation of evoked thumb twitch. *Br J Anaesth* 1988;61:479–481.
4. O'Hara DA, Fragen RJ, Shanks CA. Reappearance of the train-of-four after neuromuscular blockade induced with tubocurarine, vecuronium, or atracurium. *Br J Anaesth* 1986;58:1296–1299.
5. Ostergaard D, Engbaek J, Ording H, Viby-Mogensen J. A new infusion design for atracurium and vecuronium. *Eur J Anaesth* 1987;4:87–92.
6. Rowlands DE. Simple atracurium infusions. *Br J Anaesth* 1985;57:542.
7. Ridley SA, Braude N. Post-tetanic count and intense neuromuscular blockade with vecuronium in children. *Br J Anaesth* 1988;61:551–556.
8. Chauvin M, Lebrault C, Duvaldestin P. The neuromuscular blocking effect of vecuronium on the human diaphragm. *Anesth Analg* 1987;66:117–122.
9. Donati F, Antzaka C, Bevan DR. Potency of pancuronium at the diaphragm and the adductor pollicis muscle in humans. *Anesthesiology* 1986;65:1–5.
10. Caffrey RR, Warren ML, Becker KE Jr. Neuromuscular blockade monitoring comparing the orbicularis oculi and adductor pollicis muscles. *Anesthesiology* 1986;65:95–97.
11. Brand JB, Cullen DJ, Wilson NE, Ali HH. Spontaneous recovery from nondepolarizing neuromuscular blockade: correlation between clinical and evoked responses. *Anesth Analg* 1977;56:55–58.
12. Viby-Mogensen J, Jensen NH, Engbaek J, Ording H, Skovgaard LT, Chraemmer-Jorgensen B. Tactile and visual evaluation of the response to train-of-four nerve stimulation. *Anesthesiology* 1985;63:440–443.
13. Pavlin EG, Holle RH, Schoene RB. Recovery of airway protection compared with ventilation in humans after paralysis with curare. *Anesthesiology* 1989;70:381–405.

14. Savarese JJ, Kitz RJ. Does clinical anesthesia need new neuromuscular blocking agents? *Anesthesiology* 1975;42:236–239.
15. Wierda JMKH, van den Broek L, Smeulers NJ. Dose requirements, reversibility and pharmacokinetics of Org 9487. *Br J Anaesth* 1994;72(Suppl 1):A154(abst).
16. Stenlake JB, Hughes R. In vitro degradation of atracurium in human plasma. *Br J Anaesth* 1987;59: 806–807.
17. Kitts JB, Fisher DM, Canfell PC, et al. Pharmacokinetics and pharmacodynamics of atracurium in the elderly. *Anesthesiology* 1990;72:272–275.
18. Ward S, Neill EAM. Pharmacokinetics of atracurium in acute hepatic failure (with acute renal failure). *Br J Anaesth* 1983;55:1169–1172.
19. Parker CJR, Jones JE, Hunter JM. Disposition of infusions of atracurium and its metabolite, laudanosine, in patients in renal and respiratory failure in an ITU. *Br J Anaesth* 1988;61:531–540.
20. Lawhead RG, Matsumi M, Peters KR, et al. Plasma laudanosine levels in patients given atracurium during liver transplantation. *Anesthesia & Analgesia* 1993;76:569–573.
21. Savarese JJ, Ali HH, Basta SJ, Embree PB, Scott RP, Sunder N, et al. The clinical neuromuscular pharmacology of mivacurium chloride (BW B1090U): a short-acting nondepolarizing ester neuromuscular blocking drug. *Anesthesiology* 1988;67:723–732.
22. Cook DR, Freeman JA, Lai AA, et al. Pharmacokinetics of mivacurium in normal patients and in those with hepatic or renal failure. *Br J Anaesth* 1992;69:580–585.
23. Fisher DM, Hale V. Pharmacokinetic modelling of mivacurium. *Br J Anaesth* 1993;71:328–329.
24. Lien CA, Schmith VD, Embree PB, et al. The pharmacokinetics and pharmacodynamics of the stereoisomers of mivacurium in patients receiving nitrous oxide/opioid/barbiturate anesthesia. *Anesthesiology* 1994;80:1296–1302.
25. Goudsouzian N, Chakavorti S, Denamn W, de Bros F, Patel S. Lack of accumulation of the cis-cis isomer of mivacurium in patients with low plasma cholinesterase activity. *Anesthesiology* 1994;81: A1060(abst).
26. deBros F, Goudsouzian N, Chakavorty S, Patel S, Cook DR. Pharmacokinetic evaluation of thc cis-cis isomer, alcohol, and ester metabolites of mivacurium during prolonged infusions in neurosurgical patients. *Anesthesiology* 1994;81:A1085(abst)
27. Viby-Mogenssen J. Correlation of succinylcholine duration with plasma cholinesterase activity in subjects with the genotypically normal enzyme. *Anesthesiology* 1980;53:517–520.
28. Cook DR, Wingard LB, Taylor FH. Pharmacokinetics of succinylcholine in infants, children and adults. *Clin Pharmacol Ther* 1976;20:493–498.
29. Ramzan MI, Somogyi AA, Walker JS, Shanks CA, Triggs EJ. Clinical pharmacokinetics of the nondepolarising muscle relaxants. *Clin Pharmacokinet* 1981;6:25–60.
30. Shanks CA. Pharmacokinetics of the nondepolarizing neuromuscular relaxants applied to calculation of bolus and infusion dosage regimens. *Anesthesiology* 1986;64:72–86.
31. Bencini AF, Scaf AHJ, Sohn YJ, Kersten-Kleef UW, Agoston SA. Hepatobiliary disposition of vecuronium bromide in man. *Br J Anaesth* 1986;58:988–995.
32. Goldfarb G, Ganeau P, Ang ET, Lassale B, Jolis P. Hepatic extraction and clearance of vecuronium in humans. *Anesthesiology* 1988;69:A480(abst).
33. Arden JR, Lynam DP, Castagnoli KP, Canfell PC, Cannon JC, Miller RD. Vecuronium in alcoholic liver disease: a pharmacokinetic and pharmacodynamic analysis. *Anesthesiology* 1988;68:771–776.
34. Lebrault C, Berger JL, d'Hollander AA, Gomeni R, Henzel D, Duvaldestin P. Pharmacokinetics and pharmacodynamics of vecuronium (ORG NC45) in patients with cirrhosis. *Anesthesiology* 1985;62: 601–605.
35. Segredo V, Caldwell JE, Matthay MA, Sharma ML, Gruenke LD, Miller RD. Pharmacokinetics of vecuronium after long-term administration. *Anesth Analg* 1990;70:S450.
36. Gibaldi M, Levy G. Dose-dependent decline of pharmacologic effects of drugs with linear pharmacokinetic characteristics. *J Pharm Sci* 1972;61:567–569.
37. Hull CJ. Pharmacodynamics of non-depolarizing neuromuscular blocking agents. *Br J Anaesth* 1982; 54:169–182.
38. Sheiner LB, Stanski DR, Vozeh S, Miller RD, Ham J. Simultaneous modeling of pharmacokinetics and pharmacodynamics: application to d-tubocurarine. *Clin Pharmacol Ther* 1979;25:358–371.
39. Weatherley BC, Williams SG, Neill EA. Pharmacokinetics pharmacodynamics and dose-response relationships of atracurium administered i.v. *Br J Anaesth* 1983;55(Suppl 1):39S–45S.
40. Sohn YJ, Bencini AF, Scaf AH, Kersten UW, Agoston S. Comparative pharmacokinetics and dynamics of vecuronium and pancuronium in anesthetized patients. *Anesth Analg* 1986;65:233–239.

41. Ward S, Boheimer N, Weatherley BC, Simmonds RJ, Dopson TA. Pharmacokinetics of atracurium and its metabolites in patients with normal renal function, and in patients with renal failure. *Br J Anaesth* 1988;59:697–706.
42. Fisher DM, Rosen JI. A pharmacokinetic explanation for increasing recovery time following larger or repeated doses of nondepolarizing muscle relaxants. *Anesthesiology* 1986;65:286–291.
43. Feldman SA. Vecuronium—a variable dose technique. *Anaesthesia* 1987;42:199–201.
44. Fahey MR, Morris RB, Miller RD, Nguyen TL, Upton RA. Pharmacokinetics of Org NC45 (norcuron) in patients with and without renal failure. *Br J Anaesth* 1981;53:1049–1053.
45. Norman J. Pharmacokinetics of non-depolarizing muscle relaxants. *Clin Anaesthesiol* 1985;3:273–282.
46. Mitenko PA, Ogilvie RI. Rapidly achieved plasma concentration plateaus, with observations on theophyllin kinetics. *Clin Pharmacol Ther* 1972;13:329–335.
47. Brandom BW, Woelfel SK, Cook DR, Weber S, Powers DM, Weakly JN. Comparison of mivacurium and suxamethonium administered by bolus and infusion. *Br J Anaesth* 1989;62:488–493.
48. Futter ME, Donati F, Bevan DR. Prolonged suxamethonium infusion during nitrous oxide anaesthesia supplemented with halothane or fentanyl. *Br J Anaesth* 1983;55:947–953.
49. Bevan JC, Donati F, Bevan DR. Prolonged infusion of suxamethonium in infants and children. *Br J Anaesth* 1986;58:839–843.
50. DeCook TH, Goudsouzian NG. Tachyphylaxis and phase II block development during infusion of succinylcholine in children. *Anesth Analg* 1980;59:639–643.
51. Lee C. Dose relationships of phase II tachyphylaxis and train-of-four fade in suxamethonium-induced dual neuromuscular block in man. *Br J Anaesth* 1975;47:841–845.
52. Donati F, Bevan DR. Effect of enflurane and fentanyl on the clinical characteristics of long-term succinylcholine infusion. *Can Anaesth Soc J* 1982;29:59–64.
53. Donati F, Bevan DR. Long-term succinylcholine infusion during isoflurane anesthesia. *Anesthesiology* 1983;58:6–10.
54. Caldwell JE, Kitts JB, Heier T, Fahey MR, Lynam DP, Miller RD. The dose-response relationship of mivacurium chloride in humans during nitrous oxide-fentanyl or nitrous oxide-enflurane anesthesia. *Anesthesiology* 1989;70:31–35.
55. Shanks CA, Fragen RJ, Pemberton D, Katz JA, Risner ME. Mivacurium-induced neuromuscular blockade following single bolus doses and with continuous infusion during either balanced or enflurane anesthesia. *Anesthesiology* 1989;71:362–366.
56. Ali HH, Savarese JJ, Embree PB, Basta SJ, Stout RG, Bottros LH, et al. Clinical pharmacology of mivacurium chloride (BW B1090U) infusion: comparison with vecuronium and atracurium. *Br J Anaesth* 1988;61:541–546.
57. Powers DM, Brandom BW, Cook DR, et al. Mivacurium infusion during nitrous oxide-isoflurane anesthesia: a comparison with nitrous oxide-opioid anesthesia. *J Clin Anesth* 1992;4:123–126.
58. Caldwell JE, Heier T, Kitts JB, et al. Comparison of the neuromuscular block induced by mivacurium, suxamethonium or atracurium during nitrous oxide-fentanyl anaesthesia. *Br J Anaesth* 1989; 63:393–399.
59. Diefenbach C, Mellinghoff H, Lynch J, et al. Mivacurium: dose-response relationship and administration by repeated injection or infusion. *Anesth Analg* 1992;74:420–423.
60. Brandom BW, Sarner JB, Woelfel SK, et al. Mivacurium infusion requirements in pediatric surgical patients during nitrous oxide-halothane and during nitrous oxide-narcotic anesthesia. *Anesth Analg* 1990;71:16–22.
61. Meretoja OA, Olkkola KT. Pharmacodynamics of mivacurium in children, using a computer-controlled infusion. *Br J Anaesth* 1993;71:232–237.
62. Maddineni VR, Mirakhur RK, McCoy EP. Recovery of mivacurium block with or without anticholinesterase administration. *Anesthesiology* 1994;81:A1065(abst).
63. Brandom BW, Cook DR, Woelfel SK, Rudd GD, Fehr B, Lineberry CG. Atracurium infusion requirements in children during halothane, isoflurane, and narcotic anesthesia. *Anesth Analg* 1985;64:471–477.
64. Vanlithout LEH, de Wolff MH, van Egmond J, Booij LHDH, Robertson EN. The effect of isoflurane and sevoflurane on the potency and the recovery of neuromuscular blockade by vecuronium, pancuronium, and atracurium. *Anesthesiology* 1994;81:A1113(abst).
65. d'Hollander AA, Hennart DA, Barvais L, Baurain M. Administration of atracurium by infusion for long surgical procedures: simple techniques for routine use. *Br J Anaesth* 1986;58(Suppl 1):56S–59S.
66. d'Hollander AA, Luyckx C, Barvais L, De Ville A. Clinical evaluation of atracurium besylate requirement for a stable muscle relaxation during surgery: lack of age-related effects. *Anesthesiology* 1983;59:237–240.

67. Eager BM, Flynn PJ, Hughes R. Infusion of atracurium for long surgical procedures. *Br J Anaesth* 1984;56:447–452.
68. Gramstad L, Lilleaasen P. Neuromuscular blocking effects of atracurium, vecuronium and pancuronium during bolus and infusion administration. *Br J Anaesth* 1985;57:1052–1059.
69. Goudsouzian N, Martyn J, Rudd GD, Liu LM, Lineberry CG. Continuous infusion of atracurium in children. *Anesthesiology* 1986;64:171–174.
70. Withington DE, Donati F, Bevan DR, et al. Potentiation of atracurium neuromuscular blockade by enflurane: time-course of effect. *Anesth Analg* 1991;72:469–473.
71. Griffiths RB, Hunter JM, Jones RS. Atracurium infusions in patients with renal failure on an ITU. *Anaesthesia* 1986;41:375–381.
72. Eriksson LI, Staun P, Cederholm I, Lennmarken C, Lofstrom JB. Experience with vecuronium during long-lasting surgery. *Acta Anaesthesiol Scand* 1988;32:619–622.
73. Haraldsted VY, Nielsen JW, Madsen JV, Hasselstrom L. Maintenance of constant 95% neuromuscular blockade by adjustable infusion rates of pancuronium and atracurium. *Br J Anaesth* 1988;60: 491–494.
74. Hunter JM, Kelly JM, Jones RS. Atracurium infusions in major ophthalmic surgery. *Eur J Anaesthesiol* 1987;4:9–15.
75. Madsen JV, Andersen BN, Schurizek BA, Jensen OV, Juhl B. Atracurium administered by infusion for long neurosurgical procedures. *Br J Anaesth* 1986;58:605–615.
76. MacLeod AD, Asbury AJ, Gray WM, Linkens DA. Automatic control of neuromuscular block with atracurium. *Br J Anaesth* 1989;63:31–35.
77. Nilsson A, Tamsen A, Persson MP. Atracurium infusion in total intravenous anesthesia. *Acta Anaesthesiol Scand* 1987;31:205–208S.
78. Martineau RJ, St. Jean B, Kitts JB, et al. Cumulation and reversal with prolonged infusions of atracurium and vecuronium.*Can J Anaesth* 1992;39:670–676.
79. Rees DI, Howell ML. Ketamine-atracurium by continuous infusion as the sole anesthetic for pulmonary surgery. *Anesth Analg* 1986;65:860–864.
80. Wait CM, Goat VA, Blogg CE. Feedback control of neuromuscular blockade: a simple system for infusion of atracurium. *Anaesthesia* 1987;42:1212–1217.
81. Olkkola KT, Schwilden H, Apffelstaedt C. Model-based adaptive closed-loop feedback control of atracurium-induced neuromuscular blockade. *Acta Anaesthesiol Scand* 1991;35:420–423.
82. O'Hara DA, Derbyshire GJ, Overdyk FJ, et al. Closed-loop infusion of atracurium with four different anesthetic techniques. *Anesthesiology* 1991;74:258–263.
83. Kalli I, Meretoja OA. Infusion of atracurium in neonates, infants and children: a study of dose requirements. *Br J Anaesth* 1988;60:651–654.
84. Wait CM, Goat VA. Atracurium infusion during paediatric craniofacial surgery: closed loop control of neuromuscular block. *Anaesthesia* 1989;44:567–570.
85. Fisher DM, Canfell C, Miller RD. Stability of atracurium administered by infusion. *Anesthesiology* 1984;61:347–348.
86. Farman JV, Turner JM, Blanloeil Y. Atracurium infusion in liver transplantation. *Br J Anaesth* 1986;58 Suppl 1:96S–102S.
87. Denny NM, Kneeshaw JD. Vecuronium and atracurium infusions during hypothermic cardiopulmonary bypass. *Anaesthesia* 1986;41:919–922.
88. Flynn PJ, Hughes R, Walton B, Jothilingam S. Use of atracurium infusions for general surgical procedures including cardiac surgery with induced hypothermia. *Br J Anaesth* 1983;55(Suppl 1): 135S–136S.
89. Lepage JY, Malinovskyy JM, Malinge M, Cozian A, Pinaud M. Comparison of equipotent doses of 51W89 and atracurium. *Anesthesiology* 1994;81:A1090(abst).
90. Shanks CA, Fragen RJ, Ling D. Continuous intravenous infusion of rocuronium (ORG 9426) in patients receiving balanced, enflurane, or isoflurane anesthesia. *Anesthesiology* 1993;78:649–651.
91. Olkkola KT, Tammisto T. Quantifying the interaction of rocuronium (Org 9426) with etomidate, fentanyl, midazolam, propofol, thiopental, and isoflurane using closed-loop feedback control of rocuronium infusion. *Anesth Analg* 1994;78:691–696.
92. Cannon JE, Fahey MR, Castagnoli KP, et al. Continuous infusion of vecuronium: the effect of anesthetic agents. *Anesthesiology* 1987;67:503–506.
93. d'Hollander AA, Czerucki R, Deville A, Cuvelier F. Stable muscle relaxation during abdominal surgery using combined intravenous bolus and demand infusion: clinical appraisal with ORG NC45. *Can Anaesth Soc J* 1982;29:136–141.

94. d'Hollander A, Agoston S, Barvais L, Massaut J, Baurain M. Evolution of vecuronium requirements for stable mechanical effect: comparison with or without previous succinylcholine administration. *Anesth Analg* 1985;64:319–322.
95. Mirakhur RK, Ferres CJ. Muscle relaxation with an infusion of vecuronium. *Eur J Anaesthesiol* 1984; 1:353–359.
96. Newton DEF. Vecuronium-continuous infusion in general clinical practice. *Excerpta Medica Curr Clin* 1983;11:109–114.
97. Noeldge G, Hinsken H, Buzello W. Comparison between the continuous infusion of vecuronium and the intermittent administration of pancuronium and vecuronium. *Br J Anaesth* 1984;56:473–477.
98. Shanks CA, Avram MJ, Fragen RJ. Pharmacokinetics and pharmacodynamics of vecuronium administered by bolus and infusion during halothane or balanced anesthesia. *Clin Pharmacol Ther* 1987; 42:459–464.
99. de Vries JW, Ros HH, Booij LH. Infusion of vecuronium controlled by a closed-loop system. *Br J Anaesth* 1986;58:1100–1103.
100. d'Hollander A, Massaux F, Nevelsteen M, Agoston S. Age-dependent dose-response relationship of ORG NC45 in anaesthetized patients. *Br J Anaesth* 1982;54:653–657.
101. Swen J, Gencarelli PJ, Koot HW. Vecuronium infusion dose requirements during fentanyl and halothane anesthesia in humans. *Anesth Analg* 1985;64:411–414.
102. Meretoja OA. Vecuronium infusion requirements in pediatric patients during fentanyl-N_2O–O_2 anesthesia. *Anesth Analg* 1989;68:20–24.
103. Fitzpatrick KT, Black GW, Crean PM, et al. Continuous vecuronium infusion for prolonged muscle relaxation in children. *Can J Anaesth* 1991;38:169–174.
104. Woelfel SK, Dong ML, Brandom BW, et al. Vecuronium infusion requirements in children during halothane-narcotic-nitrous oxide, isoflurane-narcotic-nitrous oxide, and narcotic-nitrous oxide anesthesia. *Anesth Analg* 1991;73:33–38.
105. Smith CL, Hunter JM, Jones RS. Vecuronium infusions in patients with renal failure in an ITU. *Anaesthesia* 1987;42:387–393.
106. Coursin DB, Klasek G, Goelzer SL. Increased requirements for continuously infused vecuronium in critically ill patients. *Anesth Analg* 1989;69:518–521.
107. Darrah WC, Johnston JR, Mirakhur RK. Vecuronium infusions for prolonged muscle relaxation in the intensive care unit. *Crit Care Med* 1989;17:1297–1300.
108. Asbury AJ, Linkens DA. Clinical automatic control of neuromuscular blockade. *Anaesthesia* 1986; 41:316–320.
109. Somogyi AA, Shanks CA, Triggs EJ. Combined i.v. bolus and infusion of pancuronium bromide. *Br J Anaesth* 1978;50:575–582.
110. Bradlow HS, Uys PC, Rametti LB. On-line control of atracurium induced muscle relaxation. *J Biomed Eng* 1986;8:72–75.
111. Cass NM, Lampard DG, Brown WA, Coles JR. Computer controlled muscle relaxation: a comparison of four muscle relaxants in the sheep. *Anaesth Intens Care* 1976;4:16–22.
112. Ritchie G, Ebert JP, Jannett TC, Kissin I, Sheppard LC. A microcomputer based controller for neuromuscular block during surgery. *Ann Biomed Eng* 1985;13:3–15.
113. Webster NR, Cohen AT. Closed-loop administration of atracurium. Steady-state neuromuscular blockade during surgery using a computer controlled closed-loop atracurium infusion. *Anaesthesia* 1987; 42:1085–1091.
114. Kong KL, Cooper GM. Recovery of neuromuscular function and postoperative morbidity following blockade by atracurium, alcuronium and vecuronium. *Anaesthesia* 1988;43:450–453.
115. Lennmarken C, Lofstrom JB. Partial curarization in the postoperative period. *Acta Anaesthesiol Scand* 1984;28:260–262.
116. Viby-Mogensen J, Jorgensen BC, Ording H. Residual curarization in the recovery room. *Anesthesiology* 1979;50:539–541.
117. Pedersen T, Viby-Mogensen J, Ringsted C. Anaesthetic practice and postoperative pulmonary complications. *Acta Anaesthesiol Scand* 1992;36:812–818.
118. Gordon KL, Reilly CS. Recovery of neuromuscular function after infusion or intermittent bolus doses of atracurium or vecuronium. *Br J Anaesth* 1989;62:269–273.
119. Dupuis JY, Martin R, Tetrault JP. Clinical, electrical and mechanical correlations during recovery from neuromuscular blockade with vecuronium. *Can J Anaesth* 1990;37:192–196.
120. Katz RL. Neuromuscular effects of d-tubocurarine, edrophonium, and neostigmine in man. *Anesthesiology* 1967;28:327.

121. Baraka A. Irreversible tubocurarine neuromuscular block in the human. *Br J Anaesth* 1967;39:891.
122. Astley BA, Hughes R, Payne JP. Antagonism of atracurium-induced neuromuscular blockade by neostigmine or edrophonium. *Br J Anaesth* 1986;58:1290.
123. Caldwell JE, Robertson EN, Baird WL. Antagonism of profound neuromuscular blockade induced by vecuronium or atracurium: comparison of neostigmine with edrophonium. *Br J Anaesth* 1986;58:1285–1289.
124. Caldwell JE, Robertson EN, Baird WLM. Antagonism of vecuronium and atracurium: comparison of neostigmine and edrophonium administered at 5% twitch height recovery. *Br J Anaesth* 1987;59:478–481.
125. Kopman AF. Recovery times following edrophonium and neostigmine reversal of pancuronium, atracurium, and vecuronium steady-state infusions. *Anesthesiology* 1986;65:572–578.
126. Rupp SM, McChristian JW, Miller RD, Taboada JA, Cronnelly R. Neostigmine and edrophonium antagonism of varying intensity neuromuscular blockade induced by atracurium, pancuronium, or vecuronium. *Anesthesiology* 1986;64:711–717.
127. Donati F, Ferguson A, Bevan DR. Twitch depression and train-of-four ratio after antagonism of pancuronium with edrophonium neostigmine or pyridostigmine. *Anesth Analg* 1983;62:314.
128. Engbaek J, Ostergaard D, Skovgaard LT, Viby-Mogensen J. Reversal of intense neuromuscular blockade following infusion of atracurium. *Anesthesiology* 1990;72:803–806.
129. Klessig HT, Geiger HJ, Murray MJ, Coursin DB. A national survey of anesthesiologist intensivists in the use of muscle relaxants. *Crit Care Med* 1992;20:1341–1345.
130. Segredo V, Caldwell JE, Matthay MA, et al. Persistent paralysis in critically ill patients after long-term administration of vecuronium. *New Engl J Med* 1992;327:524–528.
131. Watling SM, Dasta JF. Prolonged paralysis in intensive care unit patients after the use of neuromuscular blocking agents: a review of the literature. *Crit Care Med* 1994;22:884–893.
132. Kushimo OT, Darowski MJ, Morris P, et al. Dose requirements of atracurium in paediatric intensive care patients. *Br J Anaesth* 1991;67:781–783.
133. Wadon AJ, Dogra S, Anand S. Atracurium infusion in the intensive care unit. *Br J Anaesth* 1986;58(Suppl 1):64S–647S.
134. Yate PM, Flynn PJ, Arnold RW, Weatherly BC, Simmonds RJ, Dopson T. Clinical experience and plasma laudanosine concentrations during the infusion of atracurium in the intensive therapy unit. *Br J Anaesth* 1987;59:211–217.
135. Walker JS, Triggs EJ, Shanks CA. Clinical pharmacokinetics of alcuronium chloride in man. *Eur J Clin Pharmacol* 1980;17:449–457.
136. Basta SJ, Savarese JJ, Ali HH, et al. Clinical pharmacology of doxacurium chloride: a new long-acting nondepolarizing muscle relaxant. *Anesthesiology* 1988;69:478–486.
137. Ramzan MI, Triggs EJ, Shanks CA. Pharmacokinetic studies in man with gallamine triethiodide II single 4 and 6 mg/kg iv doses. *Eur J Clin Pharmacol* 1980;17:145–152.
138. Matteo RS, Brotherton WP, Nishitateno K, Khambatta HJ. Pharmacodynamics and pharmacokinetics of metocurine in humans: Comparison to d-tubocurarine. *Anesthesiology* 1982;57:183–190.
139. Duvaldestin P, Saada J, Berger JL, d'Hollander A, Desmonts JM. Pharmacokinetics pharmacodynamics and dose-response relationships of pancuronium in control and elderly subjects. *Anesthesiology* 1982;56:36–40.
140. Caldwell JE, Castagnoli KP, Canfell PC, et al. Pipecuronium and pancuronium: comparison of their pharmacokinetics and duration of action. *Br J Anaesth* 1988;61:693–697.
141. Shanks CA, Ramzan MI, Triggs EJ. Studies in man with a constant-rate infusion of tubocurarine. *Anaesth Intens* Care 1979;7:209–214.
142. Lien CA, Schmith VD, Belmont MR, Kisor D. Pharmacokinetics/dynamics of 51W89 in healthy patients during opioid anesthesia. *Anesthesiology* 1994;81:A1082(abst).
143. Matteo RS, Ornstein E, Schwartz AE, et al. Pharmacokinetics and pharmacodynamics of rocuronium (Org 9426) in elderly surgical patients. *Anesth Analg* 1993;77:1193–1197.
144. Walker JS, Shanks CA, Triggs EJ. Alcuronium kinetics and plasma concentration-effect relationship. *Clin Pharmacol Ther* 1983;33:510–516.
145. Ramzan IM, Shanks CA, Triggs EJ. Relationship between gallamine plasma concentration and neuromuscular paralysis in surgical patients. *J Clin Pharmacol* 1983;23:243–251.
146. Evans MA, Shanks CA, Brown KF, Triggs EJ. Pharmacokinetic and pharmacodynamic modelling with pancuronium. *Eur J Clin Pharmacol* 1984;26:243–250.
147. Shanks CA, Matteo RS, Ornstein E, Dee CM, Kim KS. Pharmacodynamic modelling of rocuronium in young and elderly. *Anesthesiology* 1994;81;A1073(abst).

Drug Infusions in Anesthesiology, Second Edition,
edited by R. J. Fragen. Lippincott-Raven Publishers,
Philadelphia © 1996.

6

Total Intravenous Anesthesia

Robert J. Fragen

Department of Anesthesia, Northwestern University Medical School, Chicago, Illinois 60611

Total intravenous anesthesia (TIVA) implies that all the components of general anesthesia are injected intravenously: Unconsciousness and amnesia are produced by sedative-hypnotic drugs; reflex response to surgery is decreased or abolished by analgesic drugs; and muscle relaxation is provided, when needed, by nondepolarizing muscle relaxants. The lungs are ventilated with oxygen-enriched air. TIVA can simply be two syringes with a hypnotic drug in one and an analgesic drug in the other (one syringe if ketamine is given for somatic pain or if a hypnotic and analgesic are mixed in the same syringe). A system involving three drugs given by computer-controlled infusion pumps is much more sophisticated but possibly just as simple.

ADVANTAGES

Total IV anesthesia overcomes some of the disadvantages of traditional inhalational anesthesia in the following ways: First, the components of TIVA can be regulated independently as the need for each component changes during surgery. Both somatic and autonomic responses to varying degrees of surgical stimulation can be controlled.

Second, precision vaporizers are unnecessary. Currently used vaporizers have no mechanism to prevent drug delivery of lethal concentrations of anesthetics to patients; thus, a separate gas-analysis monitor is necessary to determine the concentration of volatile agent delivered from the vaporizer.

Third, anesthetized areas remain unpolluted by trace concentrations of nitrous oxide (N_2O) or volatile anesthetic agents. Although the evidence is unclear or controversial, inhalation of these gases may cause bone marrow depression (1), an increased incidence of miscarriages in pregnant operating room personnel (2), and a decrease in the alertness of the anesthesiologist (3). To alleviate these potential problems caused by trace concentrations of anesthetic agents, scavenging systems are installed in operating rooms at additional expense. These systems divert waste gases from the operating theater to a remote place, usually the atmosphere. Although halothane, enflurane, and isoflurane are considered "ozone friendly," N_2O has ozone-depleting potential (4). Fluorohydrocarbons also are considered to be atmospheric pollutants, and all the volatile anesthetic wastes may contribute. Pollution of the atmosphere by waste anesthetic gases is small compared to industrial pollution, but its importance should not be ignored.

Fourth, it is unnecessary to depend on the lungs as a transport mechanism to achieve an effective drug concentration in the blood and eventually in the target receptor. Finally, TIVA prevents delivery of hypoxic mixtures because oxygen-enriched air is delivered to the lungs.

DISADVANTAGES

TIVA also has disadvantages: First, a free-flowing IV infusion must be available for drug administration. This may necessitate a separate IV infusion site from that used to administer maintenance fluid therapy or blood products.

Second, precision infusion devices that accurately deliver the chosen dose are needed in most cases. The infusion pump should have the safety devices described in Chapter 2. Some anesthesiologists prefer an infusion pump that can be programmed for each drug, matching drug delivery to the pharmacokinetic profile. This allows the pump to deliver drugs rapidly to achieve and maintain set blood or effect site concentrations.

Third, no convenient measure of depth of anesthesia is available. Blood concentrations are unobtainable on a "stat" basis and are poorly correlated with clinical effects. The electroencephalogram (EEG) or its descriptors, spectral edge, or median frequency may correlate with anesthetic depth in a laboratory but correlate poorly in the operating room.

Fourth, drug effects are terminated by redistribution and eventually by metabolism and excretion. Conditions that slow blood flow and metabolism in the liver and slow renal function may prolong the action of IV anesthetics, particularly their residual effects. Volatile agents and N_2O can be exhaled to promote recovery.

Fifth, currently available drugs may not be specific enough or have the best pharmacokinetic profile for ensuring a fast, safe recovery. Possibly, the introduction of esterase-metabolized drugs will improve this situation.

Sixth, information about the proper doses of IV anesthetic drug combinations for various types of surgery and different patient medical conditions is not as abundant as that available for volatile and gaseous anesthetic agents. Additional information is needed about interactions among IV agents.

Finally, to help avoid a patient's awareness under anesthesia, muscle relaxants should be dosed so that some movement is possible if anesthesia becomes inadequate (presence of one or two twitch responses to train-of-four stimulation).

IDEAL DRUG PROPERTIES

Ideally, drugs used for TIVA should be water soluble to avoid solvent toxicity, be capable of being given in a concentrated solution to avoid excess fluids, be stable in solution, not be absorbed by plastics, and be nonirritating to tissue if extravasated. They should be lipid soluble, potent, nonallergenic, and nontoxic. They should have a fast equilibration time, have a short context-sensitive half-time even with long infusions, and be inexpensive. Metabolites should be inactive and not accumulate to prolong drug action. The drugs used in combination should be chemically compatible with each other and with commonly used IV carrier solutions so that they can be delivered from multiple infusion devices through a common channel to the patient.

INDICATIONS

In some situations, TIVA is preferable to inhalational anesthesia, but it can be used for any anesthetic that can be administered intravenously. Nitrous oxide and volatile agents interfere with the interpretation of somatosensory evoked potentials because they depress the amplitude and change the latency of the evoked responses. Thus, TIVA may be indicated for intracranial and spinal cord neurosurgery where monitoring of somatosensory or motor evoked potentials is indicated. Once the quality of the signal is known, N_2O or a volatile agent such as isoflurane can be added gradually because its effect on the signal will be immediately apparent and, if the signal is adversely affected, the inhalational agent can be stopped.

For thoracic surgery, TIVA allows delivery of a high inspired-oxygen concentration and averts the negative effects of volatile agents on pulmonary circulation, respiratory drive, and breathing patterns. It is beneficial for anesthetizing patients with a compromised airway when ventilation is possible, but achieving an anesthetizing concentration of inhalational anesthetic agents in the lung is difficult. TIVA is useful for otolaryngologic procedures, usually endoscopy, requiring jet ventilation. It is an option in all situations for which N_2O is contraindicated or undesirable, such as pneumocephalus, pneumothorax, middle ear surgery, and intestinal surgery for closed-loop obstruction. It is useful for open heart anesthesia, military anesthesia, and veterinary anesthesia.

The drugs that are most appropriate to combine for TIVA are propofol, methohexital, and midazolam as sedative-hypnotics; remifentanil, alfentanil, sufentanil and fentanyl as opioid analgesics; and mivacurium, atracurium, vecuronium, and rocuronium for muscle relaxation. Dose regimens mentioned in this chapter are to serve as guidelines; regimens must be individualized by titrating the dose according to the patient's response or lack of response during surgery or in the intensive care unit. Because the individual drugs are discussed in the chapters on hypnotics, analgesics, and muscle relaxants, this chapter mainly presents known data about various drug combinations used for TIVA.

SPECIFIC TECHNIQUES

In its simplest form, TIVA consists of one syringe of a hypnotic drug and one syringe of an analgesic drug, both of which are administered intravenously by intermittent injection for a brief surgical procedure, usually less than 30 minutes. When done in this manner, any of the hypnotic or analgesic drugs listed above, with the addition of etomidate, ketamine, or thiopental, can be injected. The trachea can be intubated without muscle relaxants 90 seconds after giving at least 40 μg/kg of alfentanil and 2 mg/kg of propofol (5). Indications for repeat bolus doses are signs of awakening and response to surgical stimuli. Recovery is usually rapid. For longer procedures, intermittent drug injection is cumbersome and apt to produce peaks and troughs in the blood concentration of the injected drug, possibly evoking side effects at the peaks and inadequate anesthesia at the troughs. An easier approach is drug administration by continuous infusion.

The best drugs to give by infusion are those with the smallest context-sensitive half-time over the duration of the anesthetic. When a calculator pump is used, drug doses are based on a μg/kg/min or mg/kg/hr dosing schedule. If a computer-assisted continuous infusion is used, the computer is programmed to a specific target blood or effect site concentration and the units are μg/ml or ng/ml. Therefore, the infusion schemes mentioned in this chapter can be described by either infusion rates or target concentrations. In either case, these are dosing guidelines—starting points that should be adjusted according to anesthetic requirements.

The muscle relaxant part of TIVA can easily be given by intermittent injection of a nondepolarizing relaxant, the duration of action of which is appropriate for the duration of the surgical procedure. However, if one wants a steady degree of relaxation that satisfies surgical requirements but keeps one-to-two twitches of the train-of-four response present (movement is the best sign of inadequate anesthesia), administration by infusion is better.

Propofol, because of its context-sensitive half-time profile, is the best drug to infuse for the hypnotic component of TIVA if fairly rapid recovery is desirable. When hypnotics are infused for 3 hours and stopped, the propofol blood concentration decreases below the therapeutic range more rapidly than the blood concentration of etomidate or thiopental (Fig. 1). Plasma decay curves of methohexital, midazolam, and ketamine would also be to the right of the propofol curve in the figure.

The best opioid analgesic to use in TIVA depends on the length of the infusion and how far the effect site concentration must decrease to achieve recovery of adequate respiration and consciousness. Also remember that equilibration half-time for fentanyl and sufentanil is 5–6 minutes, whereas it is 1.5 minutes for alfentanil and remifentanil. After a brief infusion that maintains peak effect site concentrations for 10 minutes, the effect site concentrations of alfentanil, fentanyl, and sufentanil decrease at the same rate. The time required for a 50% decrease in effect site opioid concentration after an infusion of 30 minutes or less is similar for all three drugs. Thereafter, the curve for fentanyl increases rapidly, making it a

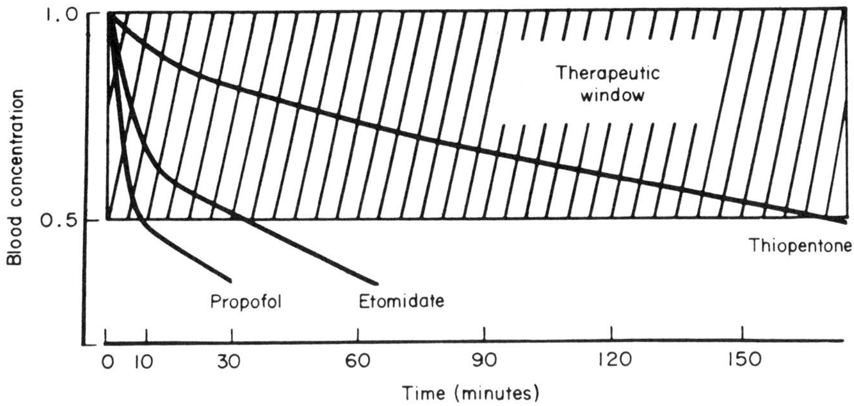

FIG. 1. Simulated blood-level decay from optimal to minimal therapeutic concentrations after a 3-hr infusion of propofol, etomidate, and thiopental. Concentrations are given as fractions of the optimal therapeutic concentration for each drug at the end of infusion. (Data from Schüttler et al., ref. 9, with permission.)

less desirable drug to use for longer infusions. For infusions shorter than 8 hours, the decreases in effect site concentration will be faster after sufentanil than after equivalent analgesic doses of alfentanil, but alfentanil will have the advantage thereafter (6). Therefore, for most operating room use of TIVA, the combination of propofol and alfentanil or sufentanil have been the most popular; however, most articles have been written about propofol and alfentanil. Perhaps remifentanil will replace them when it becomes available for general use.

Remifentanil has a context-sensitive half-time that plateaus at 3–4 minutes for at least 8 hours. When propofol (or another hypnotic agent) is infused simultaneously with an opioid, one should probably keep the infusion rate of one drug constant and vary the other. It is my opinion that the opioid should be varied because surgical stimuli vary in severity, but seldom does the drug concentration necessary to produce unconsciousness vary. Vuyk et al. (7) also point out that alfentanil has a shorter equilibration time than propofol (1.5 versus 2.9 min), so one can treat responses during surgery faster. It would also make sense to keep the drug with the longest context-sensitive half-time as close to the threshold as possible so that when the infusions are stopped recovery will be prompt. With currently available drugs, this means keeping the propofol infusion rate constant and varying the infusion rate of opioid analgesic. When remifentanil is available, it may be the best one to keep constant, but that needs validation. In reported TIVA techniques, each of the components has been varied while the other has been kept constant, and the recovery results have been satisfactory. Monk et al. (8) treated "light" anesthesia with either supplemental propofol or alfentanil. They found a faster response time and earlier awakening when they used supplemental alfentanil, but more of those patients required early postoperative antihypertensive therapy than did those treated with supplemental propofol.

Schüttler et al. (9) first described the administration of alfentanil and propofol using a computer-assisted infusion. They programmed the computer to produce a theoretical target blood propofol concentration of 2.5 μg/ml after administering 2 mg of vecuronium just before induction in patients premedicated with a benzodiazepine an hour earlier. The alfentanil infusion was started 30 seconds after propofol to achieve an alfentanil plasma concentration of 100 ng/ml. This was increased to 200 ng/ml before surgical incision and then adjusted according to the patient's response. The alfentanil infusion was stopped 30 minutes before the end of surgery, and the propofol infusion continued until the last skin suture was placed. Awakening occurred 8 ± 3.4 minutes after propofol was stopped at the plasma concentrations shown in Fig. 2. Extubation was possible about 4 minutes later. Figure 3 shows the plasma concentrations of alfentanil and the blood concentrations of propofol at various times during anesthesia.

Gepts et al. (10) found that propofol caused unconsciousness at blood concentrations of 2.3 ± 0.84 μg/ml and recovery occurred at 1.29 ± 0.44 μg/ml. They believed that the specific activities of propofol and alfentanil were potentiated by each other. Schüttler et al. (9) had similar findings.

Vuyk et al. (7), in a study of females undergoing lower abdominal surgery, found that less alfentanil was required to suppress the response to tracheal intubation,

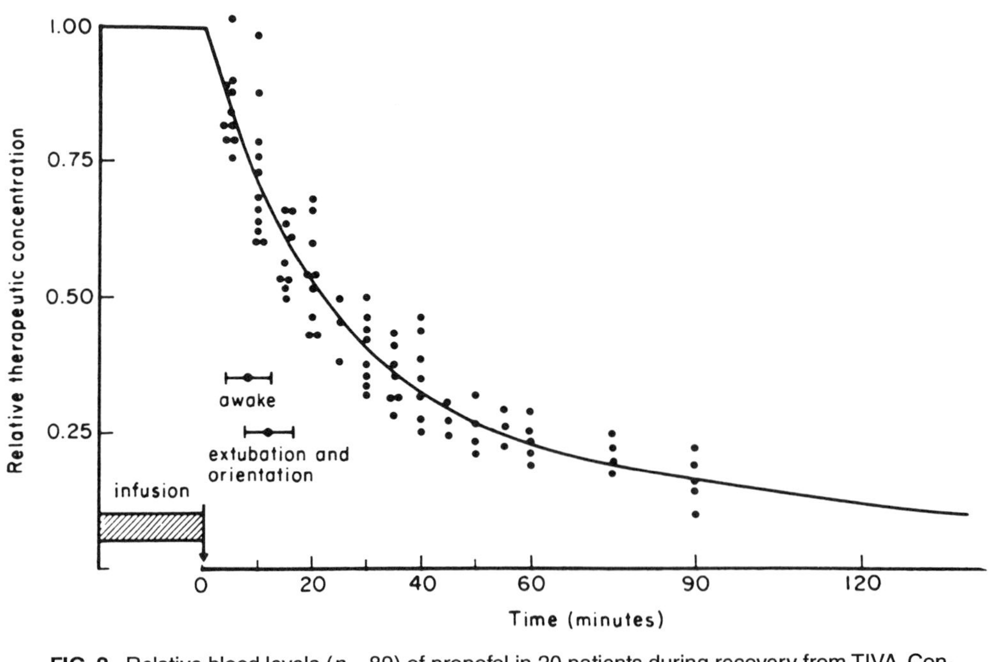

FIG. 2. Relative blood levels ($n = 89$) of propofol in 20 patients during recovery from TIVA. Concentrations are given as fractions of the individual concentrations at the end of infusion. (Data from Schüttler et al., ref. 9, with permission.)

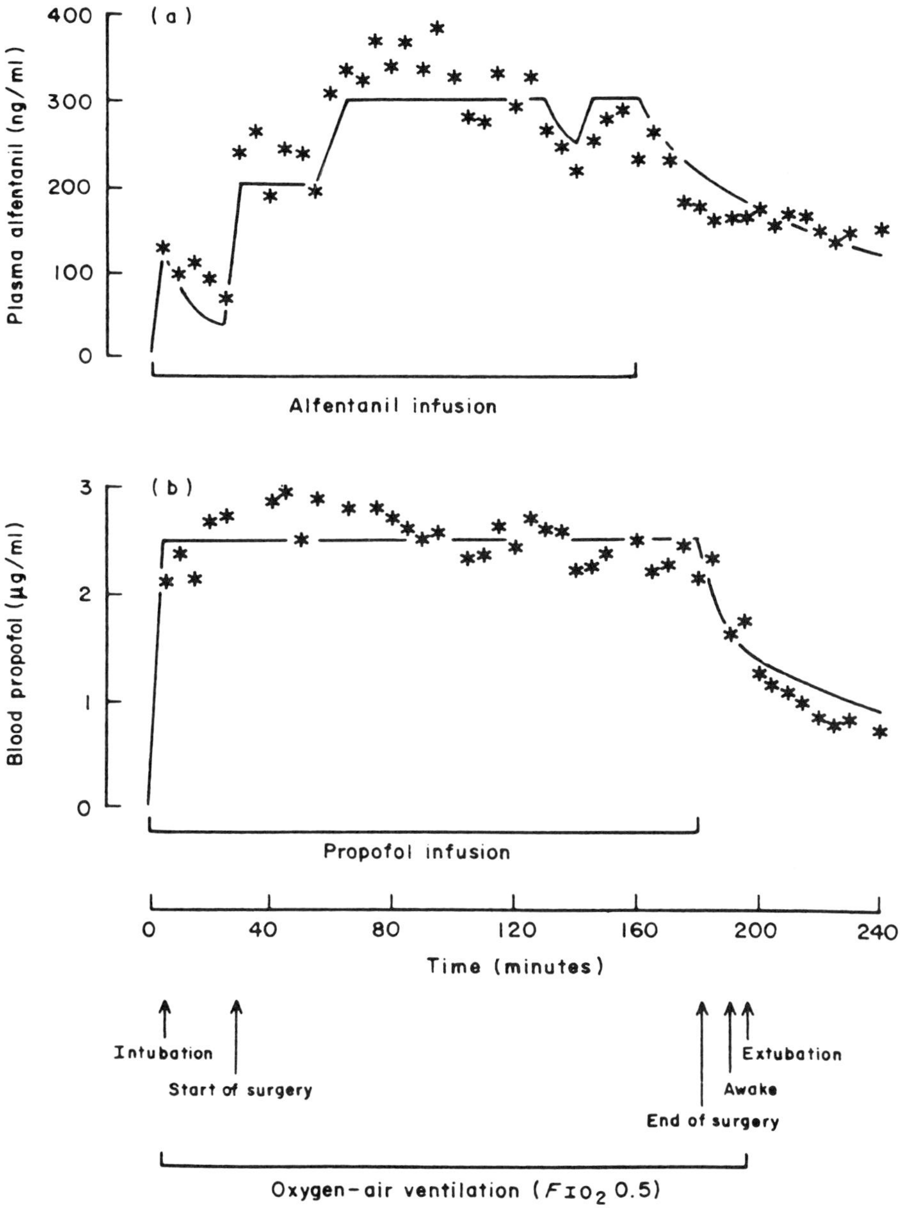

FIG. 3. A: Plasma levels of alfentanil and **B:** blood levels of propofol, as predicted (–) by computer-assisted infusions (solid line) and as actually measured (asterisks) in one representative patient who received the described anesthetic technique. (Data from Schüttler et al., ref. 9, with permission.)

skin incision, and intraabdominal surgery when given with a target propofol concentration of 4 ± 0.6 μg/ml in TIVA than when it was infused with 67% N_2O (Figs. 4–7). Their results with N_2O are similar to those reported previously by Lemmens et al. (11) and Ausems et al. (12).

Wessen et al. (13) reported that a higher target concentration was necessary to keep patients asleep when propofol was infused with epidural anesthesia than when it was given with alfentanil for TIVA, 2.5 μg/ml versus 2.1–2.3 μg/ml. Their TIVA technique consisted of 1.5 mg/kg of propofol, followed by an infusion of 8 mg/kg/hr for 15 minutes that was decreased to 6 mg/kg/hr until the end of surgery. An initial alfentanil dose of 25 μg/kg was followed by an infusion rate of 3 μg/kg/min for 15 minutes that was decreased to 1 μg/kg/min until the start of the

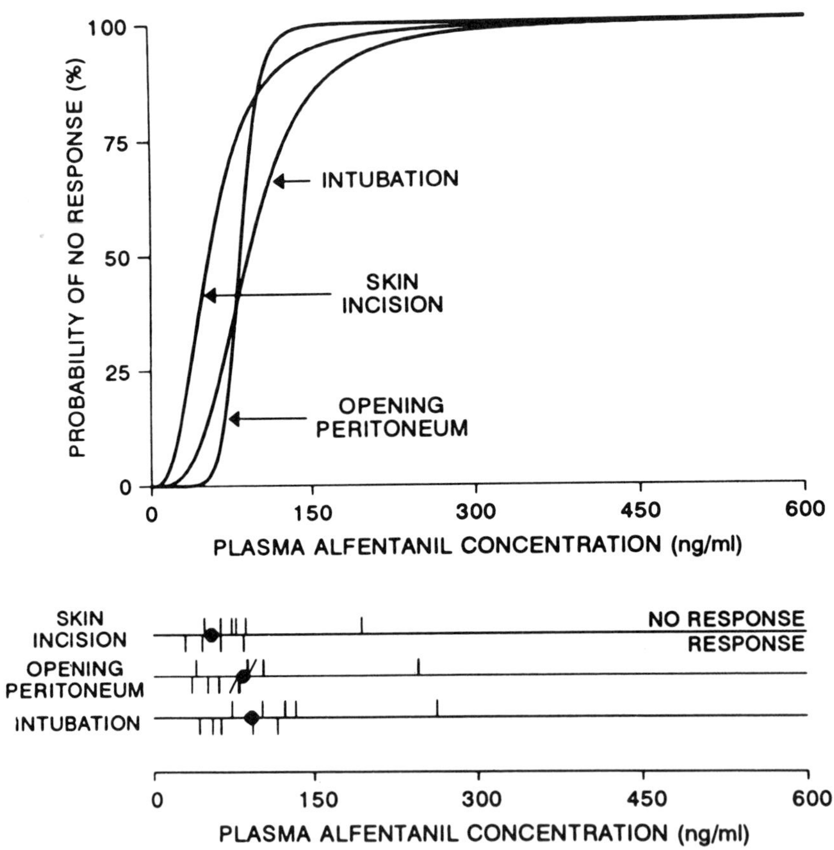

FIG. 4. The alfentanil concentration-effect relationships for intubation, skin incision, and the opening of the peritoneum when given as a supplement to propofol. The curves were determined by fitting a sigmoid E_{max} model to response/no response data versus the corresponding measured plasma alfentanil concentrations, as displayed underneath the curves. Dots represent EC_{50}. (Data from Vuyk et al., ref. 7, with permission.)

abdominal closure. A 50 μg/kg bolus dose was given just before skin incision. This infusion scheme theoretically produced a target blood propofol concentration of 3 μg/ml and an alfentanil plasma concentration of 300 ng/ml.

Propofol, alfentanil, muscle relaxant TIVA has been used for various surgical procedures and patient populations. It produces good brain relaxation during surgery and rapid awakening after craniotomy for brain tumors (14). Both propofol and midazolam TIVA decrease the cerebral vasomotor effect of carbon dioxide and decrease cerebral blood flow (15). It provides better surgical conditions, more stable anesthesia, and faster recovery than when etomidate was the hypnotic component for microlaryngeal surgery with jet ventilation (16). Slower recovery occurs in burn patients than in healthy patients (17), but TIVA can produce

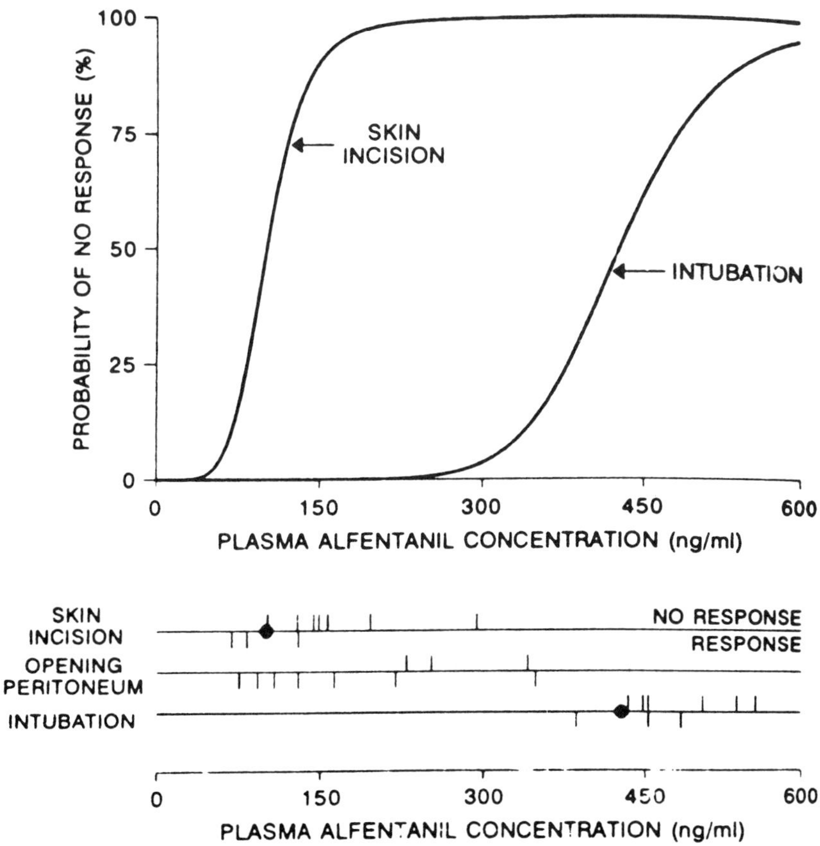

FIG. 5. The alfentanil concentration-effect relationships for intubation and skin incision when given as a supplement to nitrous oxide. The curves were determined by fitting a sigmoid E_{max} model to response/no response data versus the corresponding measured plasma alfentanil concentrations, as displayed underneath the curves. Dots represent EC_{50}. (Data from Vuyk et al., ref. 7, with permission.)

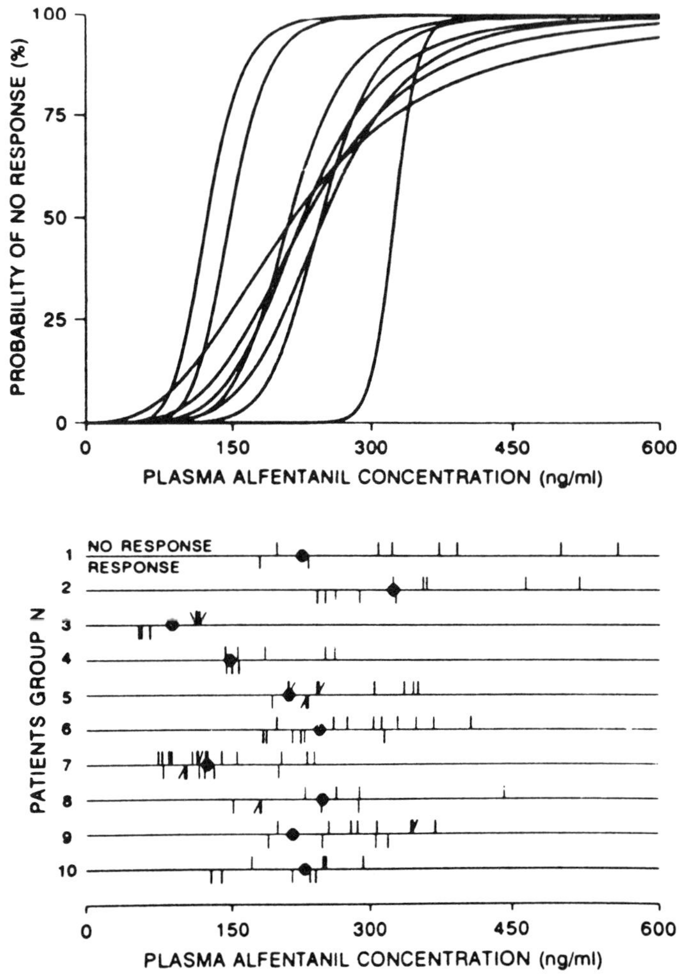

FIG. 6. The alfentanil concentration-effect relationships in the individual patients for the intraabdominal part of surgery when given by fitting a sigmoid E_{max} model to response/no response data versus the corresponding measured plasma alfentanils, as displayed underneath the curves. In patient N3, no overlap between response and no-response data occurred. In this patient the EC_{50} was determined by the midrange between the highest plasma alfentanil concentration with a response and the lowest plasma alfentanil concentration without a response. Dots represent EC_{50}. (Data from Vuyk et al., ref. 7, with permission.)

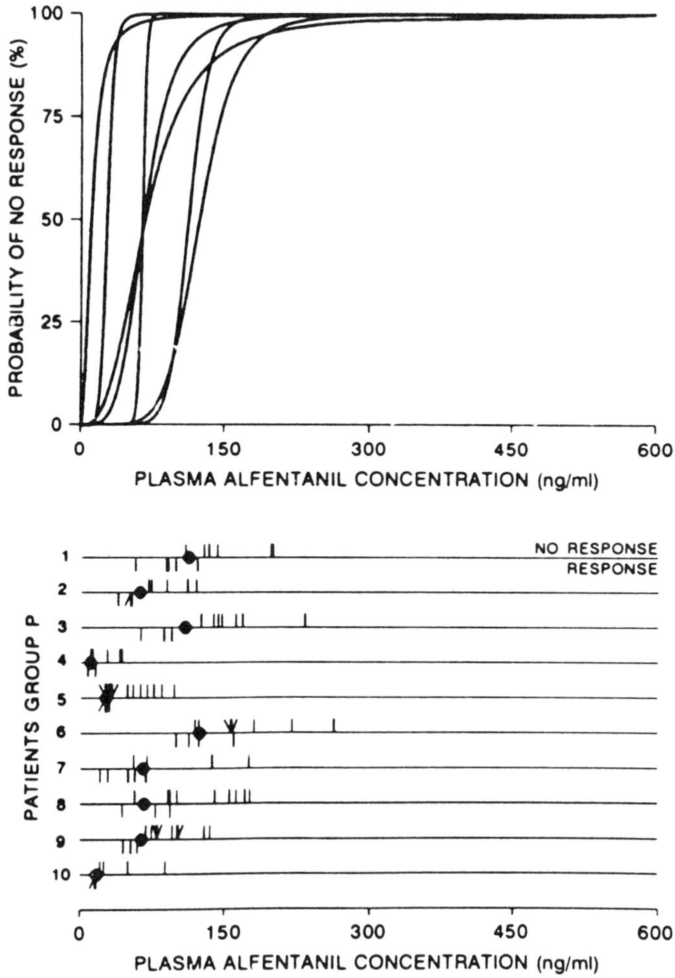

FIG. 7. The alfentanil concentration-effect relationships in the individual patients for the intraabdominal part of surgery when given as a supplement to propofol. The curves were determined by fitting a sigmoid E_{max} model to response/no response data versus the corresponding measured plasma alfentanil concentrations, as displayed underneath the curves. In patients P2, P3, and P10, no overlap between response and no-response data occurred. In these patients, the EC_{50} was determined by the midrange between the highest plasma alfentanil concentration with a response and the lowest plasma alfentanil concentration without a response. Dots represent EC_{50}. (Data from Vuyk et al., ref. 7, with permission.)

faster recovery than can the same IV drugs given with N_2O and isoflurane in healthy patients (18).

TIVA has been used for children. An average infusion rate of 474 μg/kg/min of propofol was needed for anesthesia, producing a mean blood concentration of 6.6 μg/ml (range, 3–11 μg/ml). At awakening, which was slower than expected because of the high dose requirements, mean blood concentrations of propofol were 0.86 μg/ml (range, 0.4–1.45 μg/ml) (19). They used different rate constants (Table 1) to design their model-controlled infusion because they found that those of Marsh et al. (20) had less precision and more bias and underestimated the blood concentration of propofol by 18.5%.

When propofol is given by infusion to unpremedicated patients in two different age groups, 16–40 years or 41–65 years, the ED_{50} and the ED_{95} for loss of response to verbal command is 5 mg/kg/hr and 8 mg/kg/hr in the younger group and 4.2 mg/kg/hr and 5.8 mg/kg/hr in the older group. (See Fig. 9, Chapter 3). When propofol alone was infused at target blood concentrations of 3 μg/ml, 4 μg/ml, or 5 μg/ml in 60 patients premedicated with temazepam, 40%, 75%, and 90% of the patients, respectively, lost consciousness (21). Therefore, in premedicated adults, an initial target propofol concentration of 5 μg/ml will produce unconsciousness in most patients, whereas 6 μg/ml would be a better initial target concentration in unpremedicated adults. A 6 μg/ml concentration corresponds closely to the initial infusion rate of 12 mg/kg/hr when a calculator pump is used.

When designing an infusion scheme for target plasma concentrations of alfentanil, there appears to be less discrepancy between theoretical and measured alfentanil concentrations (22,23) when using the pharmacokinetic data of Scott and Stanski (24) rather than that of Maitre et al. (25).

Our initial study with propofol and alfentanil TIVA used a constant maintenance infusion for propofol and a variable rate infusion for alfentanil (26). By frequently adjusting the alfentanil infusion on the basis of response or nonresponse to surgical stimuli, the drug level was generally close to threshhold values at the end of surgery, resulting in rapid recovery. Propofol, 2 mg/kg, was given over 2 minutes, followed by an initial infusion of 200 μg/kg/min for 20 minutes that was lowered to 80 μg/kg/min until 5 minutes before the end of surgery. Depending on

TABLE 1. *Rate constants for a pharmacokinetic model program to drive a computer pump to deliver propofol in children*

Parameter	Rate constants
Vc ml/kg	432.0
K10 min	0.0967
K12 min	0.1413
K13 min	0.0392
K21 min	0.1092
K31	0.0049

From Short et al., ref. 19.

the anticipated severity of the surgical stimulus, either 50 μg/kg or 100 μg/kg of alfentanil was given over 10 minutes, and then an infusion of 50 μg/kg/hr was started. This was adjusted by 25 μg/kg/hr increments within the limits of 25–150 μg/kg/hr. An increase in infusion rate was preceded by a 1-mg bolus dose. This produced satisfactory anesthesia, except that it was difficult to control hypertension when a leg tourniquet was inflated longer than 30 minutes.

Usually, anesthetic techniques involving opioids as a major component are associated with a high incidence of emetic symptoms. When a TIVA technique for egg harvesting was compared with an inhalational anesthetic technique using N_2O and enflurane, the incidence of nausea and vomiting was about 40% less when TIVA was given (27). It is also my experience that TIVA is associated with a low incidence of nausea and vomiting when propofol is the hypnotic component. In a study combining propofol and remifentanil, only one patient (N = 17) was nauseated and none vomited when a target blood propofol concentration of 2 μg/ml or 4 μg/ml was combined with a remifentanil infusion for outpatient anesthesia (28). We also observed a rapid return of adequate ventilation and the ability to maintain normal oxygen saturation after the remifentanil-propofol technique. When alfentanil was given by infusion with N_2O for lumbar laminectomy, the carbon dioxide (CO_2) response curve was depressed up to 1 hour postoperatively (29). The same could occur after TIVA with alfentanil or longer-acting opioids.

One advantage of TIVA is the independent regulation of each anesthetic component. However, combining propofol and alfentanil in the same syringe and administering the mixture with a single infusion pump has some appeal. The mixture is chemically compatible and can produce a pharmacodynamically stable anesthetic (30). One group mixed 50 ml of propofol (500 mg) and 5 ml of alfentanil (2.5 mg) in a 60-ml syringe. The final concentration was 9 mg/ml of propofol and 45 μg/ml of alfentanil. For anesthetic induction, they gave a volume of the mixture that would give 0.2 mg/kg of propofol and, for maintenance, an infusion rate that would deliver propofol at a rate of 0.4 ml/kg/hr. Bolus doses of 10–15% of the induction dose was given for light anesthesia. The infusion was tapered toward the end of the surgical procedure, and the outpatients awoke 5–7 minutes after the infusion was stopped (31). Because this mixture was given with 70% N_2O, it was technically not a TIVA technique. A TIVA technique with the same propofol-alfentanil mixture was used in the military (32). After injecting 10 μg/kg of alfentanil, followed by propofol, titrated until loss of the eyelash reflex, succinylcholine was given and the trachea was intubated. The mixture was infused at a rate that would deliver 10 mg/kg/hr of propofol for the first 10 minutes and then 5 mg/kg/hr. Vecuronium was used as the maintenance muscle relaxant.

Fentanyl also can be combined with propofol for TIVA. The effect of fentanyl on the dose requirements of propofol for loss of consciousness and obliteration of the response to skin incision, as measured by the CP_{50}, was determined by investigators at Duke University (33). Their computer was programmed using the pharmacokinetic values in Table 2 to deliver both propofol and fentanyl. They gave 1.5 times the final target fentanyl concentration for 2 minutes because of the

TABLE 2. *Pharmacokinetic values (rate constants) used for a program for computer assisted continuous infusion of propofol and fentanyl in adults (33)*

Parameter	Rate constants for propofol	Rate constants for fentanyl
Vc l/kg	0.0767	0.356
K10 min	0.3035	0.041
K12 min	0.2846	0.185
K21 min	0.0866	0.103
K13 min	0.2730	0.141
K31 min	0.0036	0.020

From Smith et al., ref. 33.

drug's slow equilibration time. After determining the CP_{50} and CP_{95} of propofol for both events, they simultaneously infused fentanyl to a specific target concentration and examined its effect on the CP_{50} of propofol. Fentanyl, 3 ng/ml, decreased the CP_{50} of propofol for loss of consciousness, 3.3 μg/ml, by 40%. Fentanyl, 1 ng/ml, reduced the CP_{50} of propofol for nonreaction to skin incision by 63% and 3 ng/ml decreased it by 89%. That fentanyl decreased the CP_{50} for skin incision more is not surprising because skin incision is a painful stimulus and fentanyl is a potent μ-opioid receptor analgesic. Their CP_{50} of 3.3 μg/ml and CP_{95} of 5.4 μg/ml are similar to those that Vuyk et al. (7) found: 3.4 μg/ml and 4.3 μg/ml, respectively, for the CP_{50} and CP_{90} of propofol. This study shows the interaction between the two drugs until skin incision, but does not consider the maintenance phase during surgery.

Vermeyen et al. (34) found that a mean infusion of 4.48 mg/kg/hr of propofol after a 1.5 mg/kg bolus dose, plus 30 μg/kg of fentanyl, caused myocardial depression and peripheral vasodilation. However, coronary sinus flow, myocardial oxygen metabolism, and myocardial lactate extraction did not change when these investigators used the technique for anesthesia for coronary artery bypass surgery. The same investigators had previously published an article showing no detrimental effects of propofol-fentanyl TIVA for patients with good left-ventricular function who were undergoing the same operation (35). Other investigators, however, found that this drug combination decreased left-ventricular function because hypotension was related to a decrease in cardiac output and no change in systemic vascular resistance (36).

Mora et al. (37) and Russell et al. (38) used propofol in addition to a basic fentanyl-oxygen anesthetic to control the hypertensive episodes that occur with cardiac surgery. Mora et al. gave an initial 10–20 mg dose of propofol and started a continuous infusion at a rate of 5 mg/min. This rate was adjusted to maintain mean arterial pressure within 10% of baseline values before coronary bypass. Their final infusion rate over time was 7 ± 4 mg/min for 64 ± 21 minutes. Plasma propofol concentrations were 2.7 ± 1.2 μg/ml before bypass, 0.9 ± 0.6 μg/ml after bypass, and 0.5 ± 0.4 μg/ml after surgery—a concentration that should allow rapid recovery of psychomotor function. Russell et al. (38) gave propofol 10 mg/kg/hr from 10 minutes before skin incision until after sternotomy and sternal spread, then decreased the rate to 3 mg/kg/hr. The resulting blood concentrations of propofol are shown in Fig. 8. The addition of propofol decreased the amount of fentanyl needed to maintain anesthesia, and the patients were hemodynamically stable. The positive results of these studies in patients with good ventricular function cannot be applied to patients with coronary artery disease and poor ventricular function in whom propofol should only be used with caution.

In noncardiac patients, Billard et al. (39) gave either 0, 2, or 4 μg/kg of fentanyl and 5 minutes later gave 2.0, 2.5, 3.0, or 3.5 mg/kg of propofol to examine their blood pressure effects at anesthetic induction and tracheal intubation. At anesthetic induction, there was no difference in the degree of hypotension produced as the propofol dose increased. Increasing the dose of fentanyl, however, caused greater hypotension on induction and less blood pressure increase at the time of tracheal intubation. Adding opioid analgesics to propofol can cause hypotension and bradycardia, putting hypovolemic and cardiac compromised patients at risk. Fluid loading and preinduction administration of glycopyrrolate can lessen these effects.

For elective supratentorial craniotomy procedures, a propofol-fentanyl TIVA technique had no short-term outcome differences compared to a technique using isoflurane/N_2O or isoflurane/oxygen but gave satisfactory anesthesia (40). Propofol, combined with fentanyl for anesthesia for thoracic surgery with one-lung ven-

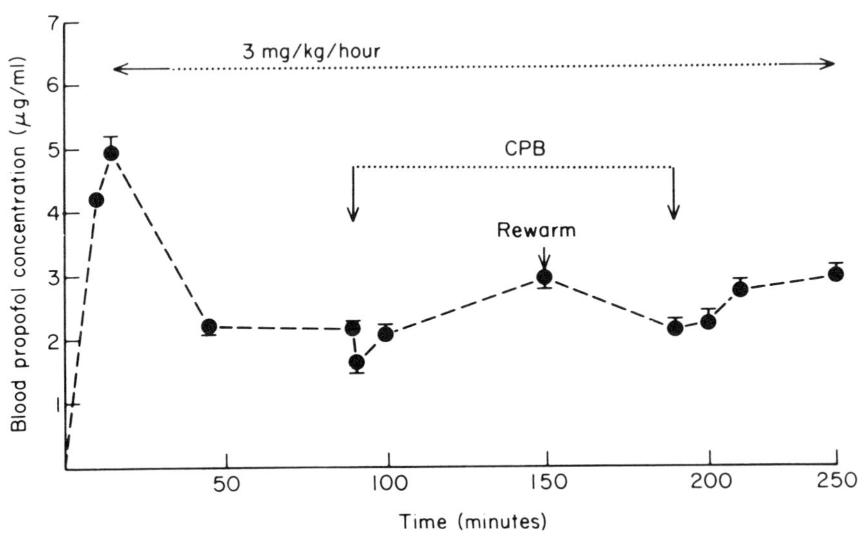

FIG. 8. The fluctuations in blood propofol concentration throughout the operative procedure. The time scale shows the mean time taken to specific events such as the onset of cardiopulmonary bypass (CPB), induced hypothermia, and the end of bypass. Bars represent SEM. (Data from Russell et al., ref. 38, with permission.)

tilation, preserved hypoxic pulmonary vasoconstriction and allowed a more rapid return of consciousness compared to anesthesia with volatile agents (41). This combination was also used successfully for thymectomy to treat myasthenia gravis, so that both volatile anesthetic agents and muscle relaxants could be avoided (42).

A propofol-fentanyl technique for outpatient kidney-stone lithotripsy in outpatients used 1.5 μg/kg of fentanyl and a propofol infusion of 50 mg/kg/min after a bolus dose of 0.5 mg/kg (43). It provided smoother anesthesia than did 0.05 mg/kg of midazolam and an alfentanil infusion of 1 μg/kg/min after a bolus dose of 10 μg/kg. When propofol was used by infusion with intermittent fentanyl doses for surgical procedures of about 150 minutes duration, spontaneous ventilation, extubation, and eye opening occurred 5.3 ± 3.9, 7.5 ± 5.2, and 8.6 ± 5.9 minutes, respectively. Veselis et al. (45) showed memory impairment in volunteers when the plasma fentanyl concentration was about 2.5 ng/ml, a concentration that could easily occur in the recovery room when patients receive a fentanyl-propofol anesthetic. Therefore, with the combination, even if the patient appears awake, some impaired memory function could exist. Shorter-acting opioid analgesics, especially remifentanil, should obviate this potential problem in outpatients.

Since the first edition of this book, there are, as yet, no published studies of sufentanil-propofol TIVA. It has been our practice to give a slow bolus dose of 1–1.5 μg/kg of sufentanil, followed by an initial infusion of 0.025 μg/kg/min that is subsequently adjusted to the patient's requirements (0.01–0.1 μg/kg/min) and discontinued about 20–30 minutes before the end of surgery, depending on the length of the infusion. Sufentanil has been combined with either propofol or midazolam as the hypnotic component.

Methohexital and alfentanil administered by intermittent injection for gynecological operations of less than 10 minutes duration led to faster recovery than did a thiopental-N_2O technique in patients who were premedicated with 5 mg of IV diazepam and 0.5 mg of atropine 5 minutes before anesthetic induction (46). When alfentanil was administered in 7 μg/kg or 15 μg/kg doses, the latter dose caused a greater incidence of apnea and decreased the amount of methohexital required.

TABLE 3. *Effects of benzodiazepines (BZD) and opiates administered separately and together*

Effects	BZD	Opiates	BZD plus opiates
Desirable			
Analgesia	minimal	++	+++
Sedation/hypnosis	+	Minimal	++
Anesthetic potentiation	++	++	+++
Stress protective	+	++	+++
Amnesia	++	–	++
Anxiolysis	++	+	++
Anticonvulsant threshold	Increased	Decreased	Increased
Undesirable			
Cardiac depression	Minimal	–	Little or +
Respiratory depression	Low	++	+++

Data from Vinik, ref. 48, with permission.

Schwilden et al. (47) achieved and maintained a median EEG frequency in the 2–3 Hz range with methohexital administered by computer-assisted continuous infusion with an infusion pump based on a pharmacokinetic model. By describing the dose-time and plasma-concentration relationship for methohexital, this modeling helps determine the best dose. When methohexital was given by a closed-loop feedback control technique, recovery occurred a mean of 20.6 minutes (range 10.7–44.5 min) after the infusion stopped at a median EEG frequency of 5.2 Hz (range 4.7–8.4 Hz). About 1 g of methohexital was given over 2 hours. Whether the same relationships will occur in the operating room when methohexital is given with an opiate is unknown. It is obvious, however, that propofol infusions for TIVA result in faster recovery times.

The individual and combined effects of benzodiazepines and opiates are compared in Table 3 (48). Obviously, the two drugs potentiate each other for both beneficial effects and side effects. Midazolam and fentanyl are often combined for IV sedation techniques. The combination does not depress the CO_2 response curve more than fentanyl does alone, but it can lead to hypoxemia and apnea (49). Thus, both drugs require careful titration, beginning with 0.5–1 mg increments of midazolam and 25–50 μg increments of fentanyl. The low end of the dose range is for older or sicker patients, or both.

Because midazolam prolongs recovery from opiate anesthesia (50), midazolam combinations are used mainly for longer, inpatient surgical procedures. For these procedures, midazolam infusions should be stopped at least 30 minutes before the end of surgery, or midazolam should be pharmacologically reversed to have awakening close to the end of surgery. Vinik et al. (51) used one-third of an ED_{50} for midazolam or 70 μg/kg and one-fourth of the ED_{50} or 28 μg/kg of alfentanil to induce anesthesia. Synergism also occurs between midazolam and fentanyl com-

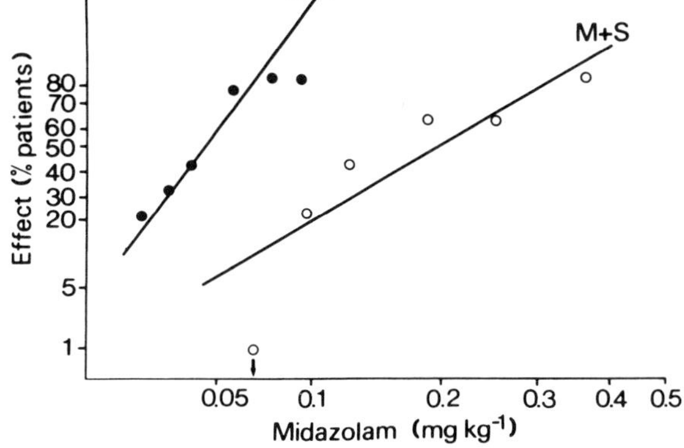

FIG. 9. Midazolam quantal dose-response curves for induction of anesthesia with the addition of fentanyl 19 μg/kg (M+F) or saline (M+S). Each point represents a subgroup of 10 patients at the indicated dosage. (Data from Ben-Shlomo et al., ref. 52, with permission.)

bined for induction of anesthesia (Fig. 9) (52). When midazolam is given to a target plasma concentration of 400 ng/ml, recovery is prolonged. However, when combined with alfentanil for lower-abdominal surgery, a target midazolam concentration of 300 ng/ml and a 200–300 ng/ml alfentanil target concentration produced good anesthesia. The plasma concentration of midazolam needed to be decreased by two-thirds to achieve a fairly alert patient postoperatively (53).

An infusion regimen that is designed to produce a stable midazolam plasma concentration of 300 ng/ml (Fig. 10) begins with a bolus dose of 0.3 mg/kg, followed by an initial infusion rate of 0.68 mg/kg/hr for 15 minutes, and then a rate of 0.125 mg/kg/hr for the remainder of the anesthetic (54).

For cardiac surgery, Reves et al. (55) described a successful midazolam-fentanyl TIVA that resulted in stability of heart rate and blood pressure (Table 4). For women undergoing a hysterectomy, Nilsson et al. (56) infused 0.42 mg/kg of midazolam over 5 minutes, followed by an infusion rate of 125 μg/kg/hr. Alfentanil was initially injected in a dose of 75 μg/kg, followed by an infusion of 300 μg/kg/hr over 15 minutes, then a final infusion rate of 65 μg/kg/hr. Atracurium was used as the muscle relaxant.

If the patient is too drowsy after a midazolam/opioid TIVA or is not breathing adequately, I would first titrate 0.2 mg doses of flumazenil incrementally until 1 mg is given. If that does not produce satisfactory results, then naloxone in 40 μg increments should be given. As Smith and Pinnock (57) pointed out, it is better not to reverse analgesia because hyperdynamic responses can occur after naloxone that are not seen after flumazenil. In one study in which flumazenil was used by the titrated method to reverse midazolam/alfentanil TIVA (50) or midazolam/fentanyl TIVA (58), patients were awake or only slightly drowsy for 30 min-

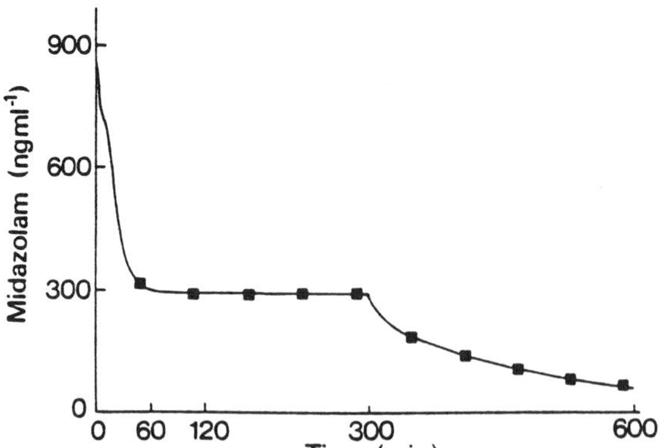

FIG. 10. Simulated concentration-time profile for midazolam after two consecutive infusion rates combined with a bolus injection. The bolus injection was 0.3 mg/kg, whereas the infusion rates were 0.68 mg/kg/hr for 15 min, followed by 0.125 mg/kg/hr over the next 285 min. (Data from Reves et al., ref. 54, with permission.)

TABLE 4. *Midazolam-fentanyl infusion scheme for cardiac surgery*

	Loading dose (μg/ml)		Maintenance dose (μg/kg/min)	
Time[a]	Midazolam	Fentanyl	Midazolam	Fentanyl
Pre-CPB	80	7	0.5	0.2
During CPB	—	—	0.4 ± 0.12	0.04
Post-CPB	—	—	0.52 ± 0.32	0.1 ± 0.07

Data from Reves et al., ref. 55, with permission.
[a] CPB = cardiopulmonary bypass.

utes and then residual drowsiness appeared and they became amnesic. Thus, to maintain complete reversal, it may be necessary to repeat flumazenil injections or give it by continuous infusion.

An etomidate infusion was designed to maintain unconsciousness and allow recovery about 10 minutes after stopping the infusion (59). Etomidate, 100 μg/kg/min, given for 3 minutes, was followed by 20 μg/kg/min for 27 minutes and by 10 μg/kg/min thereafter. Intermittent fentanyl, 50 to 150 μg, droperidol, 2.5 mg, and a muscle relaxant constituted the remainder of this TIVA regimen administered to healthy outpatients. Awakening and orientation occurred a mean of 9.3 minutes and 19.5 minutes, respectively, after the etomidate infusion was stopped; the plasma etomidate concentrations were 307 ± 76 ng/ml at awakening and 227 ± 80 ng/ml at orientation (Fig. 11). A similar etomidate infusion scheme, used for major gynecological surgery, resulted in awakening 17 minutes and orientation 30 minutes after the infusion stopped (60). Etomidate, 0.3 mg/kg, was injected over 45 seconds, and an etomidate infusion was started at a rate of 20 μg/kg/min. Fentanyl was initially given in a dose of 100 μg. A further dose of 200 μg was given before skin incision, and 50 μg increments were given as needed.

Jones et al. (61) administered an infusion of etomidate at a rate of 100 μg/kg/min and fentanyl at a rate of 1 μg/kg/min for 10 minutes before decreasing them both to one-tenth of this rate for maintenance of anesthesia. Recovery occurred less than 10 minutes after the infusion stopped in 50% of the patients. This dose regimen was satisfactory for 75% of the patients who underwent general or gynecological surgery.

When Lees et al. (62) combined 2.5 mg/ml of etomidate and 7 μg/ml of fentanyl and administered them as a single solution, patients occasionally had a prolonged recovery. This is not surprising because drug "cocktails" with fixed drug ratios have been undesirable since droperidol and fentanyl were combined as Innovar. Recovery is usually faster when the two drugs are titrated individually according to the patient's need (63).

Alfentanil and etomidate were successfully combined for TIVA for endolaryngeal microsurgery (64) and for open heart surgery (65). When etomidate/opiate combinations are unsatisfactory, the reason is the side effects of etomidate, including muscle movements, excitement phenomena, and prolonged nausea. Eto-

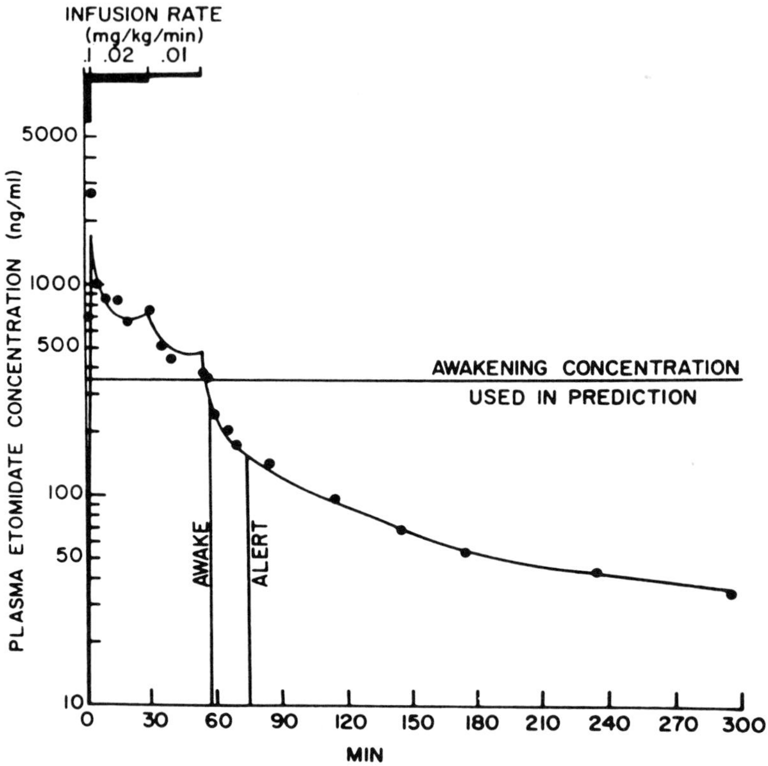

FIG. 11. Representative plasma etomidate concentration versus time relationship with the nonlinear regression line through the actual points during and after the infusion of etomidate for hypnosis in TIVA. The rates and durations of the infusion as well as the times and plasma concentrations at awakening and alertness are indicated. (Data from Fragen et al., ref. 59, with permission.)

midate infusions as a component of TIVA for surgical procedures is not associated with increased morbidity or mortality caused by adrenal cortical suppression.

Ketamine can be administered alone to provide both unconsciousness and analgesia for surgical procedures involving only somatic pain. It can be used alone or with a muscle relaxant added for TIVA while the patient breathes air/oxygen. The technique requires the addition of a benzodiazepine to prevent central nervous system or cardiovascular excitation from ketamine. Silvay et al. (66) premedicated patients who were scheduled for thoracic surgery using one-lung ventilation with 10–25 mg of diazepam by mouth and 0.4–0.6 mg of atropine intramuscularly 90 minutes before induction of anesthesia. The induction drugs were droperidol, 5–10 mg; diazepam, 10 mg; and ketamine, 2 mg/kg, administered intravenously. An infusion of 2 mg/kg/hr of ketamine was started, and muscle relaxation was provided with curare. Neither cardiovascular stimulation nor untoward emergence phenomena occurred, and anesthesia was satisfactory. When Silvay et al.

(67) compared propofol and ketamine infusions given with midazolam to pediatric patients undergoing cardiac catheterization, they found that the patients had shorter recovery times after propofol.

An IV anesthetic technique devised for military use combined 0.07 mg/kg of midazolam, 1 mg/kg of ketamine given 2 minutes later, and then 0.1 mg/kg of vecuronium (68). Midazolam, 5 mg; ketamine, 200 mg; and vecuronium, 12 mg, were added to a sufficient amount of 0.9% saline to reach a final volume of 50 ml. The infusion rate in milliliters per hour was calculated by dividing the body weight in kilograms by 2. This provided an infusion rate of 50 μg/kg/hr for midazolam, 2 mg/kg/hr for ketamine, and 120 μg/kg/hr for vecuronium. The infusion was stopped 10–15 minutes before the end of surgery. Patients breathed 35% oxygen in air. Although this technique is another example of an "anesthetic cocktail," it provided safe and fairly rapid recovery. Patients experience fewer postoperative emetic symptoms after a propofol TIVA than after a technique using ketamine (69).

Thiopental is not recommended for TIVA because of its slow metabolism, long elimination half-life, and long context-sensitive half-time. It is difficult to adjust the dose to provide an adequate level of unconsciousness yet have a safe recovery in the early postoperative period. Furthermore, no studies of TIVA using thiopental have been published.

Remember that dose schemes are only guidelines that provide starting points for titrating the drugs to each patient's needs. This review of TIVA protocols presents some of the available information. More is known now than when the first edition of this book was published. In 1991 an *International Symposium on Intravenous Anesthesia and Intensive Care Sedation* was held in Cannes, France. The proceedings of that symposium, including the 68 papers presented there, can be read by those interested in this subject (70). The Society of Intravenous Anesthesia became active in 1992 and now sponsors semiannual meetings: one held in the United States; the other held in Europe. These meetings and publications will disseminate information on specific techniques for various surgical procedures. They will increase with the introduction of more sophisticated and facile infusion pumps, new monitoring methods, and the results of studies on different drug combinations for TIVA and their effects on patients under various circumstances.

REFERENCES

1. Nunn JF, Surrock JE, Howell A. Effect of inhalational anesthetics on division of bone marrow cells in vitro. *Br J Anaesth* 1976;48:75–81.
2. Cohen EN, Brown BW, Bruce DL, et al. Occupational disease among operating personnel: a national study. *Anesthesiology* 1974;41:321–340.
3. Cook TL, Smith BA, Starkweather JA, Winter PM, Eger EI II. Behavioral effects of trace and subanesthetic halothane and nitrous oxide in man. *Anesthesiology* 1978;49:419–424.
4. Logan M, Farmer JG. Editorial I. Anaesthesia and the ozone layer.*Br J Anaesth* 1989;63:645–647.
5. Scheller MS, Zornow MH, Saidman LJ. Tracheal intubation without the use of muscle relaxants: a technique using propofol and varying doses of alfentanil. *Anesth Analg* 1992;75:788–793.

6. Shafer SL, Varvel JR. Pharmacokinetics, pharmacodynamics and rational opioid selection. *Anesthesiology* 1991;74:53–63.
7. Vuyk J, Lim T, Engbers FHM, Burm AGL, Vletter AA, Bovill JG. Pharmacodynamics of alfentanil as a supplement to propofol or nitrous oxide for lower abdominal surgery in female patients. *Anesthesiology* 1993;78:1036–1045.
8. Monk TG, Ding Y, White PF. Total intravenous anesthesia: effects of opioid versus hypnotic supplementation on autonomic responses and recovery. *Anesth Analg* 1992;75:798–804.
9. Schüttler J, Kloos S, Schwilden H, Stoeckel H. Total intravenous anaesthesia with propofol and alfentanil by computer assisted infusion. *Anaesthesia* 1988;43:2–7.
10. Gepts E, Jonckheer K, Maes V, Sonck W, Camu F. Disposition kinetics of propofol during alfentanil anesthesia. *Anaesthesia* 1988;43(Suppl):8–13.
11. Lemmens HJM, Burm AGL, Bovill JG, Hennis PJ. Phamacodynamics of alfentanil as a supplement to nitrous oxide anaesthesia in the elderly patient. *Br J Anaesth* 1988;61:173–179.
12. Ausems M, Hug CC, Stanski DR, Burm AGL. Plasma concentrations of alfentanil required to supplement nitrous oxide anesthesia for general surgery. *Anesthesiology* 1986;65:362–373.
13. Wessen A, Persson PM, Nilsson A, Hartvig P. Concentration-effect relationships of propofol after total intravenous anesthesia. *Anesth Analg* 1993;77:1000–1007.
14. Mercks L, Van Hemelrijck J, Van Aken H, Pelts C, Goffin J. Total intravenous anesthesia using propofol and alfentanil infusion in neurosurgical patients. *Anesthesiology* 1988;69:A576(abst).
15. Strebel S, Kaufmann M, Guardiola P-M, Shaefer H-G. Cerebral vasomotor responsiveness to carbon dioxide is preserved during propofol and midazolam anesthesia in humans. *Anesth Analg* 1994;78: 884–888.
16. De Grood PMRM, Mitsukuri S, Van Egmond J, Rutten JMJ, Crul JF. Comparison of etomidate and propofol for anaesthesia in microlaryngeal surgery. *Anaesthesia* 1987;42:366–372.
17. Reynecke CJ, James MFM, Johnson R. Alfentanil and propofol infusions for surgery in the burned patient. *Br J Anaesth* 1989;63:418–422.
18. Nightengale JJ, Lewis IH. Recovery from day-case anaesthesia: comparison of total I.V. anaesthesia using propofol with an inhalation technique. *Br J Anaesth* 1992;68:356–359.
19. Short TG, Aun CS T, Tan P, Wong J, Tam YH, Oh TE. A prospective evaluation of pharmacokinetic model controlled infusion of propofol in paediatric patients. *Br J Anaesth* 1994;72:302–306.
20. Marsh B, White M, Morton N, Kenny GNC. Pharmacokinetic model driven infusion of propofol in children. *Br J Anaesth* 1991;67:41–48.
21. Chaudhri S. White M, Kenney GNC. Induction of anaesthesia with propofol using a target-controlled infusion system. *Anaesthesia* 1992;47:551–553.
22. Jenstrup M, Fruergard K, Nielsen J, Moller A-M, Wilbert-Jorgensen F. Alfentanil infusions in total intravenous anaesthesia (TIVA). Population pharmacokinetics fails to predict plasma concentrations of alfentanil. *Acta Anaesthesiol Scand* 1992;36:846–847.
23. Raemer DB, Buschman A, Varvel JR, et al. The prospective use of population pharmacokinetics in a computer-driven infusion system for alfentanil. *Anesthesiology* 1990;73:66–72.
24. Scott JC, Stanski DR. Decreased fentanyl and alfentanil dose requirements with age: a simultaneous pharmacokinetic and pharmacodynamic evaluation. *J Pharm Exp Ther* 1987;240:159–166.
25. Maitre PO, Vozeh J, Heykants J, Thompson DA, Stanski DRI. Population pharmacokinetics of alfentanil: the average dose-plasma concentration relationship and interindividual variability in patients. *Anesthesiology* 1987;66:3–12.
26. Fragen RJ, Avram MJ, Henthorn TK, Asada A, Pemberton D, Correll T. Total intravenous anesthesia with propofol, alfentanil, and vecuronium for superficial surgery. *Anesth Analg* 1990;70:S112(abst).
27. Raftary S, Sherry E. Total intravenous anaesthesia with propofol and alfentanil protects against postoperative nausea and vomiting. *Can J Anaesth* 1992;39:37–40.
28. Fragen RJ, Randel GI, Librojo ES, Clarke MY, Jamerson BD. The interaction of remifentanil and propofol to prevent responses to tracheal intubation and the start of surgery for outpatient knee arthroscopy. *Anesthesiology* 1994;81:A376(abst).
29. Goldberg ME, Toyman M, Bartkowski RR, Mora CT, Boerner T, Seltzer JL. Time-course of respiratory depression after an alfentanil infusion based anesthetic. *Anesth Analg* 1992;75:965–971.
30. Taylor IN, Kenney GNC, Glen JB. Pharmacodynamic stability of a mixture of propofol and alfentanil. *Br J Anaesth* 1992;69:168–171.
31. Maurer WG, Kalhan S. Propofol and alfentanil mixture for outpatient surgery. *J Clin Anesth* 1994; 6:166–167.

32. Wilson RJT, Ridley SA. The use of propofol and alfentanil by infusion in military anaesthesia. *Anaesthesia* 1992;47:231–233.
33. Smith C, McEwan AI, Jhaveri R, et al. The interaction of fentanyl on the CP_{50} of propofol for loss of consciousness and skin incision. *Anesthesiology* 1994;81:820–828.
34. Vermeyen KM, DeHert SG, Erpels FA, Adriaensen HF. Myocardial metabolism during anaesthesia with propofol-low dose fentanyl for coronary artery bypass surgery. *Br J Anaesth* 1991;66:504–508.
35. Vermeyen KM, Erpels FA, Janssen LA, Beackman CP, Hanegreefs GH. Propofol-fentanyl anaesthesia for coronary bypass surgery in patients with good left ventricular function. *Br J Anaesth* 1987;59:1115–1120.
36. Leplage JM, Pinaud MC, Helias JH, et al. Left ventricular function during propofol and fentanyl anesthesia in patients with coronary artery disease: assessment with a radionuclide approach. *Anesth Analg* 1988;67:949–955.
37. Mora CT, Toriman M, White PF. Use of propofol during cardiac anesthesia-maintenance infusion rate and therapeutic blood levels. *Anesth Analg* 1990;70:S276(abst).
38. Russell GN, Wright EL, Fox MA, Douglas EJ, Cockshott ID. Propofol-fentanyl anaesthesia for coronary artery surgery and cardiopulmonary bypass. *Anaesthesia* 1989;44:205–208.
39. Billard V, Moulla R, Bourgoin JL, Negnigbeto A, Stanski DR. Hemodynamic response to induction and intubation. Propofol/fentanyl interaction. *Anesthesiology* 1994;81:1384–1392.
40. Todd MM, Warner DS, Sokoll MD, et al. A prospective, comparative trial of three anesthetics for elective supratentorial craniotomy: propofol/fentanyl, isoflurane/nitrous oxide, and fentanyl/nitrous oxide. *Anesthesiology* 1994;81:1384–1392.
41. Van Keer L, Van Aken H, Vandermeersch E, Vernaut G, Lerut T. Propofol does not inhibit hypoxic pulmonary vasoconstriction in humans. *J Clin Anesth* 1989;1:284–288.
42. O'Flaherty D, Pennant JH, Rao K, Gieseike AH. Total intravenous anesthesia with propofol for transsternal thymectomy in myasthenia gravis. *J Clin Anesth* 1992;4:241–244.
43. Monk TG, Boure B, White PF, Meretyk S, Clayman RV. Comparison of intravenous sedative-analgesic techniques for outpatient immersion lithotripsy. *Anesth Analg* 1991;72:616–621.
44. Galletly DC, Short TG. Total intravenous anesthesia using propofol infusion—50 consecutive cases. *Anaesth Intens Care* 1988;16:150–157.
45. Veselis RA, Reinsel RA, Geshchenko VA, et al. Impaired memory and behavioral performance with fentanyl at low plasma concentrations. *Anesth Analg* 1994;79:962–968.
46. Bernstein K, Wirpszo R, Djarv L. Anaesthesia with alfentanil and methohexitone for short gynecological surgery: a comparison with thiopentone/nitrous oxide. *Acta Anaesthesiol Scand* 1989;33:458–462.
47. Schwilden H, Schuttler J, Stoeckel H. Closed-loop feedback control of methohexitone anesthesia by quantitative EEG analysis in humans. *Anesthesiology* 1987;67:344–347.
48. Vinik HR. Midazolam infusions: introduction and overview. In: Vinik HR, ed. *Midazolam infusion for anesthesia and intensive care.* Princeton, NJ: Excerpta Medica; 1989:1–9.
49. Bailey PL, Pace NL, Ashburn MA, Moll JWB, East KA, Stanley TH. Frequent hypoxemia and apnea after sedation with midazolam and fentanyl. *Anesthesiology* 1990;73:826–830.
50. Nilsson A, Persson MP. Total intravenous anesthesia—is there a future for midazolam. *Acta Anesthesiol Scand* 1988;32(Suppl):6–10.
51. Vinik HR, Bradley EL Jr, Kissen I. Midazolam-alfentanil synergism for anesthetic induction in patients. *Anesth Analg* 1989;69:213–217.
52. Ben-Shlomo I, Abd-el-Khalim H, Ezry J, Zohar S, Tverskoy M. Midazolam acts synergistically with fentanyl for induction of anaesthesia. *Br J Anaesth* 1990;64:45–47.
53. Nilsson A, Persson MP, Hartvig P. Effects of the benzodiazepine antagonist flumazenil on postoperative performance following total intravenous anesthesia with midazolam and alfentanil. *Acta Anaesthesiol Scand* 1988;32:441–446.
54. Persson P, Nilsson A, Hartvig P, Tamsen A. Pharmacokinetics of midazolam in total IV anaesthesia. *Br J Anaesth* 1987;59:548–556.
55. Reves JG, Jacobs J, Croughwell ND, Smith LR. Continuous infusion of midazolam and fentanyl during cardiopulmonary bypass. In: Vinik HR, ed. *Midazolam infusions for anesthesia and intensive care.* Princeton, NJ: Excerpta Medica; 1989:10–13.
56. Nilsson A, Tamsen A, Persson MP. Atracurium infusion in total intravenous anesthesia. *Acta Anaesthesiol Scand* 1987;31:205–207.
57. Smith G, Pinnock C. Naloxone—paradox or panacea? *Br J Anaesth* 1985;57:547–549.

58. Klausen NO, Juhl O, Sorenson J, Ferguson AH, Neuman PB. Flumazenil in total intravenous anaesthesia using midazolam and fentanyl. *Acta Anaesthesiol Scand* 1988;32:409–412.
59. Fragen RJ, Avram MJ, Henthorn TK, Caldwell NJ. A pharmacokinetically designed etomidate infusion regimen for hypnosis. *Anesth Analg* 1983;62:654–660.
60. Rocke DA, Rubin J, Brock-Utne JG, Downey JW. Total intravenous anesthesia for major gynaecologic surgery. *Anaesth intens Care* 1981;9:119–123.
61. Jones K, Laurence AS, Thornton JA. Total intravenous anesthesia with etomidate-fentanyl: use in general and gynecological surgery. *Anaesthesia* 1983;38:29–39.
62. Lees NW, Glasser J, McGroarty FL, Miller BM. Etomidate and fentanyl for maintenance of anaesthesia. *Br J Anaesth* 1981; 53:959–961.
63. Lees NW, Antonios WRA. Two-stage infusion of etomidate for the induction and maintenance of anaesthesia. *Br J Anaesth* 1984;56:1239–1242.
64. Versichelen L, Rolly G, Beerens J. Alfentanil/etomidate anesthesia for endolaryngeal microsurgery. *Anaesthesia* 1983;38:57–60.
65. Oduro A, Tonnlinson AA, Voice A, Dawes GK. The use of etomidate infusions during anaesthesia for cardiopulmonary bypass. *Anaesthesia* 1983;38:66–69.
66. Silvay G, Weinrich AI, Lumb P, Shiang H. Continuous infusion of ketamine for thoracic surgery using one-lung ventilation. In: Adrete JA, Stanley TH, eds. *Trends in intravenous anesthesia.* Chicago: Year Book Medical Publishers; 1980:355–363.
67. Lebovic S, Reich DL, Steinberg LG, Vela FP, Silvay G. Comparsion of propofol versus ketamine for anesthesia in pediatric patients undergoing cardiac catheterization. *Anesth Analg* 1992;74:490–494.
68. Restall J, Tully AM, Ward PJ, Kidd AG. Total intravenous anesthesia for military surgery: a technique using ketamine, midazolam, and vecuronium. *Anaesthesia* 1988;43:46–49.
69. Baillie R, Craig C, Restall J. Total intravenous anesthesia for laparoscopy. *Anesthesia* 1989;44:60–63.
70. Prys-Roberts C. *Focus on infusion: intravenous anaesthesia.* London, UK: Current Medical Literature Ltd; 1991.

Drug Infusions in Anesthesiology, Second Edition,
edited by R. J. Fragen. Lippincott-Raven Publishers,
Philadelphia © 1996.

7

Infusions for the Management of Postoperative and Labor Pain

Honorio T. Benzon

Department of Anesthesia, Northwestern University Medical School, Chicago, Illinois 60611

Significant advances in postoperative pain management have been made in the last 15 years. These advances include the discovery of opiate receptors and the analgesic efficacy of intraspinal opioids and other drugs, the use of patient-controlled analgesia (PCA), and the clinical application of preemptive analgesia. The methodology used in clinical studies on postoperative pain management has generally been exemplary: Most studies have been prospective, randomized, and double blind. Studies on intrathecal neostigmine are just appearing. There is no doubt that further advances are coming.

PREEMPTIVE ANALGESIA TO REDUCE POSTOPERATIVE PAIN

"Windup" Phenomenon

The activation of C fibers from tissue injury evokes the release of transmitters from C-afferent terminals, including glutamate and certain peptides such as substance P and calcitonin gene-related peptide (1–3). This leads to depolarization of several neurons in the dorsal horn of the spinal cord, the response of which is proportional to the intensity of the stimulus. When there is a repetitive afferent barrage of C fibers, some dorsal horn neurons exhibit an exaggerated response to a given stimulus. This enhanced spinal cord response to subsequent afferent nociceptive input is called "windup," "neural plasticity," or "spinal sensitization" (4). Subsequent afferent inputs lead to an exaggerated response and an increase in the size of the receptive field (5,6).

The results of electrophysiological and behavioral animal studies support the windup phenomenon. An irritant injected into the paw of a rat causes an acute burst of C-fiber activity for about 10 minutes followed by low levels of afferent traffic for an extended period (7). In the unanesthetized animal, the procedure evokes an initial transient appearance of pain behavior corresponding to the initial C-fiber activity. This is followed by a second phase of behavior, the magnitude of which exceeds that predicted by the modest C-fiber activity recorded at that time (8,9). This discrepancy between the amount of afferent traffic and the degree of behavior is considered to reflect an exaggerated state of afferent processing. The neural and behavioral changes from the high-intensity electrical stimulation of skin nociceptors persist even when inputs from the injured region are later blocked by local anesthesia (10–12) or are interrupted by nerve section (13–15) or dorsal rhizotomy (16).

Physiologic and behavioral studies in animals show that noxious-stimulus-induced spinal sensitization can be prevented or "preempted" by the administration of analgesic or anesthetic agents before the injury. Bathing peripheral nerves in a local anesthetic solution before nerve transection reduced the incidence of pain behaviors seen after neurectomies (17,18). Pretreatment with μ-opioid receptor agonists (19,20) or local anesthetic (21) prevented the development of injury-induced spinal neuroplasticity (19,20) and pain-related behaviors (rats favoring, licking, biting, or shaking their paw) (21). Treatment was less effective when administered a few minutes after establishing the pain behaviors (19–21). For example, the dose of systemically administered morphine needed to prevent central hyperexcitability before a brief noxious electrical stimulation of the gastrocnemius-soleus nerve was one-tenth the dose required to abolish the prolonged activity once it developed (19).

Clinical Studies

Two publications in 1988 spurred clinical studies on preemptive analgesia. In a study of 929 patients who underwent orthopedic procedures, McQuay et al. (22) found that the use of a regional nerve block (e.g., spinal, epidural, axillary block, ankle block) and the use of opiate premedication reduced the time to first analgesic (TFA) request and increased the percentage of patients who did not require a postoperative analgesic. In the second study, Bach et al. (23) found that the use of epidural bupivacaine, with or without morphine, for 72 hours before limb amputation reduced the incidence of phantom limb pain.

Several publications have appeared since the studies of McQuay et al. (22) and Bach et al. (23). Several comments are relevant before discussing these studies. First, the concept of preemptive analgesia is always in the context of the presence of anesthesia (4). Second, general anesthesia, as it is practiced today, fails to alter the hyperalgesic component greatly because the smallest dose of anesthetic that is consistent with patient safety is given and immobility is produced by muscle relaxants given intraoperatively (4,24,25). In this situation, the lightly anesthetized spinal cord receives an afferent barrage of impulses produced during surgery (24). Under spinal or epidural anesthesia, the spinal cord does not receive such afferent impulses. Third, the drugs that are advocated for preemptive analgesia are effective in blocking spinal neuroplasticity, not because they are analgesic or anesthetic agents, but because they prevent the transmission of nociceptive impulses to the spinal cord or the release of transmitters that leads to the subsequent state of facilitated processing. Indeed, N-methyl-D-aspartic acid antagonists, which have little analgesic activity, block windup because of their ability to block afferent transmitter release that yields the facilitated state (26,27). Fourth, Kehlet and Dahl (28) stated that "clinical evidence of the value of preemptive analgesia must come from studies comparing the same treatment before and after the surgery." Only six studies, two on nonsteroidal antiinflammatory drugs (NSAIDs) (29,30) and four on nerve blocks (31–34) fulfill Kehlet and Dahl's criteria.

Clinical studies on preemptive analgesia can be categorized into preoperative opiate administration, preincisional local anesthetic infiltration, and preincisional nerve block/opioid administration.

Preincisional Administration of Opiates or Nonsteroidal Antiinflammatory Drugs

Two studies compared the use of opiate premedication versus no premedication. As previously mentioned, McQuay et al. (22) noted that the use of opiate premedication lengthened the interval to the first analgesic (TFA) request from less than 2 hours to 5 hours (22). This study was criticized because selection of the anesthetic technique was not randomized (4) and patients with different pain intensities such as that occurring after bunionectomy and laminectomy were grouped together. Another study showed that premedication with meperidine increased the average TFA from 219 minutes to 351 minutes in patients who had a laminectomy (35). These two studies cannot be used as an argument for the effectiveness of preemptive analgesia because there was no "postemptive" group: i.e., the same treatment was not given after the surgical incision (36)."

The two studies that looked at the preoperative use of NSAIDs showed no preemptive effect for either paracetamol (29) or diflunisal (30) in oral surgery. The paracetamol study was a randomized, double-blind, placebo-controlled, crossover study in patients who had their impacted wisdom teeth removed. The TFA interval, 4.5 hours versus 4.8 hours, and the mean pain intensity up to the TFA were similar between the two groups (29). The diflunisal study also showed no difference in pain intensity for 8 hours after removal of impacted third molars when diflunisal was given before the surgery compared to when given postoperatively (30). The lack of preemptive analgesic effect of NSAIDs may be the result of delayed release of antiinflammatory mediators: e.g., prostaglandins do not peak until 4 hours after surgical trauma (30).

Preincisional Infiltration of Local Anesthetics

Tverskoy et al. (37) showed that general anesthesia plus local anesthetic infiltration along the line of a proposed herniorrhaphy incision resulted in lower intensity of postoperative pain than did spinal or general anesthesia. Another study showed that preincisional infiltration of the tonsils with bupivacaine before tonsillectomy resulted in lower intensities of postoperative pain when compared with preincisional saline infiltration (38). On the basis of Kehlet and Dahl's criteria (28), these two studies do not support preemptive analgesia since there was no "postemptive" group.

In two studies using a preincisional local anesthetic, the same treatment was given before and after the incision (31,32), thus fulfilling Kehlet and Dahl's criteria. Both studies compared preincisional versus postincisional lidocaine infiltration in patients undergoing inguinal herniorraphy. Ejlersen et al. (31) showed a longer TFA, 3.75 hours versus 2.75 hours, and statistically fewer patients who asked for a supplementary analgesic (58% versus 94%) in the preemptive group. In contradistinction, Dierking et al. (32) showed no difference in visual analogue pain scores (VAS), verbal pain scores at rest and during mobilization, TFA, and total morphine consumption between the two groups. The different results of Ejlersen et al. and Dierking et al. are difficult to explain. While Yaksh (4) thought that the difference in the results was caused by the small amount of alfentanil given in the control group in Dierking et al.'s study, Kehlet and Dahl (28) thought the small opioid dose should make no difference. In addition, no well-defined criterion such as PCA was used to assess postoperative opioid requirements in Ejlersen et al.'s study (31).

Therefore, preincisional local anesthetic infiltration does not reliably produce preemptive analgesia. One possible explanation is that the duration of surgery outlasts the duration of the effect of lidocaine and that the transmission of nociceptive input continues after the effect of the preincisional lidocaine is gone. Alternatively, the local anesthetic may not block the nociceptive impulses completely (39).

Preoperative Administration of Nerve Block and Epidural Opioids

McQuay et al. (22) showed a longer TFA and fewer patients requiring analgesics when a nerve block was utilized for anesthesia. Bach et al. (23) noted a lower incidence of phantom limb pain when preoperative epidural local anesthetic plus morphine was given before limb amputation. There was no control or "postemptive" group in these studies.

Two studies have preemptive and "postemptive" groups. In one study, the epidural injection of bupivacaine before major abdominal surgery did not result in lower VAS at rest, during mobilization, and during coughing, compared with the same treatment given during closure of the surgical wound (33). Furthermore, the number of patients who received additional morphine was similar between the two groups. Therefore, there appears to be no preemptive effect of epidural bupivacaine. In this study, however, 0.75% bupivacaine was used in the preemptive bolus, whereas 0.25% bupivacaine was used during the intraoperative epidural infusion.

The 0.25% concentration may be inadequate to block all the nociceptive impulses during surgery. Such incomplete block of impulses during epidural anesthesia was documented using somatosensory evoked potential monitoring (40).

Another study compared epidural fentanyl given before a thoracotomy with that given after a thoracotomy incision (34). The preemptive group required less postoperative analgesic at the 6-hour postoperative period and lower patient-controlled morphine consumption between the 12 hour and 24 hour postoperative periods. Although mildly suggestive of preemptive analgesia, the study was questioned by Kehlet and Dahl (28) because a significant difference was found only at the 6-hour assessment and not at the other assessment times (2-, 4-, 12-, 24-, and 48-hr assessments). The patients in the preemptive group with decreased opioid consumption were also older. In this study, the epidural catheter was placed at the lumbar level. The preemptive effect of the preoperative epidural fentanyl may have been marked if the authors had placed their epidural catheter at the thoracic level. In addition, epidural opioids should have been infused continuously during surgery because nociceptive impulses continue to reach the spinal cord during surgery, after the effect of epidural fentanyl is gone.

Multimodal Analgesia Before Surgery

A double-blind, "placebo"-controlled study compared intramuscular (IM) morphine, IM perphenazine, and rectal indomethazine with IM midazolam and a placebo rectal suppository. After induction, the preemptive group had intercostal nerve blocks with bupivacaine while the control group received placebo blocks (41). The VAS scores at rest and after movement were similar between the two groups at any postoperative time evaluation. The treatment group required less morphine during the first 6 hours after the operation but greater amounts on the second and third days after surgery. Postoperative carbon dioxide values and the percentage changes in the forced vital capacity (FVC) and forced expiratory volume in 1 second (FEV1) were similar between the two groups.

Summary of Studies

Laboratory studies support the phenomenon of preemptive analgesia. Clinical studies, on the other hand, are not consistent in their results. Preoperative NSAIDs do not decrease the pain after oral surgery (29,30), and preincisional infiltration of local anesthetic does not reliably decrease postoperative pain (31,32). Epidural bupivacaine does not exhibit preemptive analgesia (33), whereas epidural opioids may, especially if administered segmentally (34). Finally, the combination of opiate premedication, an NSAID, and a nerve block does not result in decreased pain after surgery (41). These results are summarized in Table 1.

TABLE 1. *Effect of preemptive analgesia on postoperative pain*

Study (ref.)	Drug	Surgery	Effect[a]
I. *Preincisional opiate/NSAID administration*			
McQuay et al. (22)	Opioid	Orthopedic	Longer TFA, less analgesic
Kiss et al. (35)	Meperidine	Laminectomy	Longer TFA
Sisk et al. (30)	Diflunisal	Impacted teeth	None
Gustaffsson et al. (29)	Paracetamol	Impacted teeth	None
II. *Preincisional local anesthetic infiltration*			
Ejlersen et al. (31)	Lidocaine	Herniorrhaphy	Longer TFA, less analgesic
Dierking et al. (32)	Lidocaine	Herniorrhaphy	None
Tverskoy et al. (37)	Bupivacaine	Herniorrhaphy	Less pain
Jebeles et al. (38)	Bupivacaine	Tonsillectomy	Less pain
III. *Preoperative nerve block/opioid*			
McQuay et al. (22)	Block/local anesthetic	Orthopedic	Longer TFA
Bach et al. (23)	Epidural/bupivacaine, morphine	Amputation	Less phantom pain
Katz et al. (34)	Epidural/fentanyl	Thoracotomy	Less pain, less analgesic[b]
Dahl et al. (36)	Epidural bupivacaine	Abdominal	None
IV. *Multimodal analgesia*			
Kavanagh et al. (41)	IM morphine IM perphenazine Rectal indomethacin Intercostal bupivacaine	Thoracotomy	None

[a] TFA = time to first analgesic.
[b] Less pain at 6 hours after surgery and less patient-controlled morphine usage between 12–24 hours after surgery.

PATIENT-CONTROLLED ANALGESIA

Variability of Blood Levels and Analgesic Responses from Multiple Intramuscular Opioid Injections

Intramuscular (IM) opioid injections given at fixed intervals result in variable blood levels and inconsistent analgesia. This variability is secondary to erratic absorption from the site of injection (42). Intra- and interpatient opioid blood concentrations after an im injection vary from two- to fivefold and the time to reach peak blood concentations varies three- to sevenfold respectively (43).

PCA is a technique wherein patients can medicate themselves through a device consisting of an electronically controlled infusion pump connected to a timing device. When patients experience pain, they trigger the device by pressing a button located on the end of a cord extending from the machine. The machine then delivers a preset amount of drug into the patient's indwelling IV catheter. A timer in the machine is programmed to prevent administration of additional doses until a specific time period has elapsed.

PCA eliminates the unpredictable absorption of the analgesic from the injection site and bypasses the unavoidable delays that occur when an analgesic is requested. These delays include the slow response of a very busy nurse, screening the appropriateness of the request, signing out and preparing the drug, and finally, injecting the analgesic. With PCA, patients titrate their analgesic needs against the side effect tolerability of the given drug (44).

An ideal analgesic for PCA has a rapid onset of analgesic action, a high analgesic efficacy, no ceiling effect, and an intermediate duration of action (45). Morphine and meperidine satisfy most of these characteristics and are the most widely used drugs. Methadone and buprenorphine have long durations of action, whereas fentanyl is too short acting. The agonist-antagonist drugs have a ceiling analgesic effect, which limits their effectiveness. The guidelines for bolus doses, lock-out intervals, and continuous infusion rates for the various analgesics are listed in Table 2 (46).

Movement-associated pain is least severe with morphine (47,48) and most severe with meperidine (48). Both morphine and meperidine have a slow onset of resting analgesia, but the pain usually decreases after 4 hours with morphine and within 16 hours after meperidine (48). Oxymorphone has a rapid analgesic onset and is effective for both rest- and movement-associated pain. However, it is not as effective as morphine for prolonged use and is associated with a higher incidence of nausea and vomiting (48).

The addition of a basal opioid infusion to PCA, recommended to decrease the trough in morphine plasma concentrations during PCA use, is controversial. A basal infusion rate of morphine does not decrease resting pain but reduces move-

TABLE 2. *Guidelines regarding the bolus doses, lock-out intervals, and continuous infusions for various parenteral analgesics when using a patient-controlled analgesia system*

Drug	Bolus dose (mg)	Lock-out interval (min)	Continuous infusion ($mg \cdot hr^{-1}$)
Agonists			
Fentanyl citrate	0.015–0.05	3–10	0.02–0.1
Hydromorphone hydrochloride	0.10–0.5	5–15	0.2–0.5
Meperidine hydrochloride	5–15	5–15	5–40
Methadone hydrochloride	0.50–3.0	10–20	–
Morphine sulphate	0.50–3.0	10–20	1–10
Oxymorphone hydrochloride	0.20–0.8	5–15	0.1–1
Sufentanil citrate	0.003–0.015	3–10	0.004–0.03
Agonist — Antagonists			
Buprenorphine hydrochloride	0.03–0.2	10–20	–
Nalbupine hydrochloride	1–5	5–15	1–8
Pentazocine hydrochloride	5–30	5–15	6–40

Adapted from Lubenow et al., ref. 46, with permission.

ment-associated pain after cesarean section (49). A basal infusion of oxymorphone significantly reduces VAS scores associated with rest and movement but results in a high incidence of nausea and vomiting (49).

The addition of a nighttime basal opioid infusion did not improve patients' ability to sleep or rest comfortably. Postoperative scores for pain, sedation, fatique, discomfort, and anxiety were the same whether or not a nighttime basal infusion was added (50). The number of patient demands, supplemental bolus doses, opioid usage, and side effects were also the same. Most important, numerous programming errors were noted with the addition of a basal infusion. There was also no advantage of a background opioid infusion with epidural PCA. Patients who had a basal infusion of sufentanil consumed significantly higher amounts of the opioid, had the same number of additional analgesic demands, had higher sedation scores, and had identical VAS scores as did the patients receiving only incremental sufentanil doses (51).

EPIDURAL ADMINISTRATION OF OPIOIDS

Epidural Injections

The existence and pharmacology of spinal opiate receptors provide an attractive possibility of achieving regional analgesia with intraspinal opioid injections. Opioids were initially injected intrathecally, but a high incidence of respiratory depression caused a switch to an epidural technique.

The latency and duration of postoperative analgesia with the different epidural opioids are listed in Table 3 (52). Morphine was the first opioid used, and its efficacy and safety are established. In Reddy et al.'s (53) experience of 11,089 individual morphine injections given to 1,106 patients, no infections, neurologic in-

TABLE 3. *Epidural opioids: Latency and duration of postoperative analgesia*

		Analgesic effect			Continuous infusion	
Agent (ml·hr^{-1})	Bolus dose	Onset (min)	Peak (min)	Duration (hr)	Concentration	Rate
Meperidine	30–100 mg	5 – 10	12 – 30	4 – 6	—	—
Morphine	5 mg	24 ± 6	30 – 60	12 – 24	0.01%	1 – 6
Methadone	5 mg	12 ± 2	17 ± 3	7 ± 5	—	—
Hydromorphone	1 mg	13 ± 4	23 ± 8	11 ± 6	0.005%	6 – 8
Fentanyl	100 μg	4 – 10	20	3 ± 6	0.001%	4 – 12
Diamorphine	5 mg	5	9 – 15	12 ± 6	—	—
Sufentanil	30–50 μg	7 ± 6	26 ± 8	4 ± 7	0.0001%	10
Alfentanil	15 μg·kg^{-1}	15	—	1 – 2	—	—

juries, or deaths occurred. Catheter-related problems were minor and occurred in only 5% of their patients.

Intraspinal opioid administration causes pruritus, nausea and vomiting, urinary retention, and respiratory depression. Respiratory depression is the most feared complication, and its incidence ranges from 0.09% (53) to 0.2% (54). This is similar to the incidence of 0.9% seen after orally or parenterally administered opioids (53).

Epidural Infusions

A continuous infusion of epidural morphine, in contrast to intermittent injections, effectively reduces postoperative pain with minimal side effects (55). Epidural fentanyl infusions, compared with morphine infusions, provide comparable analgesia with a lower incidence of nausea and pruritus (56). Therefore epidural fentanyl infusions became popular. Fentanyl, 100 μg (1–1.5 μg/kg), is usually given 30–45 minutes before the end of the surgery, and an infusion is started when the patient arrives in the recovery room. In terms of its onset, analgesic efficacy, and side effects, the ideal concentration of fentanyl is 10 μg/ml (57).

Use of Local Anesthetics

Laboratory studies show synergistic analgesic effects when combinations of opioids and local anesthetics are given intrathecally. This synergism was demonstrated whether the opioid was given at the same time as the local anesthetic (58) or before (59). These studies support the clinical practice of adding bupivacaine to the epidural fentanyl infusion, theoretically to improve analgesia, reduce the amount infused, and decrease side effects. However, this practice is now controversial because the results of clinical studies with these combinations are not uniform. These studies compared the opioid/local anesthetic combination to the local anesthetic alone, the combination versus the opioid alone, or all three.

Clinical studies comparing the combination with the local anesthetic alone found superior analgesia when the two drugs were combined (60–65). There was better pain relief (60,63,65), a shorter onset of analgesia (64), and a longer duration of analgesia (60,61,64) and lower local anesthetic concentrations could be used (62).

Studies that compared epidural opioids, epidural local anesthetics, and the drug combination had different results. One study showed better analgesia with the opioid, local anesthetic, and the combination compared to epidural saline or no epidural catheter, but the investigators did not comment on the difference in analgesia among the opioid, the local anesthetic, or the combination (66). Another study showed superiority of the combination compared to the local anesthetic but showed no difference between the combination and the opioid alone (67). A third study demonstrated superior analgesia when the drugs were combined (68).

Studies that compared the combination with the epidural opioid alone also had different results (69–76). Several studies showed no advantage of the combination (69,70,73,74), whereas others showed some benefit (71,72,75,76). The advantages, however, were noted only on discharge from the recovery room (76), on the first (71) or second (76) postoperative day, or during some but not all of the observation periods (75). A prospective, randomized, double-blind study showed that the addition of 0.1%, 0.15%, or 0.2% bupivacaine did not improve the analgesia from an epidural fentanyl infusion in patients who underwent major abdominal or genitourinary surgery (77). Therefore, the routine addition of low-dose bupivacaine is not recommended.

Efficacy of Epidural Versus Intravenous Infusions

When inordinately high infusion rates of epidural fentanyl are needed to maintain adequate pain relief, some investigators theorize that the predominant mechanism of the analgesic effect of the epidural fentanyl infusion is systemic in nature. Several studies showed that epidural or intravenous (IV) opioid infusions were equally effective after knee surgery (78), cesarean section (79), hysterectomy (80), intraabdominal surgery (81), and thoracotomy (82). Both the infusion rates that produced the same levels of analgesia and the plasma opioid concentrations were similar in both the epidural and IV groups (78). However, some of these investigations studied only women, and the operations that the patients underwent were not particularly painful (78,79). Some questions also have been raised about the other studies. One study found that three patients in the IV group had inadequate pain relief and excluded them from their statistical analysis (79). In another study, although the VAS scores were similar between the two groups, there was a 25% reduction of the mean total morphine requirements and a lower incidence of drowsiness in the epidural group (81). A third study found equal analgesic efficacy between the two routes in the patients who had thoracotomy; in this study, the epidural catheter was inserted at the lumbar vertebral level (82).

Other studies showed superior efficacy of the epidural over the IV route (83–85). They dealt with more painful operations such as major abdominal surgery (83) and thoracotomy (84,85). The superiority of the epidural opioid infusion included significant reduction of the fentanyl requirements (83,84), decreased drowsiness (79,81,86), earlier onset of bowel function, better postoperative pulmonary function, and shorter hospital stay (85). The divergent results of the different studies are difficult to explain (Table 4). Possibly, the analgesic superiority of the epidural route is demonstrated only in more painful procedures (83–85).

The different results of the studies that compared epidural with IV fentanyl infusions after thoracotomy may be attributable to the vertebral level of insertion of the epidural catheter. Placement of the epidural catheter at the lumbar level resulted in comparable analgesia and a similar time course for plasma fentanyl concentrations (82). Placement of the catheter at the thoracic level resulted in lower

TABLE 4. *Comparison of epidural with intravenous opioids for postoperative pain*

Study (ref.)	Type of study[a]	Type of surgery	Routes compared[b]	Drugs used	Superior technique
Loper et al. (78)	R, DB	Knee	LE vs. IV	Fentanyl	Equal
Ellis et al. (79)	R, DB	Cesarean section	LE vs. IV	Fentanyl	Equal
Camu et al. (80)	R	Hysterectomy	LE vs. IV	Alfentanil	Equal
Miguel et al. (81)	R, DB	Abdominal	LE vs. IV	Sufentanil	Equal
Sandler et al. (82)	R, DB	Thoracotomy	LE vs. IV	Fentanyl	Equal
Geller et al. (83)	R, DB	Abdominal	LE vs. IV	Sufentanil (LE,IV), Fentanyl (LE)	Epidural
Salomaki et al. (84)	R, DB	Thoracotomy	TE vs. IV	Fentanyl	Epidural
Guinard et al. (85)	R	Thoracotomy	LE vs. TE vs. IV	Fentanyl	TE
Benzon et al. (86)	R, DB	Thoracotomy	TE vs. PCA	Fentanyl (TE), morphine (PCA)	Epidural
Grant et al. (88)	R, DB	Thoracotomy	LE vs. PCA	Fentanyl	Epidural
Allaire et al. (89)	R	RRP	LE vs. PCA	Fentanyl (LE), morphine (PCA)	Epidural
Chauvin et al. (90)	R	Abdominal	LE PCA vs. IV PCA	Alfentanil	Equal[b]
Glass et al. (92)	R, DB, C	Lower extremity, abdominal	LE PCA vs. IV PCA	Fentanyl	Equal

Adapted from HT Benzon. In: PP Raj, ed. *Comprehensive Review Book for Pain Medicine.* Chicago: Mosby Year Book; 1995, with permission.

[a]C, crossover; DB, double blind; IV, intravenous; LE, lumbar epidural; PCA, patient-controlled analgesia; R, randomized; RRP, radical retropubic prostatectomy; TE, thoracic epidural.

[b]Total alfentanil dose was higher in the IV PCA group.

infusion rates and lower plasma fentanyl concentrations than was the case with the IV technique (84). Simultaneous comparison of the lumbar (L4–5) epidural, thoracic (T4–5) epidural, and IV routes of a fentanyl infusion showed no difference in the quality of analgesia and the amount of fentanyl delivered between the three routes (85). Patients who had the thoracic epidural fentanyl infusion, however, had an earlier onset of bowel function, better postoperative forced vital capacity and FEV1, and a shorter hospital stay than did patients anesthetized by the other two routes. These results support the suggestion that highly soluble opioids should be administered at the dermatomal region of the surgical incision (87).

The epidural technique is superior to IV PCA in more painful and extensive operations. Patients who underwent thoracotomy had lower VAS (86) or required lower infusion rates to attain the same degree of analgesia (88). Patients who underwent radical retropubic prostatectomy had better pain relief (89), whereas patients who underwent major abdominal surgery (90) or cesarean section (91) required significantly less opioid. One study showed that the efficacy of the two

TABLE 5. *Lumbar versus thoracic epidural placement for postthoracotomy epidural analgesia*

Study (ref.)	Type of study	Drug used	Comparative efficacy
Guinard et al. (85)	randomized	fentanyl, infusion	equal[a]
Fromme et al. (93)	retrospective	morphine, intermittent	equal
Coe et al. (94)	randomized, blinded	fentanyl, infusion	equal[b]
Hurford et al. (95)	randomized	fentanyl with bupivacaine, infusion	equal[c]

Adapted from HT Benzon. In: *Comprehensive Review Book for Pain Medicine.* Chicago: Mosby Year Bcok; 1995, with permission.

[a] Patients in the thoracic group had earlier recovery of gastrointestinal and pulmonary functions and had shorter hospital stays.

[b] Total fentanyl requirement was higher in the lumbar group.

[c] Higher infusion rates were needed in the lumbar group to attain comparable analgesia.

routes was equal, but the small number of patients and the preponderance of less painful lower-extremity surgeries (92) may explain the lack of superiority of the epidural technique.

Lumbar Versus Thoracic Placement of the Catheter

Studies that directly compared lumbar with thoracic epidural catheter placement in thoracotomies found conflicting results. A retrospective study found lumbar placement to be as effective as thoracic placement (93). Prospective studies found significantly lower rates of fentanyl infusion but not significantly lower pain scores in the thoracic group (94,95). A randomized study comparing thoracic and lumbar epidural placements in thoracotomy showed equivalent analgesia and similar requirements for fentanyl (85). Patients receiving thoracic epidural fentanyl had earlier recovery of gastrointestinal and pulmonary functions and a shorter hospital stay (Table 5).

Outcome Studies

Most outcome studies result in better pain relief, decreased postoperative morbidity, and shortened hospital stays after the postoperative administration of epidural opioids. Compared to IM morphine, the intermittent administration of epidural morphine reduced hospital stay after gastroplasty from 9 days to 7 days (96). Hospital stays were shorter when a thoracic epidural fentanyl infusion was used after thoracotomy (85) and a shorter stay in the intensive care unit among patients who underwent major vascular surgery (97). Lower complication rates occurred in high-risk patients when epidural anesthesia and postoperative epidural analgesia were used (98). Another study confirmed better pain relief and better postoperative pulmonary function with postoperative epidural opioid analgesia but showed no reduction of pulmonary complications or shortened hospital stays (99).

CONTINUOUS INTRAPLEURAL INFUSIONS

The mechanism of action of intrapleural analgesia is not completely understood. Since the initial report of its use (100), numerous publications have described its use, mostly after thoracotomy. An indwelling epidural catheter is placed intrapleurally, and the local anesthetic is injected intermittently (101–108) or by continuous infusion (109–111). For continuous infusion, an initial bolus of 3 mg/kg of 2% lidocaine or 15–20 ml of 0.5% bupivacaine is injected. This is followed by an infusion of 1 mg/kg/hr of 2% lidocaine or 0.23–0.33 mg/kg/hr (5–10 ml/hr) of 0.25% bupivacaine. The local anesthetic should contain epinephrine to reduce systemic absorption of the anesthetic drug. The blood levels of the local anesthetic may reach a toxic range (109,110) and a significant amount may be lost in the thoracotomy drainage (109). The absence of thoracotomy drainage may lead to reduced clearance and potentially toxic levels of the local anesthetic (110). Of the three studies on continuous infusions, only one found them to be effective (111). The other two studies found that analgesia was inadequate and did not recommended this technique after thoracotomy (109,110).

AHCPR GUIDELINES FOR MANAGEMENT OF POSTOPERATIVE PAIN

Clinical practice guidelines for the management of acute pain have been published by the Agency for Health Care Policy and Research of the U.S. Department of Health and Human Services (112). One of the agency's recommendations is that mild-to-moderate postoperative pain should be managed initially with an NSAID. NSAIDs produce analgesia by decreasing levels of inflammatory mediators at the site of tissue injury. They do not cause drowsiness or respiratory depression and do not interfere with bowel or bladder function. The administration of 10 mg of oral ketorolac after gynecologic surgery was found to be comparable to 60 mg of codeine plus 600 mg acetaminophen in terms of analgesia (113). Lower incidences of nausea and somnolence and earlier return of bowel function were noted with ketorolac (113). NSAIDs also have an opioid dose sparing-effect. The addition of IM ketorolac resulted in lower usage of epidural fentanyl, less bladder spasm, and earlier recovery of gastrointestinal function (114). IV ketorolac was found to decrease the PCA usage, shorten the gastrointestinal recovery, and improve the quality of the patients' sleep pattern (115).

CONTINUOUS INFUSIONS IN OBSTETRICS

The continuous epidural infusion of local anesthetic is used to treat labor pain and provide analgesia for the delivery (116–119). Theoretical advantages include constant analgesia and a stable sensory level of blockade, lower and less variable maternal and fetal blood concentrations, fewer hypotensive episodes, a lower level of sensory blockade if the catheter migrates to the subarachnoid space, and smaller peak blood concentrations should the catheter become intravascular (120,121). An infusion of 500 ml to 750 ml of Ringer's lactate should be administered 10–15 minutes before epidural analgesia to prevent hypotension from the sympathetic block. After inserting the epidural catheter, a test dose of epinephrine containing local anesthetic is given, usually 3 ml of 1.5% lidocaine or 0.5% bupivacaine (122–124). If there are no signs of intravascular or subarachnoid injection, 6–8 ml of 0.25% bupivacaine is injected. The continuous infusion with a volumetric infusion pump is started once the sensory level is established, usually 15–20 minutes after injecting the bupivacaine (120). Useful local anesthetic concentrations range from 0.125% to 0.375% bupivacaine (121), 0.75% lidocaine (125,126), and 0.75% chloroprocaine (126). Rates vary from 10–15 ml/hr for lidocaine (125,126) and bupivacaine (120,127,128) and 27 ml/hr for 0.75% chloroprocaine (126).

Blood pressure should be measured every 2–5 minutes for the first 20 minutes after the epidural injection and at 15-minute intervals during the infusion. The sensory level and adequacy of anesthesia is checked every 30–60 minutes, and the infusion is adjusted according to the dermatome level. The patient should be placed in the lateral position throughout labor to prevent aortocaval compression and should be turned from side to side every 30 minutes to prevent a one-sided block. The patient's ability to lift her legs is checked every half-hour. If perineal anesthesia is required, the patient is placed in a semirecumbent or sitting position and given 10–20 ml of 1.5–2% lidocaine or 2–3% chloroprocaine.

Whereas high concentrations of bupivacaine used to be administered, Chestnut et al. (127) showed that lower concentrations can be administered if an opioid is added to the local anesthetic. They found that the analgesia from 0.0625% bupivacaine with 0.0002% fentanyl added was similar to that provided by 0.125% bupivacaine alone. The treatments were similar with regard to the duration of the second stage of labor, duration of pushing, position of the vertex before delivery, method of delivery, Apgar scores, and umbilical-cord blood gas and acid-base values (127). The interaction between local anesthetics and opioids was previously described in the section on the use of local anesthetic in epidural opioid infusions. The timing and the effect of the epidural infusion is controversial (123,124,129–131) and is beyond the scope of this chapter.

REFERENCES

1. Go VLW, Yaksh TL. Release of substance P from the cat spinal cord. *J Physiol* 1987;391:141–167.
2. Skilling SR, Smullin DH, Beitz AJ, Larson AA. Extracellular amino acid concentrations in the dorsal spinal cord of freely moving rats following veratridine and nociceptive stimulation. *J Neurochem* 1988;51:127–132.
3. Sorkin LS, Westluind KN, Sluka KA, et al. Neural changes in acute arthritis in monkeys. IV. Time-course of amino acid release into the lumbar dorsal horn. *Brain Res Rev* 1992;17:39–50.
4. Yaksh TL, Abram SE. Preemptive analgesia. A popular misnomer, but a clinically relevant truth? *APS Journal* 1993;2:116–121.
5. Owens CM, Zhang D, Willis WD. Changes in the response state of primate spinothalamic tract cells caused by mechanical damage of the skin or activation of descending controls. *J Neurophysiol* 1992; 67:1509–1527.

6. Pearce RA, Stringer JL, Lothman EW. Effect of volatile anesthetics on synaptic transmission in the rat hippocampus. *Anesthesiology* 1989;71:591–598.
7. Heapy CG, Jamieson A, Russel NJW. Afferent C fiber and A-delta fiber activity in models of inflammation. *Br J Pharmacol* 1987;90:164P.
8. Wheeler-Aceto H, Cowan A. Standardization of the rat paw formalin test for the evaluation of analgesics. *Psychopharmacology* 1991;104:35–44.
9. Wheeler-Aceto H, Porreca F, Cowan A. The rat paw formalin test: comparison of noxious agents. *Pain* 1990;40:229–238.
10. Woolf CJ. Evidence for a central component of post-injury pain hypersensitivity. *Nature* (London) 1983;306:686–688.
11. Woolf CJ. Long-term alterations in the excitability of the flexion reflex produced by peripheral tissue injury in the chronic decerebrate cat. *Pain* 1984;18:325–343.
12. Woolf CJ, Wall PD. Relative effectiveness of C primary afferent fibers of different origins in evoking a prolonged facilitation of the flexor reflex in the rat. *J Neurosci* 1986;6:1433–1442.
13. Coderre TJ, Melzack R. Increased pain sensitivity following heat injury involves a central mechanism. *Behav Brain Res* 1985;15:259–262.
14. Katz J, Vaccarino AL, Coderre TJ, Melzack R. Injury prior to neurectomy alters the pattern of autotomy in rats. *Anesthesiology* 1991;75:876–883.
15. Coderre TJ, Melzack R. Cutaneous hyperanalgesia: contributions of the peripheral and central nervous systems to the increase in pain sensitivity after injury. *Brain Res* 1987;404:95–106.
16. Dennis SG, Melzack R. Self-mutilation after dorsal rhizotomy in rats: effects of prior pain and pattern of root lesions. *Exp Neurol* 1979;65:412–421.
17. Gonzalez-Darde JM, Barbera J, Abellan MJ. Effects of prior anesthesia on autotomy following sciatic transections in rats. *Pain* 1986;24:87–91.
18. Seltzer Z, Beilin BZ, Ginzburg R, Paran Y, Shimko T. The role of injury discharge in the induction of neuropathic pain behavior in rats. *Pain* 1991;46:327–336.
19. Woolf CJ, Wall PD. Morphine-sensitive and morphine-insensitive actions of C-fibre input on the rat spinal cord. *Neurosci Lett* 1986;64:221–225.
20. Dickenson AH, Sullivan AF. Subcutaneous formalin-induced activity of dorsal horn neurons in the rat: differential response to an intrathecal opiate administered pre or post formalin. *Pain* 1987;30:349–360.
21. Coderre TJ, Vaccarino Al, Melzack R. Central nervous system plasticity in the tonic pain response to subcutaneous formalin injection. *Brain Res* 1990;535:155–158.
22. McQuay HJ, Carroll D, Moore RA. Postoperative orthopedic pain: the effect of opiate premedication and local anesthetic blocks. *Pain* 1988;33:291–295.
23. Bach S, Noreng MF, Tjellden NU. Phantom limb pain in amputees during the first 12 months following limb amputation, after preoperative lumbar epidural blockade. *Pain* 1988; 33:297–301.
24. Wall PD. The prevention of postoperative pain. *Pain* 1988;33:289–290.
25. Bridenbaugh PO. Preemptive analgesia—is it clinically relevant? *Anesth Analg* 1994;78:2203–2204.
26. Tverskoy M, Oz Y, Isakson AS, Finger J, Bradley EL, Kissin I. Preemptive effect of fentanyl and ketamine on postoperative pain and wound hyperalgesia. *Anesth Analg* 1994;78:205–209.
27. Woolf CJ, Thompson SWN. The induction and maintenance of central sensitization is dependent on N-methyl-D-aspartic acid receptor activation; implications for the treatment of post-injury pain hypersensitivity states. *Pain* 1991;44:293–299.
28. Kehlet H, Dahl JB. Preemptive analgesia: a misnomer and a misinterpreted technique. *APS Journal* 1993;2:122–124.
29. Gustaffsson I, Nystrom E, Quiding H. Effect of preoperative paracetamol on pain after oral surgery. *Eur J Clin Pharmacol* 1983:24:63–65.
30. Sisk AL, Mosley RO, Martin RP. Comparison of preoperative and postoperative diflunisal for suppression of postoperative pain. *J Oral Maxillofac Surg* 1989;47:464–468.
31. Ejlersen E, Andersen HB, Eliasen K, Mogensen T. A comparison between preincisional and postincisional lidocaine infiltration and postoperative pain. *Anesth Analg* 1992;74:495–498.
32. Dierking GW, Dahl JB, Kanstrup J, Dahl A, Kehlet H. Effect of pre- vs postoperative inguinal field block on postoperative pain after herniorraphy. *Br J Anaesth* 1992;68:344–348.
33. Dahl JB, Hansen BL, Hjortso NC, Erichsen CJ, Moiniche S, Kehlet H. Influence of timing on the effect of continuous extradural analgesia with bupivacaine and morphine after major abdominal surgery. *Br J Anaesth* 1992;69:4–8.
34. Katz J, Kavanah BP, Sandler AN, et al. Preemptive analgesia: clinical evidence of neuroplasticity contributing to postoperative pain. *Anesthesiology* 1992;77:439–446.

35. Kiss IE, Killian M. Does opiate premedication influence postoperative analgesia? a prospective study. *Pain* 1992;48:157–158.
36. Dahl JB, Kehlet H. The value of preemptive analgesia in the treatment of postoperative pain. *Br J Anaesth* 1993;70:434–439.
37. Tverskoy M, Oz Y, Isakson AS, Finger J, Bradley EL, Kissin I. Preemptive effect of fentanyl and ketamine on postoperative pain and wound hyperalgesia. *Anesth Analg* 1994;78:205–209.
38. Jebeles JA, Reilly JS, Gutierrez JF, Bradley EL, Kissin I. The effect of pre-incisional infiltration of tonsils with bupivacaine on the pain following tonsillectomy under general anesthesia. *Pain* 1991;47: 305–308.
39. Johansson B, Glise H, Hallerback B, Dalman P, Kristoffersson A. Preoperative local infiltration with ropivacaine for postoperative pain relief after cholecystectomy. *Anesth Analg* 1994;78:210–214.
40. Benzon HT, Toleikis JR, Dixit P, Goodman I, Hill J. Onset, intensity of blockade and somatosensory evoked potential changes of the lumbosacral dermatomes after epidural anesthesia with alkalinized lidocaine. *Anesth Analg* 1993;76:328–332.
41. Kavanagh BP, Katz J, Sandler AN, et al. Multimodal analgesia before thoracic surgery does not reduce postoperative pain. *Br J Anaesth* 1994;73:1874–1879.
42. Austin KI, Stapleton JV, Mather LE. Relationship between blood meperidine concentrations and analgesic response: a preliminary report. *Anesthesiology* 1980;53:460–466.
43. Austin Kl, Stapleton JV, Mather LE. Multiple intramuscular injections: a major source of variability in analgesic response to meperidine. *Pain* 1980;8:47–62.
44. Graves DA, Foster TS, Batenhorst RL, et al. Patient-controlled analgesia. *Ann Intern Med* 1983;99: 360–366.
45. White PD. Patient-controlled analgesia: a new approach to the management of postoperative pain. *Semin Anesth* 1985;4:255–266.
46. Lubenow TR, McCarthy RJ, Ivankovich AD. Management of acute postoperative pain. In: Barash PG, Cullen BF, Stoelting RK, eds. *Clinical anesthesia.* 2nd ed. Philadelphia: JB Lippincott; 1992: 1547–1577.
47. Bahar M, Rosen M, Vickers MD. Self-administered nalbuphine, morphine and pethidine: Comparison by intravenous route following cholecystectomy. *Anaesthesia* 1985;40:529–532.
48. Sinatra RS, Lodge K, Sibert K, et al. A comparison of morphine, meperidine, and oxymorphone as utilized in patient-controlled analgesia following cesarean delivery. *Anesthesiology* 1989;70:585–590.
49. Sinatra R, Chung KS, Silverman DG, et al. An evaluation of morphine and oxymorphone administered via patient-controlled analgesia (pca) or pca plus basal infusion in postcesarean-delivery patients. *Anesthesiology* 1989;71:502–507.
50. Parker RK, Holtmann B, White PF. Effects of a nighttime opioid infusion with pca therapy on patient comfort and analgesic requirements after abdominal hysterectomy. *Anesthesiology* 1992;76:362–367.
51. Vercauteren MP, Coppejans HC, ten Broecke PW, Van Steenberge AL, Adriaensen HA. Epidural sufentanil for postoperative patient-controlled analgesia (pca) with or without background infusion: a double-blind comparison. *Anesth Analg* 1995;80:76–80.
52. Cousins MJ, Mather LE. Intrathecal and epidural administration of opioids. *Anesthesiology* 1984;61: 276–310.
53. Ready LB, Loper KA, Nessly M, Wild L. Postoperative epidural morphine is safe on surgical wards. *Anesthesiology* 1991;75:452–456.
54. Rawal N, Arner S, Gustafsson LL, Allvin R. Present state of extradural and intrathecal opioid analgesia in Sweden: a nationwide follow-up survey. *Br J Anaesth* 1987;59:791–799.
55. El-Baz NM, Faber P, Jensik RJ. Continuous epidural infusion of morphine for treatment of pain after thoracic surgery: a new technique. *Anesth Analg* 1984;63:757–764.
56. Fisher RL, Lubenow TR, Liceaga A, McCarthy RJ, Ivankovich AD. Comparison of continuous epidural infusion of fentanyl-bupivacaine and morphine-bupivacaine in management of postoperative pain. *Anesth Analg* 1988;67:559–563.
57. Welchew EA. The optimum concentration for epidural fentanyl. *Anaesthesia* 1983;38:1037–1041.
58. Akerman B, Arwestrom E, Post C. Local anesthetics potentiate spinal morphine antinociception. *Anesth Analg* 1988;67:943–948.
59. Wang C, Chakrabarti MK, Whitman JG. Specific enhancement by fentanyl of the effects of intrathecal bupivacaine on nociceptive afferent but not on sympathetic efferent pathways in dogs. *Anesthesiology* 1993;79:766–773.
60. Hjortso NC, Lund C, Mogensen T, Bigler D, Kehlet H. Epidural morphine improves pain relief and maintains sensory analgesia during continuous epidural bupivacaine after abdominal surgery. *Anesth Analg* 1986;65:1033–1036.

61. Niv D, Rudick V, Golan A, Chayen MS. Augmentation of bupivacaine analgesia in labor by epidural morphine. *Obstet Gynecol* 1986;67:206–209.
62. Chestnut DH, Owen CL, Bates JN, Ostman LG, Choi WW, Geiger MW. Continuous infusion epidural analgesia during labor: a randomized double-blind comparison of 0.0625% bupivacaine/0.00002% fentanyl versus 0.125% bupivacaine. *Anesthesiology* 1988;68:754–759.
63. Scott NB, Mogensen T, Bigler D, Lund C, Kehlet H. Continuous thoracic extradural 0.5% bupivacaine with or without morphine: effect on quality of blockade, lung function and the surgical stress response. *Br J Anaesth* 1989;62:253–257.
64. Hunt CO, Naulty JS, Malinow AM, Datta S, Ostheimer GW. Epidural butorphanol-bupivacaine for analgesia during labor and delivery. *Anesth Analg* 1989;68:323–327.
65. King MJ, Bowden MI, Cooper GM. Epidural fentanyl and 0.5% bupivacaine for elective cesarean section. *Anaesthesia* 1990;45:285–288.
66. Cullen MJ, Staren ED, El-Ganzouri A, Logas WG, Ivankovich AD, Economou G. Continuous epidural infusion for analgesia after major abdominal operations: a randomized, prospective, double-blind study. *Surgery* 1985;98:718–728.
67. Logas WG, El-Baz N, El-Ganzouri A, et al. Continuous thoracic epidural analgesia for postoperative pain relief following thoracotomy: a randomized, prospective study. *Anesthesiology* 1987; 67:787–791.
68. Lee A, Simpson D, Whitfield A, Scott DB. Postoperative analgesia by continuous extradural infusion of bupivacaine and diamorphine. *Br J Anaesth* 1988;60:845–850.
69. Badner NH, Reimer EJ, Komar WE. Low-dose bupivacaine does not improve postoperative epidural fentanyl analgesia in orthopedic cases. *Anesth Analg* 1991;72:337–341.
70. Badner NH, Komar WE. Bupivacaine 0.1% does not improve postoperative epidural fentanyl analgesia after abdominal or thoracic surgery. *Can J Anaesth* 1992;39:330–336.
71. George KA, Wright PMC, Chisakuta A. Continuous thoracic epidural fentanyl for post-thoracotomy pain relief; with or without bupivacaine? *Anaesthesia* 1991;46:732–736.
72. Hanson AL, Hanson B, Matousek M. Epidural anesthesia for cesarean section: the effect of morphine-bupivacaine administered epidurally for intra- and postoperative pain relief. *Acta Obstet Gynecol Scand* 1984;63:135–140.
73. Douglas MJ, Mcmorland GH, Janzen JA. Influence of bupivacaine as an adjuvant to epidural morphine for analgesia after cesarean section. *Anesth Analg* 1988;67:1138–1141.
74. Parker RK, Sawaki Y, White PF. Epidural patient-controlled analgesia: influence of bupivacaine and hydromorphone basal infusion on pain control after cesarean delivery. *Anesth Analg* 1992;75:740–746.
75. Dahl JB, Rosenberg J, Hansen BL, Hjortso NC, Kehlet H. Differential analgesic effects of low-dose epidural morphine and morphine-bupivacaine at rest and during mobilization after major abdominal surgery. *Anesth Analg* 1992;74:362–365.
76. Badner NH, Bhandari R, Komar WE. 0.125% bupivacaine is the optimum concentration for continuous postoperative epidural fentanyl analgesia. *Reg Anesth* 1993;18(Suppl 2):27.
77. Benzon HT, Wong CA, Wong HY, Brooke C, Wade L. The effect of low-dose bupivacaine on postoperative epidural fentanyl analgesia and thromboelastography. *Anesth Analg* 1994;79:911–917.
78. Loper KA, Ready LB, Downey M, et al. Epidural and intravenous fentanyl infusions are clinically equivalent after knee surgery. *Anesth Analg* 1990;70:72–75.
79. Ellis DJ, Millar WA, Reisner LS. A randomized double-blind comparison of epidural versus intravenous fentanyl infusion for analgesia after cesarean section. *Anesthesiology* 1990;72:981–986.
80. Camu F, Debucquoy F. Alfentanyl infusion for postoperative pain: a comparison of epidural and intravenous routes. *Anesthesiology* 1991;75:171–178.
81. Miguel R, Barlow I, Morrell M, Scharf J, Sanusi D, Fu E. A prospective, randomized, double-blind comparison of epidural and intravenous sufentanil infusions. *Anesthesiology* 1994;81:346–352.
82. Sandler AN, Stringer D, Panos L, et al. A randomized, double-blind comparison of lumbar epidural and intravenous fentanyl infusions for postthoracotomy pain relief. *Anesthesiology* 1992;77:626–634.
83. Geller E, Chrubasik J, Graf R, Chrubasik S, Scvhulte-Monting J. A randomized, double-blind comparison of epidural sufentanil versus intravenous sufentanil or epidural fentanyl analgesia after major abdominal surgery. *Anesth Analg* 1993;76:1243–1250.
84. Salomaki TE, Laitinen JO, Nuutinen LS. A randomized double-blind comparison of epidural versus intravenous fentanyl infusion for analgesia after thoracotomy. *Anesthesiology* 1991;75:790–795.
85. Guinard JP, Mavrocordatos P, Chiolero R, Carpenter RL. A randomized comparison of intravenous versus lumbar and thoracic epidural fentanyl for analgesia after thoracotomy. *Anesthesiology* 1992; 77:1108–1115.
86. Benzon HT, Wong HY, Belavic A, et al. A randomized double-blind comparison of epidural fentanyl

infusion versus patient-controlled analgesia with morphine for postthoracotomy pain. *Anesth Analg* 1993;76:316–322.
87. Kavanagh BP, Katz J, Sandler AN. Pain control after thoracic surgery. *Anesthesiology* 1994;81:737–759.
88. Grant RP, Dolman JF, Harper JA, et al. Patient-controlled lumbar epidural fentanyl compared with patient-controlled intravenous fentanyl for postthoracotomy pain relief. *Can J Anaesth* 1992;39:214–219.
89. Allaire PH, Messick JM, Osterling JE, et al. A prospective randomized comparison of epidural infusion of fentanyl and intravenous administration of morphine by patient-controlled analgesia after radical retropubic prostatectomy. *Mayo Clin Proc* 1992;67:1031–1041.
90. Chauvin M, Hongnat JM, Mourgeon E, Lebrault C, Bellentant F, Alfonsi P. Equivalence of postoperative analgesia with patient-controlled intravenous or epidural alfentanil. *Anesth Analg* 1993;76: 1251–1258.
91. Peach MJ, Moore JS, Evans SF. Meperidine for patient-controlled analgesia after cesarean section. *Anesthesiology* 1994;1268–1276.
92. Glass PSA, Estok P, Ginsberg B, Goldberg JS, Sladen RN. Use of patient-controlled analgesia to compare the efficacy of epidural to intravenous fentanyl administration. *Anesth Analg* 1992;74:345–351.
93. Fromme GA, Steidl LJ, Danielson DR. Comparison of lumbar and thoracic epidural morphine for relief of postthoracotomy pain. *Anesth Analg* 1985;64:454–455.
94. Coe A, Sarginson R, Smith MW, Donnelly RJ, Russell GN. Pain following thoracotomy: a randomized, double-blind comparison of lumbar versus thoracic epidural fentanyl. *Anaesthesia* 1991;46: 918–921.
95. Hurford WE, Dutton RP, Alfille PH, Clement D, Wilson RTS. Comparison of thoracic and lumbar epidural infusions of bupivacaine and fentanyl for post-thoracotomy analgesia. *J Cardiothorac Vasc Anesth* 1993;7:521–525.
96. Rawal N, Sjostrand U, Christofferson E, Dahlstrom B, Arvin A, Rudman H. Comparison of intramuscular and epidural morphine for postoperative analgesia in the grossly obese: influence on postoperative ambulation and pulmonary function. *Anesth Analg* 1984;63: 583–592.
97. Tuman KJ, McCarthy RJ, March RJ, De Laria GA, Patel RV, Ivankovich AD. Effects of epidural anesthesia and analgesia on coagulation and outcome after major vascular surgery. *Anesth Analg* 1991; 73:696–704.
98. Yeager MP, Glass DD, Neff RK, Brinck-Johnsen T. Epidural anesthesia and analgesia in high-risk surgical patients. *Anesthesiology* 1987;66:729–736.
99. Jayr C, Thomas H, Rey A, Farhat F, Lasser P, Bourgain JL. Epidural analgesia using bupivacaine and opioids versus parenteral opioids. *Anesthesiology* 1993;78:666–676.
100. Kvalheim L, Reiestad F. Intrapleural catheter in the management of postoperative pain. *Anesthesiology* 1984;61:A231(abst).
101. Symreng T, Gomez MN, Rossi N. Intrapleural bupivacaine versus saline after thoracotomy: effects on pain and lung function—a double-blind study. *J Cardiothorac Anesth* 1989;3:144–149.
102. Symreng T, Gomez MN, Johnson B, Rossi NP, Chiang CK. Intrapleural bupivacaine: technical considerations and intraoperative use. *J Cardiothorac Anesth* 1989;3:139–143.
103. Scheinin B, Lindgren L, Rosenberg PH. Treatment of postthoracotomy pain with intermittent instillations of intrapleural bupivacaine. *Acta Anaesthesiol Scand* 1989;33:156–159.
104. Kambam JR, Hammon J, Parris WCV, Lupinetti FM. Intrapleural analgesia for postthoracotomy pain and blood levels of bupivacaine following intrapleural injection. *Can J Anaesth* 1989;36:106–109.
105. Ferrante FM, Chan VWS, Arthur GR, Rocco AG. Interpleural analgesia after thoracotomy. *Anesth Analg* 1991;72;105–109.
106. Mann LJ, Young GR, Williams JK, Dent OF, McCaughan BC. Intrapleural bupivacaine in the control of postthoracotomy pain. *Ann Thorac Surg* 1992;53:449–454.
107. Schneider RF, Villamena PC, Harvey J, Surick BG, Weiner SI, Beattie EJ. Lack of efficacy of intrapleural bupivacaine for postoperative analgesia following thoracotomy. *Chest* 1993;103;414–416.
108. Elman A, Debaene B, Magny-Metrot C, Murciano G. Interpleural analgesia with bupivacaine following thoracotomy: ineffective results of a controlled study and pharmacokinetics. *J Clin Anaesth* 1993:5:118–121.
109. Rosenberg PH, Barbro MA, Scheinin A, Lepantalo MJ, Lindfors O. Continuous intrapleural infusion of bupivacaine for analgesia after thoracotomy. *Anesthesiology* 1987;67:811–813.
110. Raffin L, Fletcher D, Sperandio M, et al. Interpleural infusion of 2% lidocaine with 1:200,000 epinephrine for postthoracotomy analgesia. *Anesth Analg* 1994;79:328–334.
111. McIlvaine WB, Knox RF, Fennessey PV, Goldstein M. Continuous infusion of bupivacaine via intrapleural catheter for analgesia after thoracotomy in children. *Anesthesiology*; 1988:69:261–264.

112. Agency for Health Care Policy and Research. *Acute pain management: operative or medical procedures and trauma.* (Clinical practice guidelines.) Bethesda, Maryland: U.S. Department of Health and Human Services; 1992.
113. Wong HY, Carpenter RL, Kopacz DJ, et al. A randomized, double-blind evaluation of ketorolac tromethamine for postoperative analgesia in ambulatory surgery patients. *Anesthesiology* 1993;78: 6–14.
114. Grass JA, Sakima NT, Valley M, et al. Assessment of ketorolac as an adjunct to fentanyl patient-controlled epidural analgesia after radical retropubic prostatectomy. *Anesthesiology* 1993;78:642–648.
115. Parker RK, Holtmann B, Smith I, White PF. Use of ketorolac after lower abdominal surgery: effect on analgesic requirement and surgical outcome. *Anesthesiology* 1994;80:6–12.
116. Evans KRL, Carrie LES. Continuous epidural infusion of bupivacaine in labour: a simple method. *Anaesthesia* 1979;34:310–315.
117. Davies AO, Fettes IW. A simple safe method for continuous infusion epidural analgesia in obstetrics. *Can Anaesth Soc J* 1981;28:484–487.
118. Taylor HJC. Clinical experience with continuous epidural infusion of bupivacaine at 6 ml per hour in obstetrics. *Can Anaesth Soc J* 1983;30:277–285.
119. Li DF, Rees GAD, Rosen M. Continuous extradural infusion of 0.0625% or 0.125% bupivacaine for pain relief in primigravid labour. *Br J Anaesth* 1985;57:264–270.
120. Rosenblatt R, Wright R, Denson D, Raj P. Continuous epidural infusions for obstetric analgesia. *Reg Anesth* 1983;8:10–15.
121. Morrison DH, Smedstad KG. Continuous infusion epidurals for obstetric analgesia. *Can Anaesth Soc J* 1985;32:101–104.
122. Chestnut DH, Vandewalker GE, Owen CL, Bates JN, Choi WW. The influence of continuous epidural bupivacaine analgesia on the second stage of labor and method of delivery in nulliparous women. *Anesthesiology* 1987;66:774–780.
123. Chestnut DH, Vincent RD, McGrath JM, Choi WW, Bates JN. Does early administration of epidural analgesia affect obstetric outcome in nulliparous women who are receiving intravenous oxytocin? *Anesthesiology* 1994;80:1193–1200.
124. Chestnut DH, McGrath JM, Vincent RD, et al. Does early administration of epidural analgesia affect obstetric outcome in nulliparous women who are in spontaneous labor? *Anesthesiology* 1994;80: 1201–1208.
125. Chestnut DH, Bates JN, Choi WW. Continuous infusion epidural analgesia with lidocaine: efficacy and influence during the second stage of labor. *Obstet Gynecol* 1987;69:323–327.
126. Abboud TK, Afrasiabi A, Sarkis F, et al. Continuous infusion epidural analgesia in parturients receiving bupivacaine, chloroprocaine, or lidocaine—maternal, fetal, and neonatal effects. *Anesth Analg* 1984;63:421–428.
127. Chestnut DH, Owen CL, Bates JN, Ostman LG, Choi WW, Geiger MW. Continuous infusion epidural analgesia during labor: a randomized, double-blind comparison of 0.0625% bupivacaine/0.0002% fentanyl versus 0.125% bupivacaine. *Anesthesiology* 1988;68:754–759.
128. Philipps G. Continuous infusion epidural analgesia in labor: the effect of adding sufentanil to 0.125% bupivacaine. *Anesth Analg* 1988;67:462–465.
129. Dewan DM, Cohen SE. Epidural analgesia and the incidence of cesarean section: time for a closer look. *Anesthesiology* 1994;80:1189–1192.
130. Thorp JA, Eckert LO, Ang MS, Johnston DA, Peaceman AM, Parisi VM. Epidural analgesia and cesarean section for dystocia: risk factors in nulliparas. *Am J Perinatol* 1991;8:402–410.
131. Thorp JA, Hu DH, Albin RM, et al. The effect of intrapartum epidural analgesia on nulliparous labor: a randomized, controlled, prospective trial. *Am J Obstet Gynecol* 1993;169:851–858.

Drug Infusions in Anesthesiology, Second Edition, edited by R. J. Fragen. Lippincott-Raven Publishers, Philadelphia © 1996.

8

Drug Infusions in Pediatric Anesthesia

Patrick K. Birmingham and Steven C. Hall

Department of Anesthesia, Northwestern University Medical School, and Children's Memorial Hospital, Chicago, Illinois 60614

Drug infusions are being used with increasing frequency and success in the pediatric population. A large and growing body of literature provides insight and guidance regarding the use of infusions in neonates and infants as well as older children. After reviewing physiologic differences in pediatric patients that affect drug pharmacokinetics and pharmacodynamics, we will review the use of the more commonly used narcotics, muscle relaxants, local anesthetics, and sedative/hypnotic agents in this age group. Included in the discussion will be the role that drug infusions play in the operating room as well as in diagnostic or therapeutic procedures outside the operating room, in the management of postoperative pain and other painful conditions, and for sedation or muscle relaxation in the intensive care unit (ICU).

The rational use of parenteral infusions in pediatric patients requires a recognition of the considerable differences in pharmacokinetics and pharmacodynamics in the pediatric patient compared to the adult patient. Some of these differences are related to maturational changes in both body composition and core organ function. The differences between the preterm newborn, the full-term newborn, the infant, and the child are significant. For purposes of this discussion, a neonate or newborn is defined as a patient between birth and 1 month of age, an infant is defined as one between 1 month and 1 year (although some authors use 2 yrs), and a child is defined as one between 1 year and adolescence. A premature or preterm infant is born before 37 weeks' gestation.

CHANGES IN BODY COMPOSITION

Distribution

Fluid Compartments

Body fluid compartments change during the different stages of development. Total body water represents about 80% of total body weight in the full-term newborn, decreasing to only 60% of the body weight by age 2 years. In terms of water distribution, the full-term newborn has about 45% of its body weight in extracellular water, compared with 20% of body weight at 2 years of age (1,2) This drop in extracellular fluid is dramatic. The proportionally large distribution of extracellular water in the newborn has several implications. First, water soluble drugs are diluted into a relatively larger pool. Second, most of the water-soluble drugs are then circulated through core organs such as the liver and kidney, leading to a rapid onset of action at those sites. Third, because of the high proportion of water in the extracellular space, there is relatively little (compared to older children or adults) in the intracellular space. This represents a decreased intracellular "reserve" of fluid in the presence of increased loss or reduced intake. Because the metabolic rate and consequent insensible loss of water in newborns is double the adult value, newborns are much less tolerant of unreplaced water loss. The newborn with vomiting, diarrhea, or prolonged fasting is much more likely to demonstrate hypovolemia and cardiovascular instability.

The change in the fluid compartments that occurs in the first months of life is extraordinary. A diuresis in the first few days of life decreases the total amount of interstitial fluid and is accompanied by weight loss (2). The proportion of total body water in the intracellular space stays about the same, at 35–40%, but intracellular water increases relative to total body water and extracellular water over the first two years of life. As total body water content decreases, the potential differences in volume of distribution also change.

The distribution of water-soluble drugs is extremely important when considering drug administration by infusion. Age and fluid compartments are important for infusions of muscle relaxants. The volume of distribution at steady state for muscle relaxants is much greater in newborns than in infants, children, or adults. This was demonstrated for d-tubocurarine, vecuronium, and atracurium (3–5). When steady-state levels of drug are achieved, there is a much greater volume of distribution in the neonate. This also was demonstrated for propofol (6). If the same drug dose/kg of body weight is given, the newborn will have a lower plasma concentration than will the child or adult.

Cardiac Output

Cardiac output is relatively higher in children than in adults, though this difference becomes less important after infancy. This increase is preferentially distributed to the core organs of the central nervous system (CNS) and pulmonary, cardiac, renal, hepatic, and gastrointestinal systems and leads to rapid equilibration of drug concentrations in the vessel-rich tissues. Blood flow is increased to the kidneys and liver. After these organs functionally mature in the first weeks of life, the increased cardiac output to these vessel-rich organs promotes extraction and excretion of drugs. However, this is a complex situation because hepatic and renal blood flow are only part of the components necessary for efficient functioning of these organs.

Compared to adults, more of the cardiac output is directed to the CNS, allowing rapid equilibration time between drug concentrations in the plasma and in brain tissue (effect site). This is also important when titrating drug infusions.

Children may have anatomical abnormalities that affect drug distribution (7,8). Intracardiac shunting (e.g., through a ventricular septal defect) or extracardiac shunting (e.g., through a patent ductus arteriosus) can increase circulation through the pulmonary circulation. This "left-to-right" shunting can delay and dilute the delivery of drug to other organs and tissues. Similarly, other shunts can bypass blood from the pulmonary circulation ("right-to-left") and increase the speed and concentration of drug reaching the brain and other tissues. Thus, congenital heart disease can change both the timing and degree of drug action.

Blood-Brain Barrier

The blood-brain barrier is different in pediatric patients, especially in neonates (9). This lipid-based interface that inhibits the passage of lipophobic substances into the brain and spinal cord is not fully established in the newborn, permitting rapid entrance of substances that normally would be inhibited. The classic example of this is morphine. Morphine has only limited lipid solubility; in adults, its uptake into the brain is slow and limited compared with the more lipid-soluble opiates heroin and meperidine. However, the newborn has a less intact barrier than do adults (9). Diffusion of morphine in the neonatal brain is therefore more dependent on cardiac output (since diffusion is not inhibited). With the relatively high cardiac output to this vessel-rich area, rapid equilibration of morphine occurs. Toxicity could occur at plasma concentrations that are nontoxic in adults. There is some clinical evidence to confirm this. Kupferberg and Way (10) studied morphine in both rats and humans and found that it crossed to the brain to a greater degree in neonates and produced greater ventilatory depression. Interestingly, meperidine, a more lipid-soluble opiate, caused less ventilatory depression (11).

Binding of Drugs

Plasma Proteins

Protein binding is an important determinant of drug transport, penetration into tissues, and concentration of drug at the effector site. Some anesthetic drugs, such as diazepam, are poorly bound to proteins, whereas others, such as caffeine, are highly bound.

Once all plasma protein-binding sites are occupied by a drug, any additional drug will dramatically increase the amount available for action at the effector site. Any factor that decreases the total amount of protein available or decreases the ability of a drug to bind to the protein will increase the potency of drug in that patient. Pediatric patients, especially newborns, have altered protein binding of drugs.

Newborns have lower concentrations of serum albumin than do adults (12,13). This relative difference disappears by about 6 months of age. The albumin found in newborns also has a lower protein-binding capacity than does albumin found in children or adults. This lower total binding capacity of albumin is particularly troublesome in newborns because there are naturally occurring substances that bind the few available sites. Bilirubin, maternal steroids, and products of metabolism such as free fatty acids are bound to albumin. If drugs that compete with these naturally occurring substances are present, there may be undesirable consequences. First, less drug may be bound, leading to a greater effect than expected. Second, some of the naturally occurring substances can be released into the blood stream, leading to undesirable effects such as kernicterus, increased bilirubin concentrations in the brain.

Other plasma proteins besides albumin are involved in drug binding. Specifically, alpha-1 acid glycoprotein is probably the most important. It preferentially binds drugs that are basic, such as the opiates and local anesthetics (9). Both its quantity and binding ability are reduced in newborns and infants. Drugs also may bind to hemoglobin; the high level of fetal hemoglobin is usually gone by 4–6 months of age, replaced by adult hemoglobin.

Fat and Muscle

Many drugs bind in substantial amount to the body's fat and muscle stores. Because the newborn has little fat, binding of lipid-soluble drugs is decreased. These stores increase during infancy. Similarly, the smaller amount of skeletal muscle mass decreases the amount of drug bound to inactive sites in muscle (14).

CHANGES IN ORGAN FUNCTION

Renal System

There is an increase in effective renal function over the first month of life, especially in the first two weeks (15). The glomerular filtration rate (GFR) is decreased at birth, especially in the preterm newborn. The GFR increases rapidly in the first couple of weeks of life and approaches adult levels by age 2 years. An exception to this is the preterm newborn, whose rise in GFR is much slower. The newborn kidney has a reduced ability to concentrate and respond to fluid deprivation. Therefore, fluid deprivation is a concern in newborns, not only because of the inability to concentrate, but also because of the relatively high metabolic rate and insensible water loss. On the other hand, the newborn is capable of handling free water overload by excreting large amounts of dilute urine.

The newborn kidney does not excrete an overload of sodium easily. This is especially true in the preterm newborn; these babies are difficult to manage because they have a relatively high fixed excretion of sodium and cannot respond easily to either an overload or decrease in sodium load. Newborns increase their ability to handle sodium adequately over the first weeks of life.

Similarly, the ability of the kidney to excrete water-soluble drugs changes with maturation. The muscle relaxants are the prime example of drugs that are subject to renal excretion. Although there is low clearance of d-tubocurarine via glomerular filtration in the newborn, clearance reaches adult capability by about 1 year of age (3).

There has been much concern about the ability of the newborn and infant to handle extremes of water and sodium as well as to excrete water-soluble drugs. It is now recognized that the newborn's renal function increases quickly after just a few days of life (16) and reaches adult capability in about the first year. Insulin and thiosulfate clearances, reflections of GFR, are decreased in the newborn, but they approach adult values by about age 3 months when compared relative to the infant's body surface area. Tubular function approaches adult values by 5 months of age (16). Consequently, renal function is of concern in the first days of life, but it quickly matures and reaches adult function in the first year of life.

Hepatic System

The liver is a relatively larger organ in the newborn and infant than in the child or adult. Its effectiveness is determined by both its blood flow and metabolic capacity. Liver blood flow should be high in the neonate because of its large size. However, hepatic flow can be decreased by opening of the ductus venosus, which remains patent for weeks after birth, and by shunting of portal venous blood to the vena cava (17). Other factors, such as increased intraabdominal pressure, release of vasoactive substances, or volatile agent anesthesia also may reduce hepatic blood flow.

Although the liver is a large organ, its metabolic activity is decreased in the newborn. The hepatic enzyme system is poorly developed at birth. The mixed-function oxidase system (cytochrome P450) has been studied in animals and, to a lesser extent, in humans. A study of calves showed low concentrations of P450 enzymes at birth, which increased quickly during the first month of life (18). Similar results were also found in rats and ferrets (9). The concentration of these enzyme systems is low or absent in human neonates (19). However, the activity increases quickly and can reach adult levels in the first weeks of life. These enzyme systems can be induced, especially by barbiturates (20), leading to speculation that some of the low enzyme activity may be related to lack of substrate rather than a lack of enzymes (9).

A practical example of cytochrome P450 metabolism in the neonate is the elimination of fentanyl. Fentanyl clearance largely occurs in the liver (19). Studies show a marked decrease in fentanyl clearance in human neonates (19,21). This reduced clearance was further decreased in patients undergoing intraabdominal surgery, suggesting that the surgical procedure is a confounding factor of decreased hepatic blood flow. These studies showed that hepatic clearance increases as the neonatal period progresses.

The liver metabolizes drugs by systems other than the mixed-function oxidase enzymes. Conjugation reactions, such as with acetates or glucuronic acid, are limited in the newborn but develop in the first three months of life (9). Practical examples of conjugation reactions are the conjugation of morphine to glucuronic acid and the conjugation of barbiturates to glucosides. These reactions appear to be absent at birth, but they develop in the first weeks of life (22).

Beyond the newborn period, the pediatric liver functions well. The infant and child may demonstrate enhanced hepatic metabolic activity based on increased cardiac output and hepatic function equivalent to that seen in the adult. For instance, a pharmacokinetic model for propofol infusions determined a clearance value of 34.3 ml/kg/min in children compared with 27.4 ml/kg/min in adults (6).

Gastrointestinal System

Antibiotics, antiseizure medications, mild analgesics, and antihypertensive agents are a few of the drugs often given orally to children. In anesthesia, only premedicant drugs are given orally. Two issues must be considered when giving oral medication. The first issue is absorption. Because the newborn has proportionally less gastric acid than does the older child, the change in absorption of ionized drugs is reduced (9). For example, ampicillin has a relatively greater absorption in the neonate because of decreased inactivation from gastric acid. Newborns also have a slower gastric and intestinal emptying time than do older infants and children, which can increase or decrease drug absorption, depending on the effect of the gastric pH on drug ionization.

The second issue is when one can give oral medication or fluids before an elective procedure. Our understanding of the pediatric patient's ability to empty the stomach has changed dramatically. Clear liquids are emptied from the stomach much faster than was previously recognized. There are now many studies demonstrating the ability of healthy pediatric patients to empty their stomach of clear liquids within 2 hours (23–25). This ability is independent of the child's age or the amount of clear liquid ingested. For this reason, it is now common practice in pediatric centers to allow clear liquids ad lib until 2 hours before elective surgery. Having children take their chronic oral medication with a sip of water 2 hours before elective procedures also is considered to be a safe practice.

Rectal administration of drugs also is common in children. Rectal absorption appears to be comparable in children and adults (9).

Pulmonary System

There are several important differences between the pulmonary systems of pediatric patients and adults that change uptake and distribution of volatile agents.

However, the role of pulmonary function on the distribution and elimination of parenteral agents is not well studied.

Central Nervous System

Most of the work on anesthetic requirements in children focused on two different methods of measuring "anesthesia." The majority of studies focused on the concept of minimum alveolar concentration (MAC), using patient movement in response to surgical stimulation as an end point. Generally, there is an inverse relationship between MAC and age, but the first few weeks of life form a different pattern.

During the first days of life, the observable response to pain appears to be attenuated. This is true in both the awake and anesthetized newborn. Although there is a generalized arousal pattern of response to pain, it often is not seen until significant pain has been inflicted. The reason for this is unknown, though various authors have suggested that maternal progesterone levels or neonatal plasma endorphins may be responsible for the relative insensitivity (26).

There is abundant evidence that the neonate has pain receptors, neuronal pathways to the brain and centers in the brain that respond to painful stimuli, as well as enkephalin, gamma-aminobutyric acid (GABA), and other neuroactive substance systems (27). Some of the neuronal tracts, such as the spinothalamic and thalamocortical tracts, are not fully myelinated at birth, which may slow conduction and responsiveness (28). Exciting work on the development of the GABA system as well as opiate receptors suggests that receptors in the fetus and newborn may function differently than they do in the adult (29,30). There is great interest in the possibility that the development of these systems can be altered by exposure to agonists in the fetal or neonatal periods (31,32).

Using MAC as a measure of anesthetic requirement, there is a clear pattern of decreased anesthetic requirement in the neonatal period, especially if the neonate is preterm. A study by LeDez and Lerman (33) found that isoflurane MAC in preterms under 32 weeks' gestational age was 1.28% ± 0.17%, whereas neonates between 32 weeks and 37 weeks' gestational age had a MAC of 1.41% ± 0.18% (33). In another study, Cameron et al. (34) found a MAC of 1.87% in infants up to 6 months old (33). In similar work, Lerman et al. (35) found that the MAC of halothane was 0.87% ± 0.03 in neonates and 1.2% ± 0.06% in infants. These studies are representative of many studies that demonstrate a decreased need for volatile agent anesthesia in the newborn, an increased need in infancy, and then a gradual decline in MAC until adolescence (9).

Measuring cardiovascular and hormonal stress responses are a second method of investigating the response to pain and the effectiveness of general anesthetic agents (27,36). This is a less specific measure than the response to a surgical stimulation, but it yields some interesting results.

Yaster (37) measured heart rate, blood pressure, cardiac output, and systemic vascular resistance to determine the dose of fentanyl needed to prevent hemodynamic changes to surgical stimulation. He found that 10–12.5 μg/kg of fentanyl prevented cardiac stimulation in response to surgical stimulation, suggesting that this provides reliable anesthesia. Anand et al. (38–42) performed multiple studies that evaluated the ability of opiates to block not only cardiovascular responses but also a wide variety of neuroendocrine responses to surgical stimulation. The patterns of neuroendocrine response are different in the preterm newborn, full-term newborn, and child, but all can be blocked by anesthesia (27). Neonates, including preterm neonates, can mount significant cardiovascular and neuroendocrine responses to painful stimuli. Thus, neonates should receive anesthesia to block these responses, just as older children and adults should. The challenge is in the definition of "anesthesia." It remains controversial whether blunting of cardiovascular responses or neuroendocrine responses is true anesthesia and what the consequences of profound analgesia without anesthesia are (42). This is fertile ground for future research.

Summary

The use of parenteral infusions for anesthesia in pediatric patients is a relatively new area of investigation. The increased volume of distribution, increased cardiac output, increased perfusion of vessel-rich tissues, decreased fat and muscle binding, and decreased plasma proteins clearly can affect the initial establishment of adequate plasma and end-organ drug concentrations. These factors also can alter recovery when the drug infusion is stopped. The differences of renal and hepatic function, especially in the neonate, can significantly alter metabolism and excretion, with subsequent effect on steady-state dynamics. Lastly, the differences in anesthetic potency at different ages can alter the effectiveness of a fixed drug regimen. Although pediatric patients are commonly dosed on a mg/kg basis, the tremendous variability in both pharmacokinetics and pharmacodynamics at different ages demands that the practitioner carefully titrate infusions to patients' responsiveness.

OPIATES

Exaggerated concerns about the respiratory depressant effects of opiates in children, combined with the misperception that newborn and young infants do not feel pain, led to the undertreatment of pediatric pain. That pain pathways are intact and functional by late gestation is now accepted. Cardiorespiratory, hormonal, and metabolic responses to pain in adults are also well documented in neonates (27). With evidence that opiates reduce the stress response in mechanically ventilated preterm infants in the ICU (44) and in infants undergoing surgery (45) and may reduce postoperative morbidity and mortality (46), the use of opiate infusions is increasing in both the operating room and the ICU.

Morphine

Morphine is a mainstay of narcotic therapy in pediatrics. In both adults and in children older than 1 year, the pharmacokinetics of morphine are an elimination half-life of about 2 hours and similar volumes of distribution and clearance (47). More recently, Olkkola et al. (48) demonstrated morphine kinetics comparable to those of adults in infants 5–6 months of age.

Pharmacokinetic studies of premature neonates in the first 24 hours of life (49) and between 1 day and 10 weeks of age in infants born after 36–41 weeks' gestation (50) demonstrated a longer elimination half-life and lower plasma clearance compared to adults (Table 1). Subsequent studies confirmed morphine plasma clearance in premature neonates to be one-fifth that of children aged 1 to 16 years (51). In a study of 12 infants of 1–49 days postnatal age, born at 35–41 weeks' gestation, Koren et al. (52) also found an elimination half-life that was significantly longer than in adults and older children and emphasized the large variability in plasma morphine concentrations between their study patients. Thus, for a given dose of morphine, preterm infants and infants in the first week of life will achieve a higher plasma concentration for a longer duration. Morphine plasma clearance increases with gestational age, and, at age 1 month, elimination half-life and clearance begins to approach adult values.

Lynn et al. (54) examined the respiratory effects of intravenous (IV) morphine infusions in 30 patients aged 2–570 days following cardiac surgery. They examined the $PaCO_2$ level and the CO_2 response-curve slope as a function of morphine serum level and found that steady-state morphine levels greater than 20 ng/ml resulted in significant hypercarbia and depressed CO_2 response-curve slopes in a majority of study patients, regardless of age. They did not find that newborns or young infants were more sensitive to morphine than were older infants or young children at the same blood level of drug. On the basis of arterial $PaCO_2$ and respiratory rate, Olkkola et al. (48) found no difference in sensitivity to the respiratory-depressant effect of morphine between infants and children, although the youngest patient studied was 21 weeks old.

TABLE 1. *Intravenous morphine pharmacokinetics in infants and children*

Study population (gestational age at birth) postnatal age	Steady-state volume of distribution (1/kg)	Plasma clearance (ml/kg/min)	Elimination half-life (hr)	Reference
(26–34 wks) 1 day	1.82	2.4	8.75	49
(36–41 wks) 1–4 days	3.38	6.3	6.8	50
(36–41 wks) 29–65 days	5.15	23.8	3.9	50
(?) 11–182 days	2.00	21.5	1.15	48
2–4 yrs	3.17	56.2	0.76	48
6–7 yrs	3.76	47.4	1.15	48
Adults	2.4	11.5	2	53

Continuous morphine infusions have been studied extensively and are beneficial in the treatment of postoperative pain. Bray (55) demonstrated superior pain relief following major surgery with continuous morphine infusion of 20 μg/kg/hr versus intramuscular (IM) morphine in a prospective study of 20 children between 1 year and 15 years of age. Beasley and Tibballs (56) administered morphine at rates of 10–40 μg/kg/hr in 121 spontaneously breathing children, 13 of whom were younger than 1 year, following major surgery, with good analgesia and no respiratory depression. Millar et al. (57) demonstrated effective and safe analgesia in 20 spontaneously breathing postoperative ICU patients aged 3 months to 12 years using infusion rates of 14–21 μg/kg/hr. The mean total amount of morphine used was much less than if standard time-contingent IM injections were given. In a prospective study of 46 nonventilated children aged 1 year to 16 years following major chest, abdominal, or orthopedic procedures, IV infusions between 10–40 μg/kg/hr gave better pain relief than did IM injections administered as required (PRN) and without major complications such as respiratory depression (58). Koren et al. (52) recommended that infusion rates not exceed 15 μg/kg/hr in newborn infants after two infants developed generalized seizures at rates of 32 μg/kg/hr and 40 μg/kg/hr. An infusion of 15 μg/kg/hr was used after surgery in 20 neonates between 1 day and 18 days old, born at 32–41 weeks' gestation without complication and with good pain control based on serum beta-endorphin levels and subjective nursing observations (59). Lynn et al. (60) studied the dose-response characteristics and safety of a continuous morphine infusion in 44 children between 14 months and 17 years of age after cardiac surgery. Infusion rates of 10–30 μg/kg/hr gave mean serum levels of 10–22 ng/ml, provided good analgesia, and allowed weaning from assisted ventilation. Children with cerebral palsy undergoing selective dorsal rhizotomy have been safely managed postoperatively with continuous morphine infusions of 20–40 μg/kg/hr, often with a midazolam infusion as well (61) (Table 2).

The addition of a continuous morphine infusion to patient-controlled analgesia (PCA), known as PCA-Plus, was studied because of the perception that it would improve continuity of analgesia and provide analgesia during sleep. In 40 children after appendectomy, patients receiving a 20-μg/kg/hr background infusion along with the PCA demand option suffered more nausea, sedation, and hypoxemia (62). A subsequent study of postappendectomy patients using PCA-Plus with a 4-μg/kg/hr morphine infusion demonstrated less hypoxemia than with PCA alone and a better sleep pattern (63). Compared with a control group of orthopedic patients receiving IM morphine on a PRN basis, Berde et al. (64) demonstrated better pain relief with less drowsiness in patients receiving a 15-μg/kg/hr infusion with their PCA demand doses. Subcutaneous PCA-Plus administration was as effective as the more standard IV route (65).

Continuous morphine infusions with or without bolus doses were used successfully to manage pain after pediatric burns (66), prolonged oropharyngeal mucositis pain following bone marrow transplantation (67), and for severe sickle-cell vaso-occlusive crisis (68,69). Death resulted from a morphine infusion during

TABLE 2. *Continuous intravenous morphine infusion for postoperative analgesia in infants and children*

Age range of subjects (EGA)[a]	Infusion (μg/kg/hr)	Comments[b]	Number of subjects (ref.)
1–18 days (32–40 wks)	15	Some patients mechanically ventilated	20 (59)
1–49 days (35–41 wks)	6–40	Some patients mechanically ventilated; seizures at 32 and 40 μg/kg/hr; recommend rate of 15 μg/kg/hr	12 (52)
3 mos–12 yrs	14–21	Less total morphine than with time-contingent IM morphine	20 (57)
<1–>14 yrs	10–40	Spontaneously ventilating	121 (56)
14 mos–17 yrs	10–30	Postoperative cardiac; able to wean from mechanical ventilation	44 (60)
1–15 yrs	20	Superior to IM morphine	20 (55)
1–16 yrs	10–40	Superior to IM morphine	46 (58)
3–22 yrs	20–40	Cerebral palsy patients	55 (61)

[a] EGA, estimated gestational age at birth.
[b] IM, intramuscular.

a sickle-cell crisis (70). Myoclonus was reported in a 4-year-old boy after a continuous morphine infusion of 27 μg/kg/hr for 5 hours (71).

Fentanyl

Fentanyl infusions also have been used in all age groups within the pediatric population, particularly in the ICU setting. A survey of pediatric ICUs in the United States found that fentanyl was used in 88% of the units, compared with 35% of adult units (72). Advantages of fentanyl include its high potency, rapid onset, short duration of action, minimal histamine release compared with morphine, minimal hemodynamic effects (73), and ablation of pulmonary vascular responsiveness (74).

A pharmacokinetic study in nine premature infants between 29 weeks and 43 weeks of age postconception (gestational age at birth + postnatal age) following a bolus dose of 30 μg/kg of fentanyl demonstrated a mean elimination half-life of 17.7 hours compared to the adult value of 2–3 hours (75). Plasma concentrations of fentanyl decrease more rapidly by 3–10 months of age compared to adults based on both an increased volume of distribution and increased clearance (76) (Fig. 1). In a pharmacodynamic study measuring ventilatory pattern and transcutaneous CO_2, ventilatory depression in infants older than 3 months was similar to that seen in children and adults (77). Koren et al. (78) studied different bolus doses and infusion rates in infants and children with congenital heart disease and intracardiac shunting and found that a bolus of 30 μg/kg combined with an infusion of 0.3

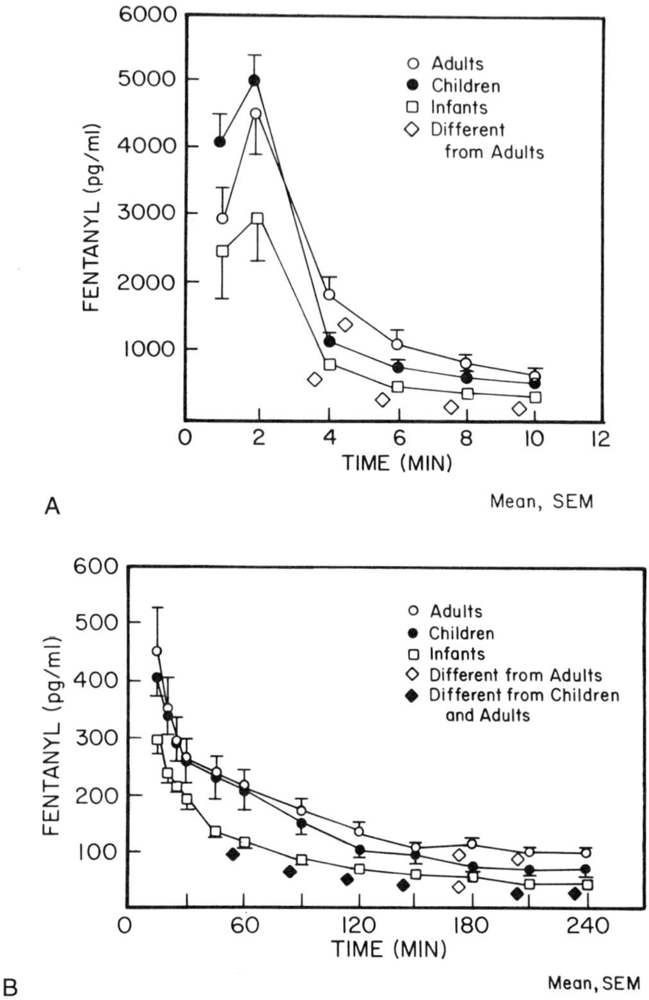

FIG. 1. Plasma fentanyl concentration per µg/kg administered following 30 µg/kg doses for infants and children, and 20 µg/kg doses for adults. Infants had lower plasma fentanyl concentrations throughout much of the 4 hr sampling period. (From Singleton et al., ref. 76, with permission.)

µg/kg/min provided effective anesthesia. Plasma fentanyl concentrations in this subpopulation were two- to threefold higher than were reported with the same regimen in adults and were explained by the lower steady-state volume of distribution observed in children with intracardiac shunts.

Improved outcome was demonstrated in infants with congenital diaphragmatic hernia treated with rapid-frequency ventilation, moderate fluid restriction, muscle relaxation, and a continuous fentanyl infusion of 3 µg/kg/hr (79). In a separate ICU study of 20 mechanically ventilated infants who were 26–40 weeks' gestational age at birth, adequate sedation was obtained using infusions of 0.25–1.50 μg/kg/hr for 1.5–10 days. Total body clearance was similar to that of adults (80). Another study of 19 mechanically ventilated patients between 17 days and 14 years of age revealed a highly variable total body clearance of fentanyl and more than a tenfold variability in fentanyl infusion rates to achieve similar rates of sedation (81). However, clearance in an individual patient was constant over time and was not influenced by the duration of administration. The development of clinical tolerance in several study patients was not the result of enhanced clearance with continued administration.

Contrary to the findings of Leuschen et al. (82), Arnold et al. (83), in a prospective study of eight neonates undergoing extracorporeal membrane oxygenation, found a rapid escalation in plasma fentanyl concentrations required for satisfactory sedation. The increase in fentanyl requirement may reflect a pharmacodynamic transition from fetal to postnatal life, such as decreases in progesterone and beta-endorphin levels. Continuous rather than intermittent fentanyl administration may also play a role in rapid development of tolerance.

Arnold et al. (84), Katz et al. (85), and others (86,87) found a high rate of dependence and narcotic withdrawal symptoms in neonates, infants, and young children following cessation of continuous fentanyl infusions (Table 3). Using the neonatal abstinence scoring system, these authors found that between 50% and 57% of the patients experienced withdrawal. The effect was dependent on both the total fentanyl dose and the duration of infusion. Symptoms included irritability, insomnia, tremors, hypertonicity, myoclonus, choreoathetosis, and increased respiratory rate and effort. Recommendations now exist for weaning the pediatric ICU patient on prolonged opiate therapy. For patients on opiate therapy for less than 1 week, a 25–50% reduction per day is suggested. For longer periods of therapy, a 20% reduction in the first 24 hours, followed by a 10% reduction every 12 hours as tolerated, is recommended. Converting to oral regimens with morphine or methadone may facilitate tapering (88).

Fentanyl-induced chest wall rigidity, a recognized phenomenon in adults, was reported in an 8-week-old infant born at 38 weeks' gestation. Chest-wall rigidity was noted 30 minutes after starting a fentanyl infusion of 5 μg/kg/hr, with no loading dose given, and ultimately required naloxone for reversal (89).

TABLE 3. *Incidence of neonatal abstinence syndrome in pediatric ICU patients following continuous fentanyl infusion*

Incidence	Comments	Number of subjects (ref.)
57%	Greater incidence if duration of extracorporeal membrane oxygenation is greater than 5 days or total fentanyl dose is greater than 1.6 mg/kg	12 (84)
57%	Duration of infusion longer than 9 days or total fentanyl dose greater than 2.5 mg/kg is 100% predictive	23 (85)
50%		12 (86)

MUSCLE RELAXANTS

Atracurium

Neuromuscular blockade from atracurium is minimally affected by age. Goudsouzian et al. (90,91) showed that the body weight-based dose of atracurium required for satisfactory intubating conditions is the same in adolescents, in children, and in infants aged 4 weeks or older. Fisher (5) subsequently confirmed and expanded upon their work. In a study comparing infants 4–11 months of age with children and adults, neither elimination half-life nor steady-state plasma concentration varied with age. The absence of age-related changes in half-life resulted from parallel decreases in volume of distribution at steady state and total clearance with increasing age (Table 4).

Atracurium infusion requirements in the operating room are fairly consistent (92–96). Using a nitrous-narcotic technique, Kalli and Meretoja (92) found that the infusion requirement to maintain steady-state neuromuscular block in all pediatric patients older than 1 month was relatively constant at 0.53 mg/kg/hr. Neonates required a 25% reduction to 0.40 mg/kg/hr. Goudsouzian et al. (92,93) found a similar infusion requirement with a nitrous-narcotic technique and a lower requirement in the presence of halothane and, particularly, enflurane. Using a closed-loop feedback-control system of neuromuscular blockade for 10 patients who were 5–36 months old and undergoing craniofacial reconstruction with a nitrous-narcotic-pentothal infusion technique, Wait and Goat (95) found a mean dose requirement of 0.40 mg/kg/hr (Table 5).

Atracurium infusion was used successfully after pancuronium failed to provide adequate muscle relaxation for a neurosurgical procedure in a 15-year-old male on chronic phenytoin for seizure control (97). Atracurium was not antagonized by phenytoin, a drug shown to induce resistance to both pancuronium and vecuronium.

Atracurium is less predictable when used for prolonged infusion in intensive care. A mean infusion rate of 1.60 mg/kg/hr, several times that required in the operating room, was needed in 12 children to facilitate mechanical ventilation (98). The mean duration of infusion was 98 hours and ranged up to 284 hours. No side effects attributable to laudanosine, a longer-acting metabolite that can cause cerebral excitation and seizures, were noted. In a study that included a child and two

TABLE 4. *Mean (SD) pharmacokinetic values for atracurium in infants, children, and adults*

	Infants	Children	Adults
$t_{1/2}B$ (min)	20.0 (5.1)	17.2 (5.1)	15.7 (2.5)
V_{ss} (ml/kg)	210 (118)	129 (44)	100 (22)
Cl (ml/kg/min)	7.9 (2.0)	6.8 (1.6)	5.3 (0.9)

Adapted from Fisher et al., ref. 5.

TABLE 5. *Atracurium infusion requirements in infants and children*

Subjects	Age	Number of subjects	Infusion rate (μg/kg/min)	Anesthetic technique	Reference
Neonates	9–30 days (full-term)	7	6.6	N_2O-narcotic	92
Infants	2–90 days	10	7.6	N_2O-halothane	94
	1–12 mos	17	8.7	N_2O-narcotic	92
Children	1–10 yrs	9	9.3	N_2O-narcotic	93
	1–17 yrs	51	8.8	N_2O-narcotic	92
	1–10 yrs	11	8.3	N_2O-halothane	93
	1–10 yrs	8	4.9	N_2O-enflurane	93

adolescents, plasma laudanosine levels were substantially below those causing seizures in dogs (99). Plasma laudanosine levels remained relatively constant in a 6-month-old infant receiving an atracurium infusion for 7 days and were well below the reported convulsive level (100).

Resistance to atracurium on the third day of an infusion occurred in a 17-year-old female ICU patient. Multiple bolus doses and increases in the infusion rate failed to prevent excessive physical movement and overriding the ventilator. The patient was adequately paralyzed within minutes of a standard dose of pancuronium, and maintained on a pancuronium infusion. The exact mechanism by which atracurium resistance occurred in this patient is unclear. Possible explanations included increased degradation of atracurium, a change in acetylcholine receptor physiology, or both (101).

Although prolonged paralysis may be more common following continuous infusions of pancuronium and vecuronium (102), it is seen with atracurium as well. Prolonged paralysis lasting 8 weeks was reported in a 17-year-old female after administration of an atracurium infusion for 13 days in the ICU (103). The use of atracurium by continuous infusion in the ICU is costly. In one study, the average cost of atracurium per patient per day was 29 times that for pancuronium (104).

Vecuronium

The initial bolus dose recommended for vecuronium in infants and children is similar to that in adults. Its onset of effect is most rapid in infants, whereas its duration and recovery times are longest in infants and shortest in children. Fisher and Miller (105) found that the time interval for supplemental doses also was longest in infants and shortest in children. The differences in duration and recovery times were subsequently explained by age-related changes in volume of distribution at steady state rather than clearance (4). Volume of distribution decreases as infants age, whereas plasma clearance does not, which results in a shortened recovery time.

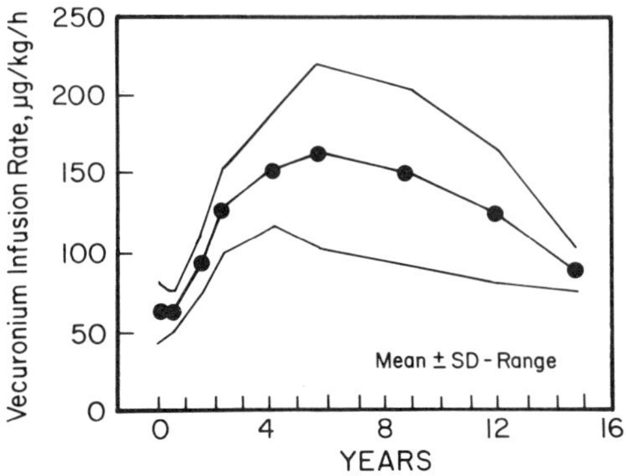

FIG. 2. The age-dependence of steady-state vecuronium infusion rate required to maintain a 90–95% neuromuscular block in pediatric patients during balanced anesthesia using a N_2O-narcotic technique. (From Meretoja, ref. 106, with permission.)

Vecuronium infusion requirements are age dependent. Neonates and infants require lower rates (62 µg/kg/hr) than do children aged 1 year to 13 years of age (106) (Fig. 2). The requirements in adolescents (89 µg/kg/hr) are comparable to infusion rates used in adults. As expected, infusion requirements decrease when halothane or isoflurane is added to a nitrous oxide (N_2O)-narcotic technique (107). Recovery from an infusion was more rapid in these children compared to adults.

Following a 90-µg/kg dose, Ridley and Braude (108) found that an infusion rate of 1.6 µg/kg/min resulted in satisfactory paralysis in 60 children receiving a halothane-N_2O anesthetic. Similar to Meretoja's (106) findings, they found a longer duration of neuromuscular blockade in neonates and young infants. They also found that vecuronium may accumulate after a 3-hour infusion.

A comparison of vecuronium given by intermittent bolus versus continuous infusion over 12 hours to infants and children in an ICU setting indicated that less vecuronium was needed to maintain adequate neuromuscular blockade when given by continuous infusion (109). The question of increasing vecuronium metabolism was raised but not actively addressed because fluctuation in the degree of blockade and breakthrough was observed in some of the study patients.

Mivacurium

Mivacurium can be used by infusion as easily and safely in children as in adults. The ED_{95} is higher in children than in adults and recovery is faster (110). In 28 children with a mean age of 6 years, a mean infusion rate of 10.4 µg/kg/min in the presence of halothane and N_2O maintained stable 90–99% muscle twitch depression (111). The infusion requirement increased to a mean of 13 µg/kg/min with a N_2O-narcotic anesthetic. No accumulation was seen with a continuous infusion of 294 minutes. After stopping the infusion, recovery was predictable and occurred in approximately 13 minutes.

In 62 children aged 2–10 years, higher levels of pseudocholinesterase activity were generally associated with a higher mivacurium infusion requirement and were a major factor influencing the infusion rate (112). Younger age was associated with a higher infusion requirement when calculated according to body weight but not body surface area. This suggests that the influence of age on infusion requirements is related to developmental changes in extracellular fluid volume. No evidence of accumulation was seen with prolonged infusion.

SEDATIVE/HYPNOTIC AND DISSOCIATIVE AGENTS

Propofol

Propofol is a useful agent for induction and maintenance of anesthesia in adults, with a short half-life, short context-sensitive half-time, and rapid recovery. It has more recently been investigated in children. Compared with adults, the volume of the central compartment in children is approximately 50% greater (6) and the elimination half-life is shorter (113).

Multiple studies have determined the induction dose at different ages of childhood. Hannallah et al. (114) studied 90 unpremedicated 3–12-year-olds and recommended a dose of 2.5–3.0 mg/kg. Subsequent studies involving larger groups of children came to similar conclusions (115,116). Westrin (117) studied 22 infants 1 month to 6 months old and found an ED_{50} of 3.0 mg/kg versus 2.4 mg/kg in children 10–15 years old. The minimum effective dose of lidocaine to prevent injection pain from propofol is 0.2 mg/kg—more than twice the adult value (118).

The use of propofol infusion techniques in pediatric surgical patients has had mixed results. One study found no difference in recovery time, defined as time to spontaneous eye opening after a propofol infusion compared with after halothane (119). Others found significantly slower recovery times using a propofol infusion for induction and maintenance (120). Postural stability (assessed by computerized posturography) and clinical recovery time were similar following propofol-alfentanil-N_2O versus thiopental-halothane-N_2O anesthesia (121).

Although they found no difference in extubation time, Hannallah et al. (122) found faster recovery and discharge times and less postoperative vomiting in 3–12-year-old children following propofol induction and maintenance with N_2O and an average propofol infusion rate of 267 μg/kg/min versus propofol-halothane, thiopental-halothane, and halothane-halothane anesthesia. A faster time to extubation and to discharge from the recovery room, as well as less nausea and vomiting, was noted in 40 children undergoing ear, nose, and throat procedures under propofol induction-infusion versus thiopental-halothane (123). In children undergoing strabismus surgery who received no postoperative opiates, the incidence of vomiting in the first 24 hours after surgery was 24% in patients receiving a maintenance propofol infusion (300 μg/kg/min for 15 minutes and 150 μg/min thereafter) versus 71% in a halothane control group (124). Others found a similar decrease in postoperative vomiting but noted more pain and spontaneous movement on induction (125), a higher frequency of oculocardiac reflex-induced bradycardia during maintenance infusion (125,126), and greater apprehension scores in the early postoperative period (126). A nontriggering anesthetic using a propofol infusion of 100–150 μg/kg/min after a 2.0 mg/kg bolus was used successfully for emergency surgery in a 10-year-old boy with Duchenne's muscular dystrophy (127).

Propofol infusions are used extensively outside the operating room, most notably to facilitate magnetic resonance imaging (MRI) in children. Following a 2-mg/kg loading dose, a 100-μg/kg/min infusion effectively prevented movement in all patients (128), though lower rates of 50 and 75 μg/kg/min were associated with some patient movement. No episodes of desaturation occurred during image acquisition. Vangerven et al. (129), using a bolus and infusion technique, also found that propofol was safe and reliable for sedation during MRI; movement artifact occurred in only 1 of the 49 children studied. Lebovic et al. (130) found that propofol compared favorably with ketamine for infants and children undergoing cardiac catheterization. Time to full recovery was 24 minutes in the propofol group versus 139 minutes in the ketamine group. The only hemodynamic difference in the two groups was a higher incidence of transient hypotension with propofol induction. Propofol has also been used for sedation for computerized axial tomography (131), multiple radiation therapy procedures (131,132), outpatient transesophageal echocardiography (133), and pulsed-dye laser treatment of port-wine stains (134) (Table 6).

TABLE 6. *Propofol infusion rates for anesthesia outside the operating room*

Site	Subjects' age	Infusion rate (μg/kg/min)	Comments	Number of subjects (ref.)
Magnetic resonance imaging	1–10 yrs	100	Patient movement with rates of 50 and 75 μg/kg/min	30 (128)
Magnetic resonance imaging	1 mo–12 yrs	100–133		20 (129)
Pulsed-dye laser treatment	8 mos–12 yrs	100–400	Higher rates for more sensitive treatment areas	48 (134)
Cardiac catheterization	7 mos–6 yrs	133	Includes bolus doses given	20 (130)
Transesophageal echocardiography	3–19.5 yrs	100–300		10 (133)
Computerized axial tomography, myelography	4 yrs	150		1 (131)
Body molds for cranial radiation	3 yrs	150	Electively intubated	1 (131)
Craniospinal radiation	14 mos	50–300	16 treatments	1 (131)

Propofol was used successively for up to 44 hours of sedation in pediatric ICU patients when more commonly used sedatives and analgesics failed (135), but a propofol withdrawal syndrome involving generalized twitching, choreiform movements, and possible grand mal seizures was subsequently described in two children (136,137). An article examining the possible contribution of propofol sedation to the clinical deterioration and death of five children in the ICU prompted much controversy and led to decreased use of propofol in the pediatric ICU setting (138).

Midazolam

Although the use of propofol is limited in the ICU for the above-mentioned reasons, there is increasing use of midazolam for continuous sedation. Pharmacokinetic studies in 15 1- to 5-day-old infants born at 29–41 weeks' gestation found a plasma clearance of 1.7 mg/kg/min and an elimination half-life of 12.0 hours (139). Midazolam clearance did not increase during therapy in these patients, who received infusions for an average of 60 hours. Hypotension was seen in 4 patients, 3 of whom also received fentanyl.

Midazolam was used successfully for postoperative sedation following open heart surgery. Forty-seven of 50 children between the ages of 6 months and 8 years were well sedated with infusion rates of 2–6 μg/kg/min for up to 197 hours and met the requirements for extubation within 4 hours of cessation of the infusion (140). The same authors measured serum midazolam levels in 10 of the patients, and concluded that midazolam clearance in these older infants and children was similar to that in adults. Elimination half-life also is either in the same range as in adults or slightly prolonged (141). Rosen and Rosen (142) and Silvasi et al. (143) also reported good results with midazolam sedation, using an initial bolus of 0.20–0.25 mg/kg and infusions of 0.4–4.0 μg/kg/min. They noted that 1% benzyl alcohol is a preservative in midazolam. "Gasping baby syndrome" is a fatal consequence of benzyl alcohol poisoning reported in low-birth-weight premature infants. However, the infusion level needed to accumulate toxic levels of benzyl alcohol would be 24 times the therapeutic dose observed in their youngest patient.

Hartwig et al. (144) reported changes in midazolam clearance with continuous infusion after several days. Clearance measured between 80–120 hours after initiation of continuous infusion in 11 patients was more than twice that measured in the same patients between 24–48 hours. An increase in distribution volume, enzyme induction by midazolam, or increasing hepatic blood flow during treatment may have caused the measured increase in clearance.

Midazolam bolus and infusion successfully treated status epilepticus in seven patients, including three children, who did not respond to other benzodiazepines, barbiturates, or additional anticonvulsants. After a single injection, a mean continuous infusion rate of 2.8 μg/kg/min was used for an average of 31 hours (145).

Severe reversible encephalopathy lasting 5 days to 4 weeks and attributed to benzodiazepine withdrawal was seen in three patients aged 3–15 months following 5–10 days of continuous midazolam infusion (32). The authors did not observe abstinence symptoms after use of other benzodiazepines in large and frequent doses.

Ketamine

The dissociative agent ketamine has many pediatric applications. The dose of intravenously administered ketamine necessary to maintain surgical anesthesia is age related, with infants and younger children requiring larger doses per unit weight (146). Grant et al. (147) found that plasma concentrations in 4–9 year-old children after both IV and IM doses were similar to concentrations in adults receiving the same dose per unit weight. The plasma concentrations at which children awakened were greater than in adults, implying that the greater dose requirements in children may be attributable to pharmacodynamic rather than pharmacokinetic factors. The absence of a significant difference in half-life and clearance may be the result of the relatively short sampling period (5 hrs).

In children, as in adults, ketamine can induce respiratory depression. The effects of ketamine on ventilatory response were studied in nine children between 6 years and 10 years old following a 2 mg/kg IV ketamine dose and a continuous infusion of 40 μg/kg/min (147) (Table 7, Fig. 3). Although ketamine did not affect resting respiratory rate, tidal volume, end-tidal CO_2, or minute ventilation, it decreased the slope of the CO_2 response curve. Apnea and cyanosis were not observed in the study, but arterial oxygen saturation was not measured.

The effect of ketamine on pulmonary vascular resistance (PVR) and systemic vascular resistance (SVR) was studied in children with congenital heart disease with and without elevated PVR (149,150). The investigators found no changes (150) or minimal, clinically insignificant changes (149). Hickey et al. (150) emphasized that the airway and ventilation were supported in their patients and that lack of such support could lead to increases in pulmonary vascular resistance.

Ketamine infusion with or without supplemental benzodiazepines was used for interventional cardiology in children (151,152). Malviya et al. (151) reported that

TABLE 7. *Mean (SD) resting respiratory variables before ketamine (control), 5 minutes after intravenous (IV) bolus, and 30 minutes after continuous IV infusion of ketamine*

		Ketamine	
Variables	Control	Bolus	Infusion
Resting f (breaths/min)	26.0 (7.2)	23.3 (4.6)	25.1 (6.1)
Resting V_T (ml·kg^{-1})	8.7 (1.3)	9.0 (2.1)	7.7 (2.1)
Resting V_E (ml·kg^{-1}·min^{-1})	207 (65)	185 (45)	175 (60)
Resting positron emission tomography CO_2 (mmHg)	34.5 (4.2)	36.7 (3.8)	36.3 (3.9)

From Sarner et al., ref. 110, with permission.

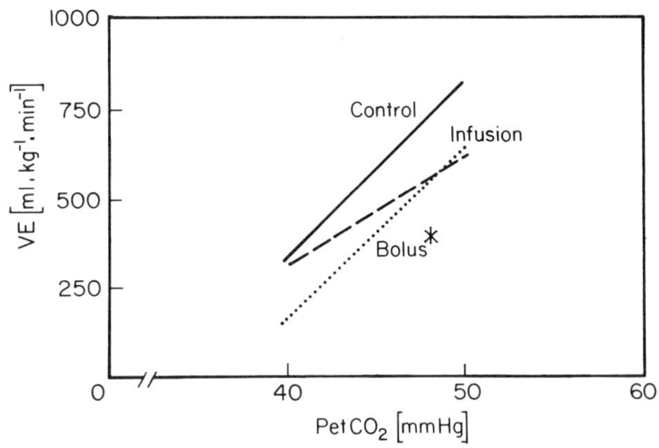

FIG. 3. Changes in the CO_2 response-curve slope in children, following ketamine bolus of 2 mg/kg, followed by continuous infusion of 40 μg/kg/min. (From Hamza et al., ref. 148, with permission.)

respiratory complications were more common after ketamine than after other sedation techniques. All patients who developed airway problems and 67% of patients with hypercarbia were anaesthetized with ketamine as the sole or primary anesthetic. Five of 87 patients receiving ketamine required emergency intubation. Hickey et al. (152) used a mean ketamine dose of 1 mg/kg/hr (16.6 μg/kg/min), which was much lower than the mean dose of 6.1 mg/kg/hr in Malviya's group, combined with a midazolam infusion for transcatheter closure of atrial septal defects. Fewer complications were described with this technique. Three of 93 patients receiving ketamine required intubation for "ventilatory compromise" or lack of immobility.

Ketamine also has been used in the pediatric ICU. Tobias et al. (153) described successful sedation in five patients when ketamine was used because other means of sedation failed or because of concerns about hemodynamic or respiratory side effects from other sedatives. A bolus dose of 0.5–1.0 mg/kg, followed by an infusion of 10–15 μg/kg/min, was used. Ketamine infusion also was used successfully to treat status asthmaticus in children, with and without mechanical ventilation, after more conventional therapy failed (154,155).

POSTOPERATIVE EPIDURAL ANALGESIA

Because of the popularity of continuous epidural infusions of local anesthetics, opiates, or both for postoperative pain relief in infants and children, a separate section is devoted to their use.

The pharmacokinetic parameters of epidural morphine in children between the ages of 2 and 15 years are similar to those observed in adults except for a shorter terminal half-life attributed to a greater total body clearance of morphine in

TABLE 8. *Pharmacokinetics of epidural morphine*

Age of subjects	C_l (ml/min/kg)	V_d (1/kg)	$t_{1/2}\beta$(min)	Number of subjects (ref.)
4.5–15 yrs	28.3 (3.4) *M* (*SD*)	2.94 (0.93) *M* (*SD*)	73.8 (41.6) *M* (*SD*)	7 (156)
Adults	Range, 14–21	Range, 2.9–5.5	200 (60) SEM	20 (157)

SEM, standard error of measurement.

children (156) (Table 8). This greater body clearance may be related to increased hepatic mass relative to body weight or to an absolute increase in hepatic microsomal activity. Effective and prolonged analgesia was obtained at plasma morphine levels that were lower than those described for systemic analgesia, indicating a nonsystemic analgesic effect of epidural morphine. Although no significant resting respiratory changes occurred in the children studied, the CO_2 ventilatory-response slope was decreased for 22 hours after morphine injection.

Ecoffey et al. (158) found similar pharmacokinetics for bupivacaine among children aged 5–10 years and adults (Table 9). Maximum bupivacaine levels were similar to those reported in adults given comparable doses based on body weight. The volume of distribution was larger in children than in adults, which explained the slightly longer elimination half-life in children. Peak plasma levels in this and subsequent studies were well below the toxic levels reported for adults (159,160). A pharmacokinetic profile similar to that of adults was also demonstrated in 1–6-month-old infants, but alpha-1 acid glycoprotein concentrations were lower and the free fraction of bupivacaine was markedly increased compared with published values for adults (161,162). No clinical evidence of CNS toxicity was seen in these patients.

Desparmet et al. (163) found that plasma concentrations of bupivacaine remained stable, without evidence of accumulation after 48 hours of infusion, in children aged 3–11 years. Total body clearance of bupivacaine was in the range of the ranges reported by others (158) and was similar to adult values. Wolf et al. (164), however, noted considerable variability in plasma bupivacaine concentrations in infants and young children; some of the patients showed accumulation after 24 hours of continuous infusion.

A hemodynamic study of 74 children using 0.25% bupivacaine with 1:200,000 epinephrine showed minimal changes in heart rate and systolic blood pressure in children younger than 8 years (165). Tobias et al. (166) found more stable cardiorespiratory responses with a continuous epidural infusion versus an intermittent bolus technique.

The effectiveness of continuous epidural analgesia (CEA) has been studied extensively in all pediatric age groups, including premature infants. In 20 infants born at 25–40 weeks' gestation, Murrell et al. (167) used CEA with great success for surgical procedures done when the infants were between 4 hours and 5 months old. Catheters were placed and dosed after induction of general anesthesia and intubation. All patients were extubated at the end of operations lasting as long as 5

TABLE 9. *Pharmacokinetics of caudal epidural bupivacaine*

Age of subjects	C_l (ml/min/kg) ±±	Vd_{ss} (1/kg) ±±	$t_{1/2}\beta$(hrs)	Number of subjects (ref.)
1–6 mos	7.1 (3.2) *M* (*SD*)	3.9 (2.0) *M* (*SD*)	7.7 (2.4) *M* (*SD*)	13 (161)
5.5–10 yrs	10 (0.7) (SEM)	2.7 (0.2) (SEM)	4.6 (0.6) (SEM)	6 (158)
Adults[a]	6.3	1.0	2.7	—(162)

SEM, standard error of measurement
[a]Assuming body weight of 75 kg.

hours. Bupivacaine, 0.1%, with 1 μg/ml fentanyl was infused via lumbar epidural catheters at 0.2 ml/kg/hr for 18–69 hours postoperatively. Effective analgesia was achieved, as assessed by physiological variables and a simplified pain scale, and no complications were encountered. Continuous caudal anesthesia using 3% 2-chloroprocaine was used safely and effectively for repair of inguinal hernia in ten former preterm infants who were 35–49 weeks of age postconception age at the time of surgery (168). Despite low plasma cholinesterase activity in some of the infants, no evidence of toxicity from 2-chloroprocaine was detected.

In a comparison between continuous epidural bupivacaine and IV morphine infusion for postoperative pain relief in patients aged 3– 46 months, patients in both groups had adequate and comparable analgesia, but those receiving morphine experienced more drowsiness, respiratory depression, and oxygen desaturation (169). CEA with bupivacaine blunted the stress response to surgery more effectively than did an IV morphine infusion (170). Perioperative increases in epinephrine, glucose, and adrenocorticotropic hormone were significantly greater in the opiate group. Modifying the stress response may be of potential benefit to postoperative recovery.

In children, continuous epidural infusion of fentanyl provided analgesia comparable to that of daily epidural morphine boluses and with fewer side effects such as itching, nausea, and vomiting (171). Continuous epidural fentanyl infusion was combined with patient-controlled epidural analgesia in children as young as 6 years (172). Good or excellent analgesia was obtained in 78% of the patients with a mean infusion rate of 0.56 μg/kg/hr, a mean bolus dose of 0.53 μg/kg, and a 15-minute lockout period. Patients with thoracic catheters placed for thoracic or upper abdominal procedures benefitted the most. Continuous infusion of 0.1–0.2% bupivacaine with 2–5 μg/ml of fentanyl provided excellent analgesia in pediatric oncology patients ranging in age from 4 months to 19 years who were undergoing major surgery (173).

Berde (174) cautioned against attempting to provide analgesia at upper abdominal or thoracic dermatomes with low-lying lumbar or caudal catheters. In infants and younger children, it is possible to thread catheters from the caudal space to mid or lower thoracic dermatomes (175–177). The technique is not as successful in preadolescents and adolescents, possibly because of increased epidural fat (177). Tobias et al. (178) found that the technique of threading caudal catheters to tho-

TABLE 10. *Suggested maximum bupivacaine dosage guidelines*

Age group	Initial bolus (mg/kg)	Infusion (mg/kg/hr)
Neonates	1.5	0.2–0.25
Children	2.0–2.5	0.4–0.5

Adapted from Berde, refs. 174, 188, and 191.

racic levels was unreliable. They and other authors (159) described placement of catheters directly at the thoracic level with ease and without complication.

Other successful alternatives to more conventional insertion and positioning of catheters have been described. Loennqvist and Olsson (179) found that continuous thoracic paravertebral blockade provided superior pain relief compared with lumbar epidural blockade in children who were undergoing renal surgery (179). A modification of the Taylor approach, with midline insertion of catheters at the L5–S1 interspace, was used successfully in 97 children undergoing abdominal urologic surgery, including infants as young as 1 month (180). Cooper and Sethna (181) reported that epidural analgesia was achieved in six patients with congenital lumbosacral spinal anomalies, including myelomeningocele, intra- or postoperatively or both using catheters placed above the level of the anomaly.

Although there are appropriately sized epidural needles and catheters for infants and children (182), technical complications such as catheter occlusion, leakage, or disconnection still resulted in early discontinuation of 11% to 16.7% of infusions in two recent audits of pediatric pain services (183,184). More serious complications such as high block (185), convulsions (186,187), and respiratory depression (183,184) led to recommendations to further improve the safety of pediatric regional anesthetic techniques (174,188) (Tables 10–12). In particular, Berde (174) emphasized that infants and children are probably no more resistant than adults to local anesthetic toxicity. Neonates have a diminished plasma concentration of alpha-1 acid glycoprotein, which binds bupivacaine, and a slower bupivacaine clearance (161). In a study of the cardiovascular toxicity of IV bupivacaine in dogs, the toxic dose and plasma concentrations associated with toxicity were both significantly lower in younger than in older dogs (189). Using the guideline limiting bupivacaine infusion rates to no more than 0.4 mg/kg/hr, Berde (190) reported no convulsions in more than 1,900 infants and children receiving postoperative epidural infusions.

TABLE 11. *Epidural morphine dosing guidelines*

Age group	Bolus (q 6–12 hrs) (μg/kg)	Infusion rate (μg/kg/hr)
Infants older than 6 mos and children	30–50	5.0
Infants younger than 6 mos	15–25	2.5

Adapted from Berde, refs. 188 and 191.

TABLE 12. *Initial epidural infusion rates*[a]

Solution	Infusion rate (ml/kg/hr)
0.1% bupivacaine with 2–5 μg/ml fentanyl	0.2–0.4
0.1% bupivacaine with 10 μg/ml hydromorphone	0.15–0.2

Adapted from Tobias, et al., ref. 173, and Berde, ref. 191.
[a] Infusion rates should be reduced about 50% in neonates. Infusion rate depends in part on the position of the catheter tip relative to the site of surgical incision. Hydromorphone may produce less pruritus than morphine.

CONCLUSION

An understanding of basic physiologic differences between infants, children, and adults, combined with knowledge of the commonly used opiates, muscle relaxants, and sedative/hypnotic agents, allows use of continuous drug infusions to provide intraoperative anesthesia and sedation, muscle relaxation, or analgesia outside the operating room. Infusion techniques will undergo further evolution and refinement and will continue to play an essential role in the care of pediatric patients.

REFERENCES

1. Friis-Hansen B. Water distribution in the foetus and newborn infant. *Acta Paediatr Scand* 1983; 305:7–11.
2. Bauer K, Bovermann, Roithmaier A, et al. Body composition, nutrition, and fluid balance during the first two weeks of life in preterm neonates weighing less than 1500 grams. *J Pediatr* 1991;118:615–620.
3. Fisher DM, O'Keefe C, Stanski DR, et al. Pharmacokinetics and pharmacodynamics of d-tubocurarine in infants, children, and adults. *Anesthesiology* 1982;57:203–208.
4. Fisher DM, Castagnoli K, Miller RD. Vecuronium kinetics and dynamics in anesthetized infants and children. *Clin Pharmacol Ther* 1985;37:402–406.
5. Fisher DM, Canfell PC, Spellman MJ, Miller RD. Pharmacokinetics and pharmacodynamics of atracurium in infants and children. *Anesthesiology* 1990;73:33–37.
6. Marsh B, White M, Morton N, Kenny GNC. Pharmacokinetic model driven infusion of propofol in children. *Br J Anaesth* 1991;67:41–48.
7. Burrows FA, Lerman J, LeDez KM, Strong A. Pharmacokinetics of lidocaine in children with congenital heart disease. *Can J Anaesth* 1991;38:196–200.
8. Hall SC. Children with congenital heart disease undergoing noncardiac surgery. *Semin Anesth* 1993; 12:8–17.
9. Cook DR, Marcy JH. Pediatric anesthetic pharmacology. In: Cook DR, Marcy JH, eds. *Neonatal anesthesia*. Pasadena, CA: Appleton Davies; 1988:87–125.
10. Kupferberg HJ, Way EL. Pharmacologic basis for the increased sensitivity of the newborn rat to morphine. *J Pharmacol Exp Ther* 1963;141:105–112.
11. Way WL, Costley EC, Way EL. Respiratory sensitivity of the newborn infant to meperidine and morphine. *Clin Pharmacol Ther* 1965;6:454–461.
12. Meistelman C, Benhamou D, Varre J, et al. Effects of age on plasma protein binding of sufentanil. *Anesthesiology* 1990;72:470–473.
13. Notarianni LJ. Plasma protein binding of drugs in pregnancy and in neonates. *Clin Pharmacokinet* 1990;18:20–36.
14. Petersen S, Gorfredsen A, Knudsen FU. Lean body mass in small for gestational age and appropriate for gestational age infants. *J Pediatr* 1988;113:886–889.

15. Aperia A, Broberger O, Herlin P, et al. Postnatal control of water and electrolyte homeostasis in preterm and full-term infants. *Acta Paediatr Scand* 1982;305:61–65.
16. Cook DR, Rowe MI. Parenteral fluid therapy. In: Cook DR, Marcy JH, eds. *Neonatal anesthesia.* Pasadena, CA: Appleton Davies; 1988:71–85.
17. Edelstone DI, Rudolph AM, Hemann MA. Liver and ductus venosus blood flows in fetal lambs in utero. *Circ Res* 1978;42:426–433.
18. Shoaf SE, Schwark WS, Guard CL, Babish JG. The development of hepatic drug-metabolizing enzyme activity in the neonatal calf and its effect on drug disposition. *Drug Metab Dispos* 1987;15:676–681.
19. Gauntlett IS, Fisher DM, Hertzka RE, et al. Pharmacokinetics of fentanyl in neonatal humans and lambs: effects of age. *Anesthesiology* 1988;69:683–687.
20. Sereni F, Mandelli M, Principi N, et al. Induction of drug metabolizing enzyme activities in the human fetus and in the newborn infant. *Enzyme* 1973;15:318–329.
21. Koehntop DE, Rodman JH, Brundage DM, et al. Pharmacokinetics of fentanyl in neonates. *Anesth Analg* 1986;65:227–232.
22. Bhargava VO, Garrettson LK. Development of phenobarbital glucosidation in the human neonate. *Dev Pharmacol Ther* 1988;11:8–13.
23. Splinter WM, Schaffer JD Zunder IH. Clear fluids three hours before surgery do not affect the gastric fluid contents of children. *Can J Anaesth* 1990;37:498–501.
24. Schreiner MS, Triebwasser A, Keon TP. Ingestion of liquids compared with preoperative fasting in pediatric outpatients. *Anesthesiology* 1990;72:593–597.
25. Phillips S, Daborn AK, Hatch DJ. Preoperative fasting for paediatric anaesthesia. *Br J Anaesth* 1994; 73:529–536.
26. Moss R, Conner H, Yee WPH, et al. Human beta-endorphin-like immunoreactivity in the perinatal/ neonatal period. *J Pediatr* 1982;101:443-446.
27. Anand KJS, Hickey PR. Pain and its effects in the human neonate and fetus. *N Engl J Med* 1987;317: 1321–1329.
28. Emhardt JD, Vasko MR. Do nconatcs nccd ancsthcsia? *Adv Anesth* 1990;7:45–81.
29. Tobin AJ, Khrestchatisky M, MacLennan AJ, et al. Structural, developmental and functional heterogeneity of rat GABAA receptors. *Adv Exper Med Biol* 1991;287:365–374.
30. Kinney HC, White WF. Opiod receptors localize to the external granular cell layer of the developing cerebellum. *Neuroscience* 1991;45:13–21.
31. Crozier TA, Flamm C, Speer CP, et al. Effects of etomidate on the adrenocortical and metabolic adaptation of the neonate. *Br J Anaesth* 1993;70:47–53.
32. Bergman I, Steeves M, Burckart G, Thompson A. Reversible neurologic abnormalities associated with prolonged intravenous midazolam and fentanyl administration. *J Pediatr* 1991;119:644–649.
33. LeDez KM, Lerman J. The minimal alveolar concentration (MAC) of isoflurane in preterm neonates. *Anesthesiology* 1987;67:301–307.
34. Cameron CB, Robinson S, Gregory GA. The minimum anesthetic concentration of isoflurane in children. *Anesth Analg* 1984;63:418–420.
35. Lerman J, Robinson S, Willis MM, et al. Anesthetic requirements for halothane in young children 0-1 month and 1-6 months of age. *Anesthesiology* 1983;59:421–424.
36. Bhat R, Gulati A, Aldana O, et al. Pharmacokinetics of a single dose of morphine in preterm infants during the first week of life. *J Pediatr* 1990;117:477–481.
37. Yaster M. The dose response of fentanyl in neonatal anesthesia. *Anesthesiology* 1987;66:433–435.
38. Anand KJS, Ward-Platt MP. Neonatal and pediatric stress responses to anesthesia and operation. *Int Anesth Clin* 1988;26:218–225.
39. Anand KJS, Brown MJ, Bloom SR, et al. Studies on the hormonal regulation of fuel metabolism in the human newborn infant undergoing anesthesia and surgery. *Hormone Res* 1985;22:115–128.
40. Anand KJS, Brown MJ, Causon RC, et al. Can the human neonate mount an endocrine and metabolic response to surgery? *J Pediatr Surg* 1985;20:41–48.
41. Anand KJS, Sippell WG, Aynsley-Green A. Randomized trial of fentanyl anaesthesia in preterm babies undergoing surgery: effects on the stress response. *Lancet* 1987;1:243–248.
42. Anand KJS, Sippell WG, Schofield NM, Aynsley-Green A. Does halothane anaesthesia decrease the stress response of newborn infants undergoing operation? *Br Med J* 1988;296:668–672.
43. Pokela M. Pain relief can reduce hypoxemia in distressed neonates during routine treatment procedures. *Pediatrics* 1994;93:379–383.
44. Quinn MW, Wild J, Dean HG, et al. Randomized double-blind controlled trial of effect of morphine on catecholamine concentrations in ventilated pre-term babies. *Lancet* 1993;342:324–327.

45. Anand KJS, Sippel WG, Aynsley-Green A. Randomized trial of fentanyl anesthesia in preterm babies undergoing surgery. *Lancet* 1987;1:62–66.
46. Anand KJS, Hickey PR. Halothane-morphine compared with high-dose sufentanil for anesthesia and postoperative analgesia in neonatal cardiac surgery. *N Engl J Med* 1992;326:1–9.
47. Dahlstrom B, Bolme P, Feychting H, Noack G, Paalzow L. Morphine kinetics in children. *Clin Pharmacol Ther* 1979;26:354–365.
48. Olkkola KT, Maunuksela EL, Korpela R, Rosenberg PH. Kinetics and dynamics of postoperative intravenous morphine in children. *Clin Pharmacol Ther* 1988;44:128–136.
49. Hartley R, Green M, Quinn M, Levene MI. Pharmacokinetics of morphine infusion in premature neonates. *Arch Dis Child* 1993;69:55–58.
50. Lynn AM, Slattery JT. Morphine pharmacokinetics in early infancy. *Anesthesiology* 1987;66:136–139.
51. Choonara A, McKay P, Hain R, Rane A. Morphine metabolism in children. *Br J Clin Pharmacol* 1989;28:599–604.
52. Koren G, Butt W, Chinyanga H, et al. Postoperative morphine infusion in newborn infants: assessment of disposition characteristics and safety. *J Pediatr* 1985;107:963–965.
53. Stanski Dr, Paalzow L, Edlund PO. Morphine pharmacokinetics: GLC assay versus radioimmunoassay. *J Pharm Sci* 1982;71:314–317.
54. Lynn AM, Nespeca MK, Opheim KE, Slattery JT. Respiratory effects of intravenous morphine infusions in neonates, infants, and children after cardiac surgery. *Anesth Analg* 1993;77:695–701.
55. Bray RJ. Postoperative analgesia provided by morphine infusion in children. *Anaesthesia* 1983;38: 1075–1078.
56. Beasley SW, Tibballs J. Efficacy and safety of continuous morphine infusion for postoperative analgesia in the paediatric surgical ward. *Aust NZ J Surg* 1987;57:233–237.
57. Millar AJW, Rode H, Cywes S. Continuous morphine infusion for postoperative pain in children. *S Afr Med J* 1987;72:396–398.
58. Hendrickson M, Myre L, Johnson DG, et al. Postoperative analgesia in children: a prospective study of intermittent intramuscular injection versus continuous intravenous infusion of morphine. *J Pediatr Surg* 1990;25:185–191.
59. Farrington EA, McGuinness GA, Johnson GF, Erenberg Ad, Leff RD. Continuous intravenous morphine infusion in postoperative newborn infants. *Am J Perinatol* 1993;10:84–87.
60. Lynn AM, Opheim KE, Tyler DC. Morphine infusion after pediatric cardiac surgery. *Crit Care Med* 1984;12:863–866.
61. Geiduschek JM, Haberkern CM, McLaughlin JF, Jacobson LE, Hays RM, Roberts TS. Pain management for children following selective dorsal rhizotomy. *Can J Anaesth* 1994;41:492–496.
62. Doyle E, Robinson D, Morton NS. Comparison of patient-controlled analgesia with and without a background infusion after lower abdominal surgery in children. *Br J Anaesth* 1993;71:670–673.
63. Doyle E, Harper I, Morton NS. Patient-controlled analgesia with low dose background infusions after lower abdominal surgery in children. *Br J Anaesth* 1993;71:818–822.
64. Berde CB, Lehn BM, Yee JD, Sethna NF, Russo D. Patient-controlled analgesia in children and adolescents: a randomized, prospective comparison with intramuscular administration of morphine for postoperative analgesia. *J Pediatr* 1991;118:460–466.
65. Doyle E, Morton NS, McNicol LR. Comparison of patient-controlled analgesia in children by i.v. and s.c. routes of administration. *Br J Anaesth* 1994;72:533–536.
66. Gaukroger PB, Chapman MJ, Davey RB. Pain control in paediatric burns—the use of patient-controlled analgesia. *Burns* 1991;17:396–399.
67. Mackie AM, Coda BC, Hill HF. Adolescents use patient-controlled analgesia effectively for relief from prolonged oropharyngeal mucositis pain. *Pain* 1991;46:265–269.
68. Robieux IC, Kellner JD, Coppes MJ, et al. Analgesia in children with sickle cell crisis: comparison of intermittent opioids vs. continuous intravenous infusion of morphine and placebo-controlled study of oxygen inhalation. *Pediatr Hematol Oncol* 1992;9:317–326.
69. Cole TB, Sprinkle RH, Smith SJ, Buchanan GR. Intravenous narcotic therapy for children with severe sickle cell pain crisis. *AJDC* 1986;140:1255–1259.
70. Gerber N, Apseloff G. Death from a morphine infusion during a sickle cell crisis. *J Pediatr* 1993;123: 322–325.
71. de Armendi AJ, Fahey M, Ryan JF. Morphine-induced myoclonic movements in a pediatric pain patient. *Anesth Analg* 1993;77:191–192.
72. Marx CM, Rosenberg DI, Ambuel B, Hamlett KW, Blumer JL. Pediatric intensive care sedation: survey of fellowship training programs. *Pediatrics* 1993;91:369–378.

73. Hickey PR, Hansen DD, Wessel DL, et al. Pulmonary and systemic hemodynamic responses to fentanyl in infants. *Anesth Analg* 1985;64:483–486.
74. Hickey PR, Hansen DD, Wessel DL, et al. Blunting of stress responses in the pulmonary circulation of infants by fentanyl. *Anesth Analg* 1985;64:1137–1142.
75. Collins C, Koren G, Crean P, Klein J, Roy WL, MacLeod SM. Fentanyl pharmacokinetics and hemodynamic effects in preterm infants during ligation of patent ductus arteriosus. *Anesth Analg* 1985; 64:1078–1080.
76. Singleton MA, Rosen JI, Fisher DM. Plasma concentrations of fentanyl in infants, children and adults. *Can J Anaesth* 1987;34:152–155.
77. Hertzka RE, Gauntlett IS, Fisher DM, Spelman MJ. Fentanyl-induced ventilatory depression: effects of age. *Anesthesiology* 1989;70:213–218.
78. Koren G, Goresky G, Crean P, Klein J, MacLeod ST. Pediatric fentanyl dosing based on pharmacokinetics during cardiac surgery. *Anesth Analg* 1984;63:577–582.
79. Vacanti JP, Crone RK, Murphy JD, et al. The pulmonary hemodynamic response to perioperative anesthesia in the treatment of high-risk infants with congenital diaphragmatic hernia. *J Pediatr Surg* 1984;19:672–679.
80. Roth B, Schluender C, Houben F, Guenther M, Theisohn M. Analgesia and sedation in neonatal intensive care using fentanyl by continuous infusion. *Dev Pharmacol Ther* 1991;17:121–127.
81. Katz R, Kelly HW. Pharmacokinetics of continuous infusions of fentanyl in critically ill children. *Crit Care Med* 1993;21:995–1000.
82. Leuschen MP, Willett LD, Hoie EB, et al. Plasma fentanyl levels in infants undergoing extracorporeal membrane oxygenation. *J Thorac Cardiovasc Surg* 1993;105:885–891.
83. Arnold JH, Truog RD, Scavone JM, Fenton T. Changes in the pharmacodynamic response to fentanyl in neonates during continuous infusion. *J Pediatr* 1991;119:639–643.
84. Arnold JH, Truog RD, Orav EJ, Scavone JM, Hershenson MB. Tolerance and dependence in neonates sedated with fentanyl during extracorporeal membrane oxygenation. *Anesthesiology* 1990;73: 1136–1140.
85. Katz R, Kelly HW, Hsi A. Prospective study on the occurrence of withdrawal in critically ill children who receive fentanyl by continuous infusion. *Crit Care Med* 1994;22:763–767.
86. French JP, Nocera M. Drug withdrawal symptoms in children after continuous infusions of fentanyl. *J Pediatr Nurs* 1994;9:107–113.
87. Lane JC, Tennison MB, Lawless ST, Greenwood RS, Zaritsky AL. Movement disorder after withdrawal of fentanyl infusion. *J Pediatr* 1991;119:649–651.
88. Carr DB, Todres ID. Fentanyl infusion and weaning in the pediatric intensive care unit: toward science-based practice. *Crit Care Med* 1994;22:725–727.
89. Well S, Williamson M, Hooker D. Fentanyl-induced chest wall rigidity in a neonate: a case report. *Heart Lung* 1994;23:196–198.
90. Goudsouzian NG,m Liu LMP, CotÈ CJ, Gionfriddo M, Rudd GD. Safety and efficacy of atracurium in adolescents and children anesthetized with halothane. *Anesthesiology* 1983;59:459–462.
91. Goudsouzian N, Liu LMP, Gionfriddo M, Rudd GD. Neuromuscular effects of atracurium in infants and children. *Anesthesiology* 1985;62:75–79.
92. Kalli I, Meretoja OA. Infusion of atracurium in neonates, infants and children: a study of dose requirements. *Br J Anaesth* 1988;60:651–654.
93. Goudsouzian N, Martyn J, Rudd GD, Liu LMP, Lineberry CH. Continuous infusion of atracurium in children. *Anesthesiology* 1986;64:171–174.
94. Goudsouzian N. Atracurium infusion in infants. *Anesthesiology* 1988;68:267–269.
95. Wait CM, Goat VA. Atracurium infusion during paediatric craniofacial surgery. *Anaesthesia* 1989; 44:567–570.
96. Ridley SA, Hatch DJ. Post-tetanic count and profound neuromuscular blockade with atracurium infusion in paediatric patients. *Br J Anaesth* 1988;60:31–35.
97. Hickey PR, Sangwan S, Bevan JC. Phenytoin-induced resistance to pancuronium. *Anaesthesia* 1988; 43:757–759.
98. Kushimo OT, Darowski MJ, Morris P, Hollis S, Meakin G. Dose requirements of atracurium in paediatric intensive care patients. *Br J Anaesth* 1991;67:781–783.
99. Yate PM, Flynn PJ, Arnold RW, Weatherly BC, Simmonds RJ, Dopson T. Clinical experience and plasma laudanosine concentrations during the infusion of atracurium in the intensive therapy unit. *Br J Anaesth* 1987;59:211–217.

100. Tabardel Y, Paquay T, Senterre J. Prolonged infusion of atracurium in an infant. *Dev Pharmacol Ther* 1990;15:52–56.
101. Kelly KJ, Clarens DM, Kohls PH, Nahum A, Vance-Bryan K. Response to pancuronium after loss of atracurium-induced neuromuscular blockade. *Ann Pharmacother* 1993;27:862–865.
102. Watling SM, Dasta JF. Prolonged paralysis in intensive care unit patients after the use of neuromuscular blocking agents: a review of the literature. *Crit Care Med* 1994;22:884–893.
103. Branney SW, Haenel JB, Moore FA, Tarbox BB, Schreiber RH, Moore EE. Prolonged paralysis with atracurium infusion: a case report. *Crit Care Med* 1994;22:1699–1701.
104. Clarens DM, Kelly KJ, Gilliland SS, Kohls PK, Nahum A, Vance-Bryan K. A retrospective analysis of long-term use of nondepolarizing neuromuscular blocking agents in the intensive care unit, and guidelines for drug selection. *Pharmacotherapy* 1993;13:647–655.
105. Fisher DM, Miller RD. Neuromuscular effects of vecuronium (ORG NC45) in infants and children during N_2O, halothane anesthesia. *Anesthesiology* 1983;58:519–523.
106. Meretoja OA. Vecuronium infusion requirements in pediatric patients during fentanyl-N_2O-O_2 anesthesia. *Anesth Analg* 1989;68:20–24.
107. Woelfel SK, Dong ML, Brandom BW, Sarner JB, Cook DR. Vecuronium infusion requirements in children during halothane-narcotic-nitrous oxide, isoflurane-narcotic-nitrous oxide, and narcotic-nitrous oxide anesthesia. *Anesth Analg* 1991;73:33–38.
108. Ridley SA, Braude N. Post-tetanic count and intense neuromuscular blockade with vecuronium in children. *Br J Anaesth* 1988;61:551–556.
109. Eldadah MK, Newth CJL. Vecuronium by continuous infusion for neuromuscular blockade in infants and children. *Crit Care Med* 1989;17:989–992.
110. Sarner JB, Brandom W, Woelfel SK, et al. Clinical pharmacology of mivacurium chloride (BW B109OU) in children during nitrous oxide-halothane and nitrous oxide-narcotic anesthesia. *Anesth Analg* 1989;68:116–121.
111. Alifimoff JK, Goudsouzian NG. Continuous infusion of mivacurium in children. *Br J Anaesth* 1989; 63:520–524.
112. Brandom BW, Sarner JB, Woelfel SK, et al. Mivacurium infusion requirements in pediatric surgical patients during nitrous oxide-halothane and during nitrous-oxide narcotic anesthesia. *Anesth Analg* 1990;71:16–22.
113. Valtonen M, Iissalo E, Kanto J, Rosenberg P. Propofol as an induction agent in children: pain on injection and pharmacokinetics. *Acta Anaesthesiol Scand* 1989;33:152–155.
114. Hannallah RS, Baker SB, Casey W, McGill WA, Broadman LM, Norden JM. Propofol: effective dose and induction characteristics in unpremedicated children. *Anesthesiology* 1991;74:217–219.
115. Manschot HJ, Meursing AEE, Axt P, Byttebier GO, Erdmann W. Propofol requirements for induction of anesthesia in children of different age groups. *Anesth Analg* 1992;75:876–879.
116. Aun CST, Short SM, Leung DHY, Oh TE. Induction dose-response of propofol in unpremedicated children. *Br J Anaesth* 1992;68:64–67.
117. Westrin P. The induction dose of propofol in infants 1–6 months of age and in children 10–16 years of age. *Anesthesiology* 1991;74:455–458.
118. Cameron E, Johnston G, Crofts S, Morton NS. The minimum effective dose of lidocaine to prevent injection pain due to propofol in children. *Anaesthesia* 1992;47:604–606.
119. Doyle E, McFadzean W, Morton NS. I.V. anaesthesia with propofol using a target-controlled infusion system: comparison with inhalation anaesthesia for general surgical procedures in children. *Br J Anaesth* 1993;70:542–545.
120. Aun CST, Short TG, O'Meara ME, Leung DHY, Rowbottom YM, Oh TE. Recovery after propofol infusion anaesthesia in children: comparison with propofol, thiopentone or halothane induction followed by halothane maintenance. *Br J Anaesth* 1994;72:554–558.
121. Hiller A, Pyykko I, Saarnivaara L. Evaluation of postural stability by computerized posturography following outpatient paediatric anaesthesia: comparison of propofol/alfentanil/N_2O anaesthesia with thiopentone/halothane/N_2O anaesthesia. *Acta Anaesthesiol Scand* 1993;37:556–561.
122. Hannallah RS, Britton JT, Schafer PG, Patel RI, Norden JM. Propofol anaesthesia in paediatric ambulatory patients: a comparison with thiopentone and halothane. *Can J Anaesth* 1994;41:12–18.
123. Borgeat A, Popovic V, Meier D, Schwander D. Comparison of propofol and thiopental/halothane for short-duration ENT surgical procedures in children. *Anesth Analg* 1990;71:511–515.
124. Weir PM, Munro HM, Reynolds PI, Lewis IH, Wilton NCT. Propofol infusion and the incidence of emesis in pediatric outpatient strabismus surgery. *Anesth Analg* 1993;76:760–764.

125. Snellen FT, Vanacker B, Van Aken H. Propofol-nitrous oxide versus thiopental sodium-isoflurane-nitrous oxide for strabismus surgery in children. *J Clin Anesth* 1993;5:37–41.
126. Larsson S, Asgeirsson B, Magnusson J. Propofol-fentanyl anesthesia compared to thiopental-halothane with special reference to recovery and vomiting after pediatric strabismus surgery. *Acta Anaesthesiol Scand* 1992;36:182–186.
127. Ginsburg RS, Porterfield K, Lippmann M. Propofol: bolus induction plus continuous infusion in a patient with Duchenne muscular dystrophy. *Anesthesiology* 1991;75:376.
128. Frankville DD, Spear RM, Dyck JB. The dose of propofol required to prevent children from moving during magnetic resonance imaging. *Anesthesiology* 1993;79:953–958.
129. Vangerven M, Van Hemelrijck J, Wouters P, Vandermeersch E, Van Aken H. Light anaesthesia with propofol for paediatric MRI. *Anaesthesia* 1992;47:706–707.
130. Lebovic S, Reich DL, Steinberg G, Vela FP, Silvay G. Comparison of propofol versus ketamine for anesthesia in pediatric patients undergoing cardiac catheterization. *Anesth Analg* 1992;74:490–494.
131. Martin LD, Pasternak LR, Pudimat MA. Total intravenous anesthesia with propofol in pediatric patients outside the operating room. *Anesth Analg* 1992;74:609–612.
132. Setlock MA, Palmisano BW. Propofol for radiation therapy in small children. *Anesth Analg* 1992;75:860–861.
133. Marcus B, Steward DJ, Khan NR, et al. Outpatient transesophageal echocardiography with intravenous propofol anesthesia in children and adolescents. *J Am Soc Echo* 1993;6:205–209.
134. Vischoff D, Charest J. Propofol for pulsed dye laser treatments in paediatric outpatients. *Can J Anaesth* 1994;41:728–732.
135. Norreslet J, Wahlgreen C. Propofol infusion for sedation of children. *Crit Care Med* 1990;18:890–892.
136. Trotter C, Serpell MG. Neurological sequelae in children after prolonged propofol infusion. *Anaesthesia* 1992;47:340–342.
137. Imray JMcG, Hay A. Withdrawal syndrome after propofol. *Anaesthesia* 1991;46:704.
138. Parke TJ, Stevens JE, Rice AS, et al. Metabolic acidosis and fatal myocardial failure after propofol infusion in children: five case reports. *Br Med J* 1992;305:613–616.
139. Jacqz-Aigrain E, Daoud P, Burtin P, Maherzi S, Beaufils F. Pharmacokinetics of midazolam during continuous infusion in critically ill neonates. *Eur J Clin Pharmacol* 1992;42:329–332.
140. Booker PD, Bechey A, Lloyd-Thomas AR. Sedation of children requiring artificial ventilation using an infusion of midazolam. *Br J Anaesth* 1986;58:1104–1108.
141. Lloyd-Thomas AR, Booker PD. Infusion of midazolam in paediatric patients after cardiac surgery. *Br J Anaesth* 1986;58:1109–1115.
142. Rosen DA, Rosen KR. Midazolam for sedation in the paediatric intensive care unit. *Intens Care Med* 1991;17:S15–S19.
143. Silvasi DL, Rosen DA, Rosen KR. Continuous intravenous midazolam infusion for sedation in the pediatric intensive care unit. *Anesth Analg* 1988;67:286–288.
144. Hartwig S, Roth B, Theisohn M. Clinical experience with continuous intravenous sedation using midazolam and fentanyl in the pediatric intensive care unit. *Eur J Pediatr* 1991;150:784–788.
145. Kumar A, Bleck TP. Intravenous midazolam for the treatment of refractory status epilepticus. *Crit Care Med* 1992;20:483–488.
146. Lockhart CH, Nelson WL. The relationship of ketamine requirement to age in pediatric patients. *Anesthesiology* 1974;40:507–508.
147. Grant IS, Nimmo WS, McNicol LR, Clements JA. Ketamine disposition in children and adults. *Br J Anaesth* 1983;55:1107–1111.
148. Hamza J, Ecoffey C, Gross JB. Ventilatory response to CO_2 following intravenous ketamine in children. *Anesthesiology* 1989;70:422–425.
149. Morray JP, Lynn AM, Stamm SJ, Herndon PS, Kawabori I, Stevenson JG. Hemodynamic effects of ketamine in children with congenital heart disease. *Anesth Analg* 1984;63:895–899.
150. Hickey PR, Hansen DD, Cramolini GM, Vincent RN, Lang P. Pulmonary and systemic hemodynamic responses to ketamine in infants with normal and elevated pulmonary vascular resistance. *Anesthesiology* 1985;62:287–293.
151. Malviya S, Burrows FA, Johnston AE, Benson LN. Anaesthetic experience with paediatric interventional cardiology. *Can J Anaesth* 1989;36:320–324.
152. Hickey PR, Wessel DL, Streitz SL, et al. Transcatheter closure of atrial septal defects: hemodynamic complications and anesthetic management. *Anesth Analg* 1992;74:44–50.
153. Tobias JD, Martin LD, Wetzel RC. Ketamine by continuous infusion for sedation in the pediatric intensive care unit. *Crit Care Med* 1990;18:819–821.

154. Rock MJ, Reyes de la Rocha S, L'Hommedieu CS, Treumper E. Use of ketamine in asthmatic children to treat respiratory failure refractory to conventional therapy. *Crit Care Med* 1986;14:514–516.
155. Strube PJ, Hallam PL. Ketamine by continuous infusion in status asthmatics. *Anaesthesia* 1986;41: 1017–1019.
156. Attia J, Ecoffey C, Sandouk P, Gross JB, Samii K. Epidural morphine in children: pharmacokinetics and CO_2 sensitivity. *Anesthesiology* 1986;65:590–594.
157. Nordberg G, Hedner T, Mellstrand T, Dahlstroem B. Pharmacokinetic aspects of epidural morphine analgesia. *Anesthesiology* 1983;58:545–551.
158. Ecoffey C, Desparmet J, Maury M, Berdeaux A, Giudicelli JF, Saint-Maurice C. Bupivacaine in children: pharmacokinetics following caudal anesthesia. *Anesthesiology* 1985;63:447–448.
159. Ecoffey C, Dubousset AM, Sami K. Lumbar and thoracic epidural anesthesia for urologic and upper abdominal surgery in infants and children. *Anesthesiology* 1986;65:87–90.
160. Takasaki M. Blood concentrations of lidocaine, mepivacaine and bupivacaine during caudal analgesia in children. *Acta Anaesthiol Scand* 1984;28:211–214.
161. Mazoit JX, Denson DD, Samii K. Pharmacokinetics of bupivacaine following caudal anesthesia in infants. *Anesthesiology* 1988;68:387–391.
162. Tucker GT. Pharmacokinetics of local anaesthetics. *Br J Anaesth* 1986;58:717–731.
163. Desparmet J, Meistelman C, Barre J, Saint-Maurice C. Continuous epidural infusion of bupivacaine for postoperative pain relief in children. *Anesthesiology* 1987;67:108–110.
164. Wolf AR, Eyres RL, Laussen PC, et al. Effect of extradural analgesia on stress responses to abdominal surgery in infants. *Br J Anaesth* 1993;70:654–660.
165. Murat I, Delleur MM, Esteve C, Egu JF, Raynaud P, Saint-Maurice C. Continuous extradural anaesthesia in children: clinical and haemodynamic implications. *Br J Anaesth* 1987;69:1441–1450.
166. Tobias JD, Wetzel RC, Nichols DG. Cardiorespiratory responses to epidural analgesia in the awake child: a retrospective review of postoperative patients. *J Postgrad Anesth Nurs* 1993;8:257–261.
167. Murrell D, Gibson PR, Cohen RC. Continuous epidural analgesia in newborn infants undergoing major surgery. *J Pediatr Surg* 1993;28:548–553.
168. Henderson K, Sethna NF, Berde CB. Continuous caudal anesthesia for inguinal hernia repair in former preterm infants. *J Clin Anesth* 1993;5:129–133.
169. Wolf AR, Hughes D. Pain relief for infants undergoing abdominal surgery: comparison of infusions of i.v. morphine and extradural bupivacaine. *Br J Anaesth* 1993;70:10–16.
170. Wolf AR, Eyres RL, Laussen PC, et al. Effect of extradural analgesia on stress responses to abdominal surgery in infants. *Br J Anaesth* 1993;70:654–660.
171. Lejus C, Roussiere G, Testa S, Ganansia MF, Meignier M, Souron R. Postoperative extradural analgesia in children: comparison of morphine with fentanyl. *Br J Anaesth* 1994;72:156–159.
172. Caudle CL, Freid EB, Bailey AG, Valley RD, Lish MC, Azizkhan RG. Epidural fentanyl infusion with patient-controlled epidural analgesia for postoperative analgesia in children. *J Pediatr Surg* 1993;28: 554–559.
173. Tobias JD, Oakes L, Rao B. Continuous epidural anesthesia for postoperative analgesia in the pediatric oncology patient. *Am J Pediatr Hem-Onc* 1992;14:216–221.
174. Berde CB. Convulsions associated with pediatric regional anesthesia. *Anesth Analg* 1992;75:164–166.
175. Boesenberg AT, Bland BAR, Schulte-Steinberg O, Downing JW. Thoracic epidural anesthesia via the caudal route in infants. *Anesthesiology* 1988;69:265–269.
176. Rasch DK, Webster DE, Pollard TG, Gurkowski MA. Lumbar and thoracic epidural analgesia via the caudal approach for postoperative pain relief in infants and children. *Can J Anaesth* 1990;37:359–362.
177. Gunter JB, Eng C. Thoracic epidural anesthesia via the caudal approach in children. *Anesthesiology* 1992;76:935–938.
178. Tobias JD, Lowe S, O'Dell N, Holcomb GW. Thoracic epidural anaesthesia in infants and children. *Can J Anaesth* 1993;40:879–882.
179. Loennquist PA, Olsson GL. Paravertebral vs epidural block in children. Effects on postoperative morphine requirement after renal surgery.*Acta Anaesthesiol Scand* 1994;38:346–349.
180. Busoni P, Messeri A, Sarti A. The lumbosacral epidural block: a modified Taylor approach for abdominal urologic surgery in children. *Anaesth Intens Care* 1991;19:325–328.
181. Cooper MG, Sethna NF. Epidural analgesia in patients with congenital lumbosacral spinal anomalies. *Anesthesiology* 1991;75:370–374.
182. Sethna NF, Berde CB. Pediatric regional anesthesia equipment. *Int Anesth Clin* 1992;30:163–176.
183. Wilson PTJ, Lloyd-Thomas AR. An audit of extradural infusion analgesia in children using bupivacaine and diamorphine. *Anaesthesia* 1993;48:718–723.

184. Wood CE, Goresky GV, Klassen KA, Kuwahara B, Neil SG. Complications of continuous epidural infusions for postoperative analgesia in children. *Can J Anaesth* 1994;41:613–620.
185. Wolf AR, Walker SM. Development of a high block in an infant during an epidural bupivacaine infusion. *Anaesth Intens Care* 1991;19:583–586.
186. Agarwal R, Gutlove DP, Lockhart CH. Seizures occurring in pediatric patients receiving continuous infusion of bupivacaine. *Anesth Analg* 1992;75:284–286.
187. McCloskey JJ, Haun SE, Deshpande JK. Bupivacaine toxicity secondary to continuous caudal epidural infusion in children. *Anesth Analg* 1992;75:287–290.
188. Berde C. Epidural analgesia in children. *Can J Anaesth* 1994;41:555–560.
189. Riquelme CM, Bell B, Edwards J, Brown TCK. The influence of age on the cardiovascular toxicity of intravenous bupivacaine in young dogs. *Anaesth Intens Care* 1987;15:436–439.
190. Berde CB. Toxicity of local anesthetics in infants and children. *J Pediatr* 1993;122:S14–S20.
191. Berde CB. Acute postoperative pain panagement in children. ASA Refresher Course Lectures 1994; 224:1–7.

Drug Infusions in Anesthesiology, Second Edition,
edited by R. J. Fragen. Lippincott-Raven Publishers,
Philadelphia © 1996.

9

Infusions of Vasoactive Drugs

Mark F. Newman, *Edward B. McKenzie, Thomas E. Stanley III, and Joseph G. Reves

*Department of Anesthesiology, Duke University Medical Center Durham, North Carolina 22710; *Department of Cardiac Anesthesia, Durham County Medical Center, Durham, North Carolina 27706*

Recent advances in cardiovascular cellular pharmacology help explain how vasoactive drugs produce their effects. Formerly perceived receptors are now characterized. Signal transduction, which activates these receptors to produce cellular activity leading to an expected clinical effect, is less of a mystery. This chapter on the appropriate use of vasoactive drug infusions is clinically oriented, but recent advances in adrenergic pharmacology and basic information on receptor subtypes and signal transduction will be discussed.

The purpose of vasoactive drugs, including positive inotropes, vasoconstrictors, vasodilators, negative inotropes, and negative chronotropes, is to temporarily support or depress the circulatory system to maintain adequate tissue perfusion or to resume the proper balance between oxygen supply and consumption. Simplistically, the cardiovascular system, with the heart acting as a pump, circulates blood through the arterial tree to the various tissues of the body. When cardiac function and arterial size remain constant, blood pressure accurately indicates tissue perfusion. Physiologic changes, disease states, and anesthetics can significantly alter cardiac function and vascular resistance, leading to inadequate perfusion of vital organs.

Advances in monitoring, pharmacology, and drug-delivery systems increase the options for appropriate therapy and make the administration of drugs more precise. The availability of more selective and specific vasoactive drugs allows the anesthesiologist to logically and scientifically select and titrate them to optimize myocardial performance with the least increase in myocardial oxygen consumption, as demonstrated by projected alterations in the Frank-Starling curve by differing vasoactive agents in Fig. 1.

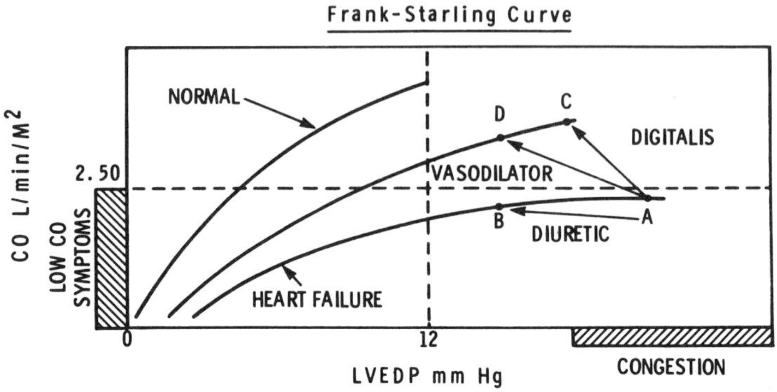

FIG. 1. Effects of different vasoactive drugs on the inotropic state in patients with congestive heart failure. (From Mason et al. Vasodilator therapy of congestive heart failure. *Drug Ther* 1978; with permission.) (1)

CARDIOVASCULAR PHYSIOLOGY

Hemodynamic Factors

Cardiac output is determined by heart rate and stroke volume. Stroke volume is determined by multiple factors, including preload, afterload, and contractility, as illustrated by the following equation:

$$\text{Cardiac output} = \text{heart rate} \times \text{stroke volume} \qquad [1]$$

Blood pressure can be expressed as a product of cardiac output and systemic vascular resistance. Vasoactive drugs exert their effects through changing heart rate, myocardial contractility, AV conduction or systemic vascular resistance, as illustrated in the following equation:

$$\text{Blood pressure} = \text{cardiac output} \times \text{systemic vascular resistance} \qquad [2]$$

These direct actions secondarily cause changes in cardiac output, stroke volume, or blood pressure to produce the desired result.

Autonomic Nervous System

The autonomic nervous system consists of two major components: the sympathetic nervous system and the parasympathetic nervous system. Sympathetic fibers that travel predominantly in thoracolumbar regions operate with norepinephrine as a neurotransmitter at the effector junction, whereas the parasympathetic efferents traveling predominantly in the cervical and sacral regions use acetylcholine as a neurotransmitter at both the ganglion and neuroeffector junction.

Both neurotransmitters and drugs interact with distinct receptors to mediate physiologic responses. This is a well-accepted theory, but the existence of these receptors is a relatively recent discovery. Currently, receptors are described as proteins that bind a single class or subclass of hormones or drugs or both. The receptor types can also be defined by virtue of their agonist potency series, binding of selective antagonists, second-messenger pathways, or distinct gene structures.

Receptor Physiology

Receptors are typically located in two primary areas: the membrane and the cytoplasm. The vast majority of drugs and indigenous hormones are hydrophilic and cannot easily pass through the lipophilic membrane. Therefore, most receptor systems that are important to clinicians are excitable membrane-bound proteins. A common transmembrane receptor-signal transduction is the interaction of the activated receptor with the intermediary guanine nucleotide protein (G protein). After hydrolysis of guanine triphosphate (GTP) to guanine diphosphate (GDP) to provide energy, this interaction activates a second messenger (Fig. 2). Then, a cascade of chemical reactions within the cell ultimately leads to desired clinical effects. In the case of the beta-adrenergic receptor, beta-adrenergic receptor agonists activate the stimulatory G proteins, which stimulate the enzyme adenylyl cyclase, resulting in the production of cyclic adenosine monophosphate (cAMP) in the cell (3). The classic adrenergic receptors—beta 1, beta 2, alpha 1, and alpha

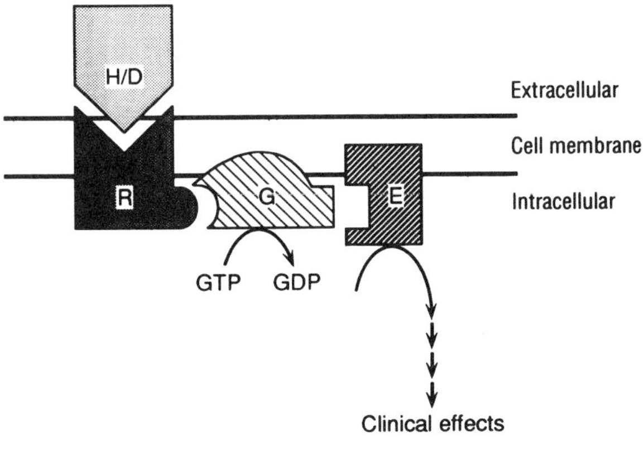

FIG. 2. Signal transduction of transmembrane receptors. Hydrophilic endogenous hormones (H) or exogenous drugs (D) bind to the extracellular surface of the transmembrane receptors (R). The activated receptor then interacts with a cytoplasmic intermediary guanine nucleotide protein (G protein) (G). Hydrolysis of guanine triphosphate (GTP) to guanine diphosphate (GDP) provides the energy required for the G protein to interact with the effector molecule (E). Effector molecule activation (or inhibition) leads to a cascade of chemical reactions within the cell, ultimately leading to the observed clinical effect. (From Schwinn DA. Cardiac pharmacology. In: Estafanous FG, et al., eds. *Cardiac anesthesia: principles and clinical practice*; 1994, with permission.) (2)

TABLE 1. *Some effects of receptor stimulation by catecholamines*

Adrenergic receptor	Site	Action
Alpha-1	Postsynaptic receptors that regulate smooth muscle arterioles (systemic and pulmonary circulation)	Vasoconstriction (increased impedance)
	Iris	Dilatation
	Heart	Increased contractility
Alpha-2	Presynaptic receptors that inhibit the release of norepinephrine of smooth muscle when stimulated	Vasodilation
Beta-1	Heart	Increased atrial and ventricular contraction
	Sinoatrial node	Increased heart rate
	Atrioventricular conduction	Increased conduction velocity or rate of conduction
	Kidney	Renin release
Beta-2	Smooth muscle arterioles (systemic and pulmonary)	Vasodilatation (decreased impedance)
	Bronchi	Bronchodilatation
	Heart	Increased rate and contractility
Dopamine-1	Vascular smooth muscle	Vasodilation
	Renal and mesentery	
Dopamine-2	Presynaptic adrenergic nerve endings	Inhibits norepinephrine release

2—represent the most important G protein coupling receptor family for cardiovascular homeostasis. Adrenergic receptors, including the dopaminergic receptors, are characterized in Table 1 and in the following paragraphs.

Most vasoactive drugs that rapidly modulate the cardiovascular system mediate their action via adrenergic receptors. Therefore, an understanding of these adrenergic receptors is essential to understand the effects of vasoactive drugs. Recent research on adrenergic receptors identified many alpha- and beta-receptor subtypes (Fig. 3). Many of these subtypes are primarily of academic interest because most currently available vasoactive drugs are not subgroup specific. However, receptor classification, receptor location in the body, and the effects of their stimulation or antagonism are used to express the effects of a drug and to guide efforts to produce new, more specific-acting drugs. Understanding receptor pharmacology allows the clinician to select appropriate drugs for manipulating the sympathetic nervous system to achieve the desired hemodynamic effect.

POSITIVE INOTROPIC DRUGS

Inotropic and chronotropic drugs can support the circulation when clinical evidence of heart failure exists. The responses to inotropic and chronotropic drugs vary with the type and amount of drug used and the pathologic state of the patient. The pharmacodynamic differences between the drugs are explained by their

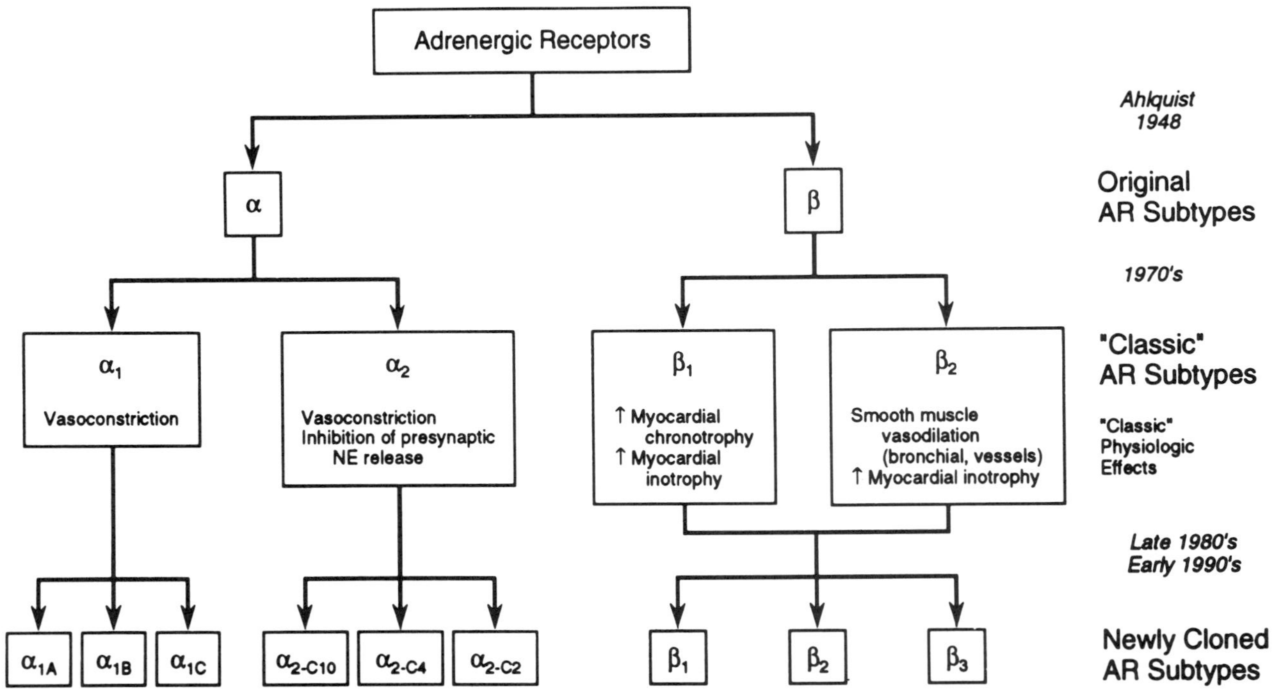

FIG. 3. History of adrenergic receptor (AR) subtypes. Individual AR subtypes are listed historically, along with associated cardiovascular responses to activation. (From Schwinn DA. Cardiac pharmacology. In: Estafanous FG, et al., eds. *Cardiac anesthesia: principles and clinical practice*; 1994, with permission.) (2)

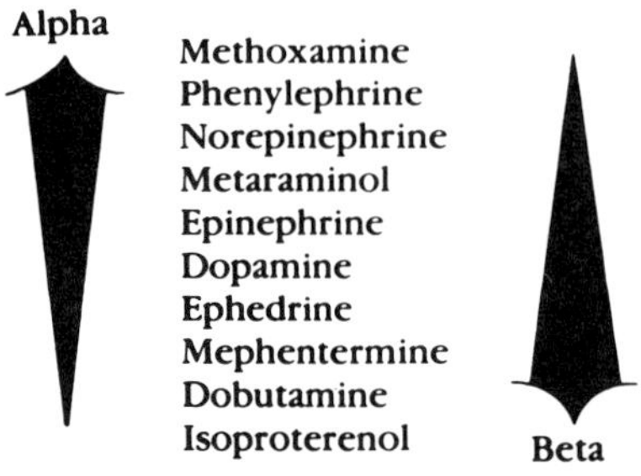

FIG. 4. Comparison of relative alpha and beta selectivity of the positive inotropic drugs and vasoconstrictors. The degree of selectivity of the mixed agonists varies with dosage. (From Reves JG, McKay RD. Cardiovascular therapy. In: Newfield P, Cottrell JE, eds. *Handbook of Neuroanesthesia.* 1983;126, with permission.) (4)

direct or indirect specificity for sympathetic nervous system receptors or second-messenger activation. The inotropic activity of the catecholamines can be determined by their degree of beta-1 stimulation. The greater the beta-1 effect, the greater inotropic activity they possess. The relative alpha and beta selectivity of the inotropes and vasoconstrictors is illustrated in Fig. 4. Inotropic agents are typically classified as catecholamines or noncatecholamines (see the list of positive inotropes in Table 2).

TABLE 2. *Pharmacological characteristics of positive inotropic drugs*

	Receptor activity[a]				
	Vascular		Cardiac		
Generic name (trade name)	Alpha-1	Beta-2	Beta-1	Adult dose (IV)	Comments
Epinephrine (Adrenalin)	+++	+	++	Infusion, 0.05–0.20 μg/kg/min	Relative alpha and beta activity is dose related: beta in low doses (1–2 μg/min); alpha in higher doses.
Dopamine (Intropin)	++	+	++	Infusion, 3–20 μg/kg/min	Like epinephrine, relative alpha and beta effects are dose related, but splanchnic and renal vasoconstriction is spared. Used in patients with compromised renal function. Renal effects seen with doses of 1–4 μg/kg/min.
Dobutamine	+	+	+++	Infusion, 5–20 μg/kg/min	Theoretically primarily beta-1 effects on myocardial contractility and little other beta-1 cardiac effect. However, tachycardia can occur.
Dopexamine	0	+	++++	Infusion, 1–10 μg/kg/min	Potent vasodilation. Used in short-term therapy in congestive heart failure.

TABLE 2. *Continued.*

Generic name (trade name)	Receptor activity[a]			Adult dose (IV)	Comments
	Vascular		Cardiac		
	Alpha-1	Beta-2	Beta-1		
Isoproterenol	0	++++	++++	Infusion, 0.025–0.05 μg/kg/min	Pure beta effects. High dosages lead to ventricular irritability and tachycardia. May be useful in pulmonary arterial hypertension.
Calcium chloride	0	0	0	Bolus, 1–10 mg/kg	Rapid-acting positive inotropic drug with effects that persist 5–10 min. Mechanism of action is direct and not beta-adrenergic. Useful in patients on propranolol to increase contractility and treat "protamine lows." May cause ventricular arrhythmias and, potentially, myocardial ischemia and accentuate pulmonary hypertension.
Amrinone (Inocor)	0	0	0	Bolus, 0.5–2.0 mg/kg, then infusion, 5–10 μg/kg/min	Causes vasodilation and may rarely produce thrombocytopenia. Mechanism of action is not adrenergic.
Milrinone (Primacor)	0	0	0	Bolus, 50–75 μg/kg, then infusion, 0.375–0.75 μg/kg/min	Causes vasodilation and occasional rhythm disturbance. More potent than amrinone.
Glucose, insulin, potassium chloride	0	0	0	Infusion, 1 ml/kg/hr (see Comments)	Solution made with 50 g glucose, 80 U insulin, and 100 mEq potassium chloride in 1 L. Close monitoring of glucose and potassium, especially with discontinuation.
Glucagon	0	0	0	Bolus, 50 mg/kg, followed by infusion, 5 mg/kg/hr	Enhances sinoatrial and atrioventricular node automaticity. Useful in intense beta blockade. May cause release of norepinephrine.
Digoxin	0	0	0	Bolus, 0.125–0.25 mg	Has delayed onset of inotropic action and low therapeutic safety ratio, which makes acute use inappropriate in most cases. Best used intraoperatively as antiarrhythmic and heart rate controller.

[a] The number of plus signs denotes increasing activity or time; 0 denotes no activity.

Mechanism of Hemodynamic Effects

Catecholamine refers to any compound composed of a catechol nucleus, a benzene ring with two hydroxyl groups, and an amine-containing side chain. The human endogenous catecholamines are dopamine, norepinephrine, and epinephrine (see the structures in Fig. 5); the synthetic catecholamines are isoproterenol and dobutamine. Catecholamines act as "first messengers" (see receptor physiology) at specific adrenergic receptors stimulating G protein, which activates adenyl cyclase. Adenyl cyclase increases the production of cAMP, which enhances excitation-contraction coupling (inotropism) by increasing calcium flux (3). A similar effect on calcium flux in pacemaker cells may explain the chronotropic effects as well.

The noncatecholamines include ephedrine, denopamine, amrinone, milrinone, calcium salts, digitalis glycosides, glucagon, and solutions containing glucose, in-

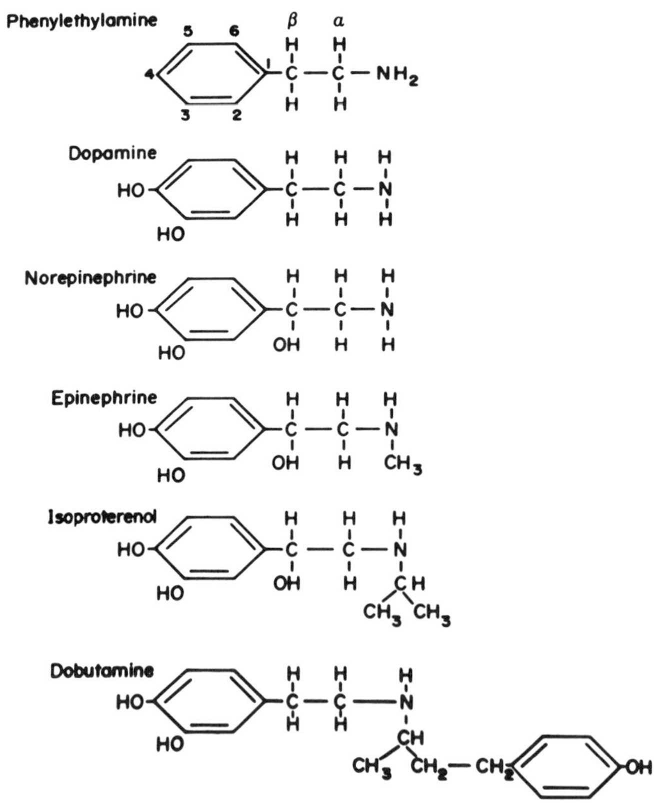

FIG. 5. The structure of commonly used catecholamines (both natural and synthetic) and their immediate precursor, phenylethylamine.

sulin, and potassium (GIK). Their diverse mechanisms of action include the changing cellular levels of cAMP by manipulating adenyl cyclase or by inhibiting phosphodiesterase and, secondarily, by increasing intracellular calcium levels.

As with other vasoactive drugs, the hemodynamic effects of each positive inotropic drug depend on the dose given and the patient's cardiovascular status. The more selective beta agents, isoproterenol and dobutamine, increase contractility, heart rate, AV conduction, and myocardial oxygen consumption and decrease systemic vascular resistance (SVR). Because SVR decreases, the effect of isoproterenol and dobutamine on blood pressure is variable. Drugs having mixed alpha and beta activity tend to increase contractility, cardiac output, and SVR, depending on the dose administered. Changes in heart rate are variable, but blood pressure is usually increased. The specific effects of each drug are discussed in the section on commonly used positive inotropic drugs.

Indications and Contraindications

Positive inotropic agents are useful primarily for low cardiac-output syndromes that are not corrected by optimizing heart rate, preload, and afterload. Particular indications include left or right ventricular failure after cardiopulmonary bypass, brief periods of myocardial dysfunction associated with anesthetic overdose, prolonged support of left ventricular function awaiting cardiac transplantation, or, occasionally, the need to increase blood pressure in patients with cerebral vasospasm.

Some drugs should be avoided because their primary hemodynamic effects will aggravate a clinical situation. For example, isoproterenol, and in some cases dopamine or dobutamine, may aggravate tachyarrhythmias. Isoproterenol will significantly increase myocardial oxygen consumption, and therefore may be contraindicated in a patient with ongoing myocardial ischemia.

Alpha-1 vasoconstriction associated with long-term use of high doses of norepinephrine and epinephrine may contribute to decreased renal function or failure, making this scenario dangerous. Finally, care must be taken with the concomitant use of sympathomimetic drugs and inhalational anesthetics because life-threatening ventricular dysrhythmias may result.

Commonly Used Agents

Catecholamines

Epinephrine

Epinephrine is a naturally occurring hormone produced primarily in the adrenal medulla and released by stimulation of the sympathetic nervous system. Epinephrine stimulates both alpha and beta adrenergic receptors. It slows digestion and shunts blood from the gastrointestinal tract to the central nervous system (CNS), heart, and musculoskeletal system. Stimulation of glycogenolysis, gluconeogenesis, and Na/K ATPase may cause insulin-resistant hyperglycemia and hypokalemia when epinephrine is given by infusion (5).

Epinephrine is a potent alpha- and beta-adrenergic receptor agonist, with a dose-dependent ratio of these effects. Given as an infusion, both inotropic and chronotropic effects occur with doses of 0.01–0.2 μg/kg/min. Beta effects usually predominate at lower doses, and alpha effects usually predominate at higher doses. As the dose is increased, tachycardia or hypertension may limit the beneficial effects. Automaticity is also enhanced with increasing beta stimulation, and arrhythmia-suppressive therapy may be necessary during high-dose epinephrine infusions. Some clinicians use epinephrine as the drug of choice for immediate support of the heart: for example, after coronary artery bypass operations. Others believe that it should be reserved for situations in which “weaker inotropes” fail.

Norepinephrine

Norepinephrine, another naturally occurring catecholamine, is the precursor of epinephrine. Like epinephrine, it is produced in the adrenal medulla; however, most norepinephrine in the body is produced and released at sympathetic nerve terminals. Norepinephrine, given at an infusion rate of 0.02 to 0.2 μg/kg/min produces some beta stimulation, but this is overshadowed by an intense alpha effect and a significant increase in systemic vascular resistance. Prolonged use of norepinephrine infusions may be associated with infarction of peripheral vascular beds and renal failure (6). This illustrates both the importance of maintaining tissue perfusion and the often poor correlation between blood pressure, obtained through alpha-adrenergic stimulation, and true tissue perfusion. The once-common practice of infusing norepinephrine with an alpha antagonist such as phentolamine has been supplanted by more specific beta-adrenergic agents (7).

Dopamine

Dopamine, the immediate metabolic precursor of norepinephrine produced in all adrenergic nerve endings, is a mixed alpha and beta agonist with beta effects occurring at lower doses of 3–7 μg/kg/min and alpha effects predominating at higher doses of 7–20 μg/kg/min. Dopamine, primarily at lower doses, also appears to interact uniquely with dopaminergic receptors in the splanchnic and renal vascular beds to increase blood flow in these areas (8). Dopamine is used clinically to improve urine output, but it is not clear if the increases in renal blood flow are the sole reason for enhanced diuresis; dopamine may inhibit tubular solute reabsorption directly (8,9). Concomitant administration of renal dose dopamine with more potent inotropes, epinephrine or norepinephrine, increases renal blood flow (Fig. 6) (10). As a result, renal-dose dopamine is used to protect the kidneys in these situations despite the lack of evidence showing improved renal outcome.

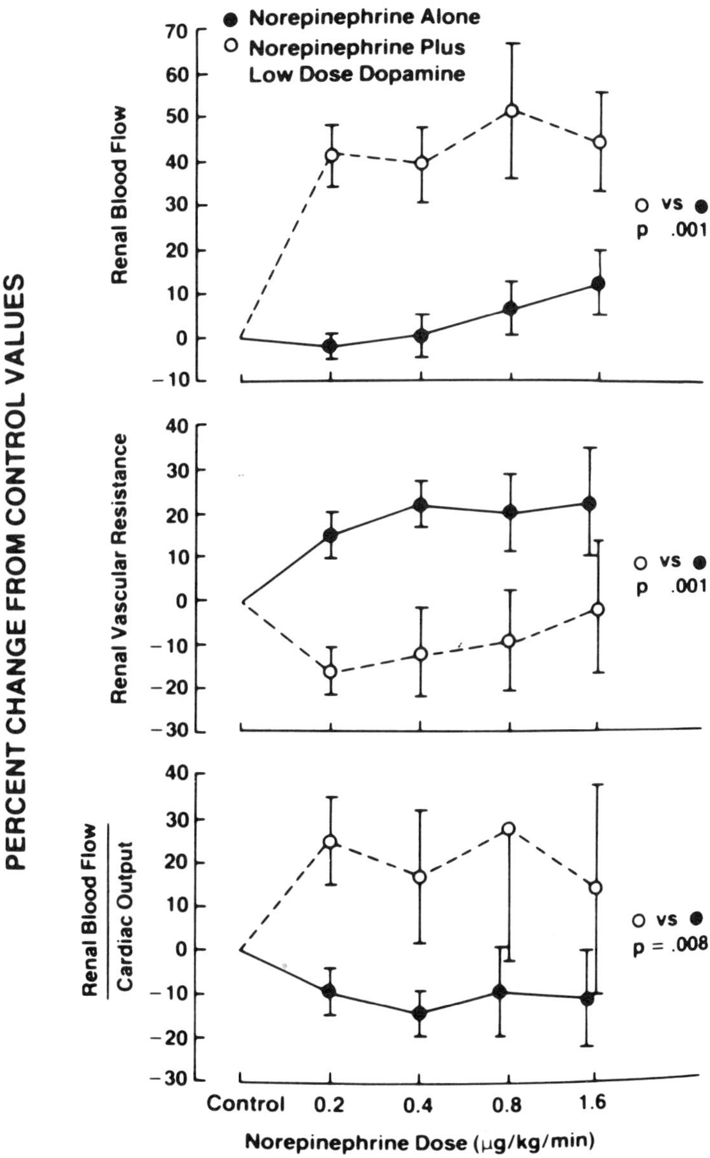

FIG. 6. Changes produced in renal blood flow and hemodynamics by the addition of renal dose dopamine to a norepinephrine infusion. (From Schaer GL, et al. Norepinephrine infusion alone versus norepinephrine plus low dose dopamine: enhanced renal blood flow with combination pressor therapy. *Crit Care Med* 1985;13:492, with permission.) (10)

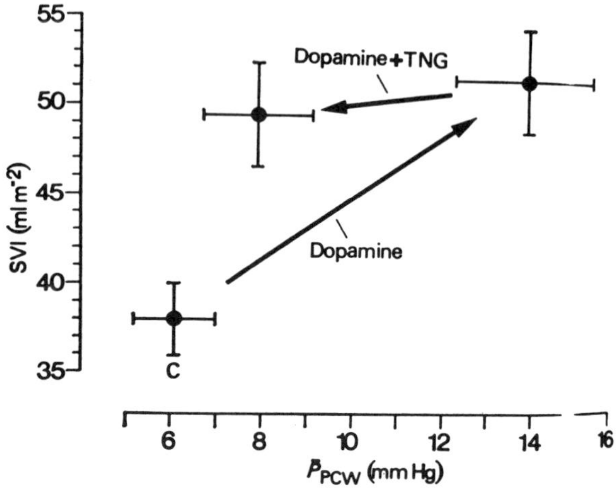

FIG. 7. Left ventricular function plots during control, dopamine infusion, and dopamine plus nitroglycerine. The left shift of the curve with dopamine infusion indicates improved left ventricular function but with increasing myocardial wall tension and oxygen demand. The addition of nitroglycerin reduced the left ventricular filling pressure without markedly affecting MAP, SVR, or stroke volume. (From Snyder and Bredt, ref. 12, with permission.)

The alpha stimulation that occurs when dopamine is infused to treat heart failure results in increased filling pressures from increased-capacitance vessel tone (11). Increased-resistance vessel tone may result in an elevated SVR. The net result may be an increase in mean pulmonary artery pressure. Increasing preload in a patient with elevated left ventricular-end diastolic pressure and left ventricular distention may worsen left ventricular function. Two different ways to counter this problem are the addition of a vasodilator such as nitroglycerin (see Fig. 7) or nitroprusside or selection of a drug that is more selective for beta receptors.

Dobutamine

Dobutamine, a synthetic catecholamine modification of isoproterenol, has almost no effect on alpha-adrenergic receptors unless the patient is receiving a beta blocker. It is more specific than dopamine for beta-1 receptors and does not interact with renal dopaminergic receptors. Given by constant infusion, dobutamine supports the failing heart by increasing inotropy and decreasing SVR and preload. Patients with elevated filling pressures and coexistent pump failure may be ideal candidates for dobutamine inotropic support (see the comparison of dopamine and dobutamine in Fig. 8). Right ventricular failure with elevated pulmonary artery pressure is another clinical situation in which dobutamine therapy may be beneficial (14). Lack of appreciable alpha-adrenergic effect is beneficial for the patient who is in cardiogenic shock, but it may be a disadvantage when dobutamine is used

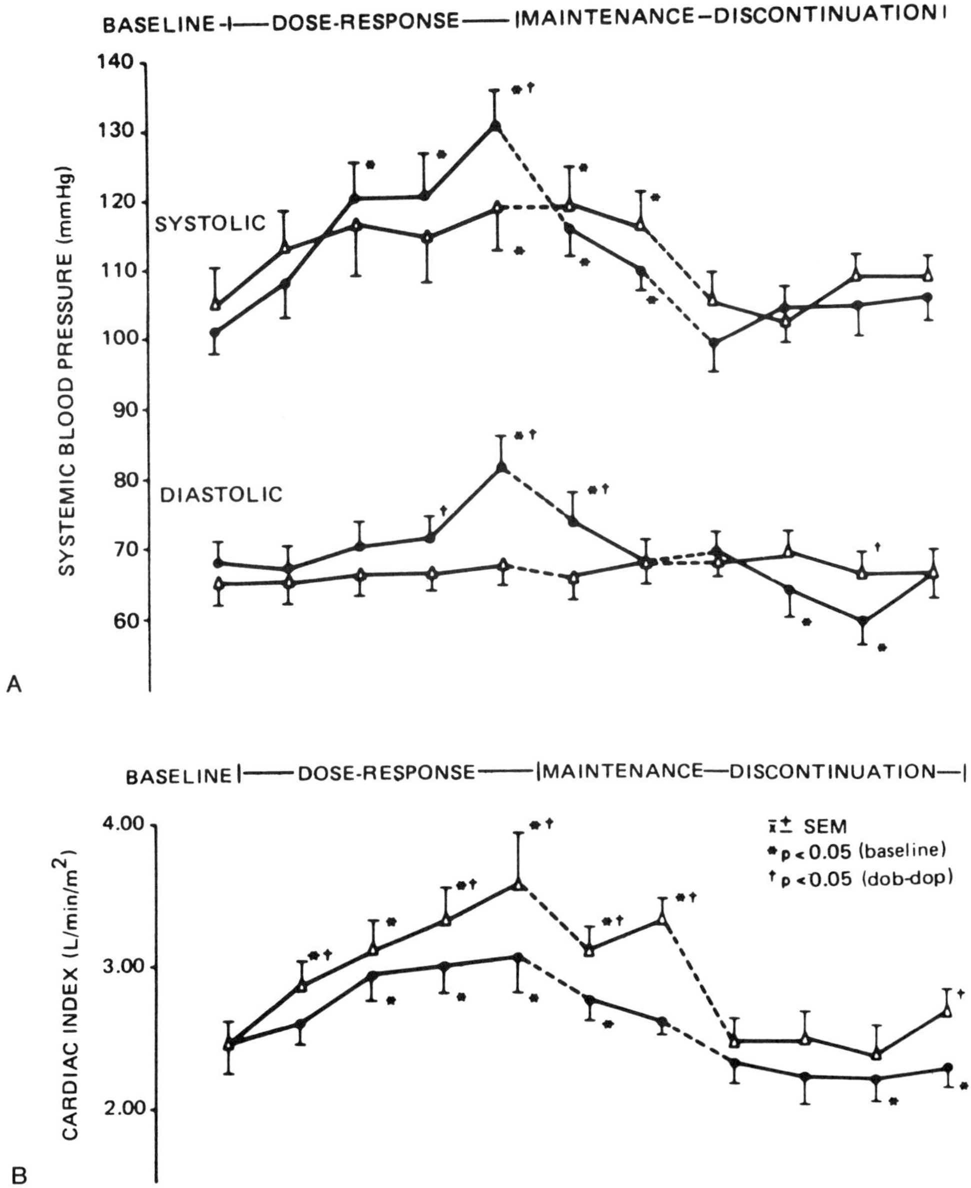

FIG. 8. Comparative hemodynamics of dopamine and dobutamine in a population with low-output congestive heart failure. (From Leier CV, et al. Comparative systemic and regional hemodynamic effects of dopamine and dobutamine in patients with cardiomyopathic heart failure. *Circulation* 1978;58:466–475, with permission.) (13)

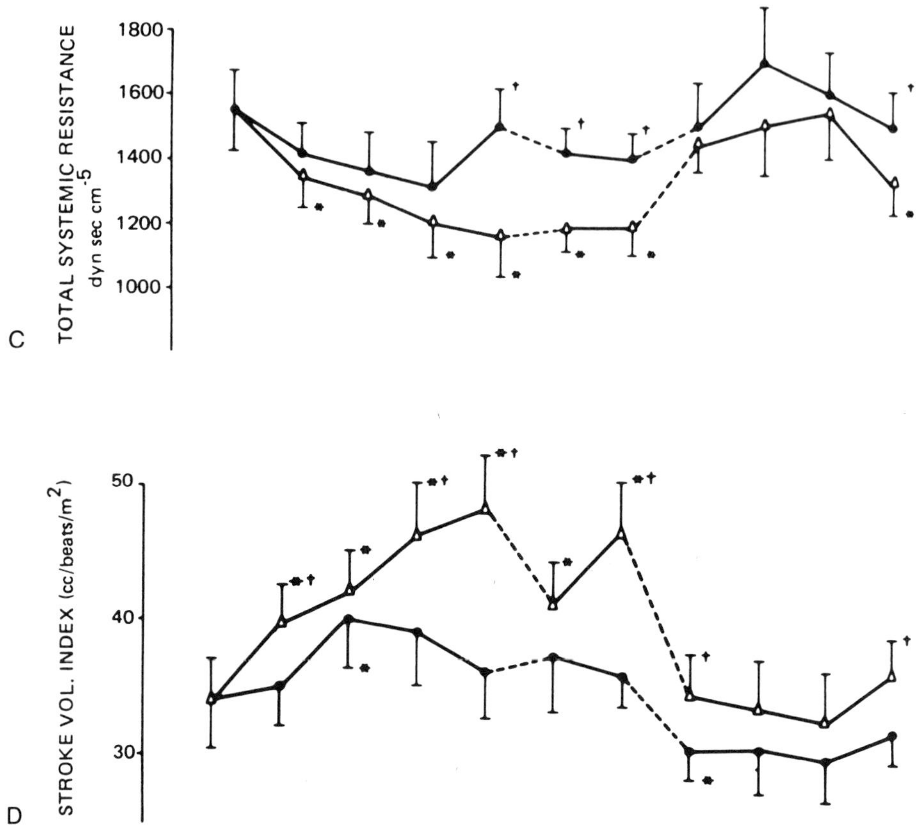

FIG. 8. *Continued.*

to support the heart in a patient with relatively low filling pressures, such as is seen after cardiac surgery (Fig. 9). There is less chronotropic effect from dobutamine than from other catecholamines, but an increased dose of dobutamine can affect automaticity and AV conduction velocity, resulting in tachycardia and arrhythmias.

Isoproterenol

Isoproterenol is a synthetic catecholamine that has mixed effects on beta-1 and beta-2 receptors. An infusion of isoproterenol increases myocardial contractility and heart rate, but strong beta-2 stimulation causes vasodilatation and, potentially, hypotension. Resultant tachycardia and hypotension may increase myocardial oxygen demand and decrease critical coronary perfusion, which makes isoproterenol poor therapy for heart failure with concomitant myocardial ischemia. Despite concerns about tachycardia and myocardial oxygen consumption, isopro-

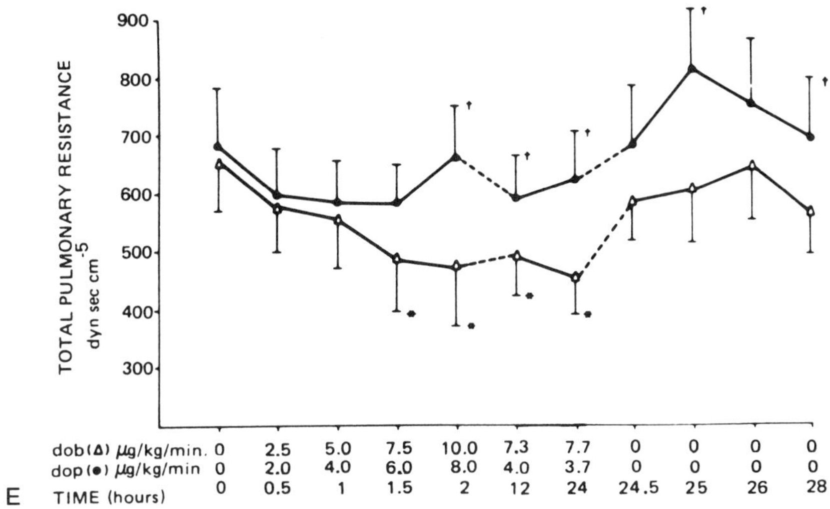

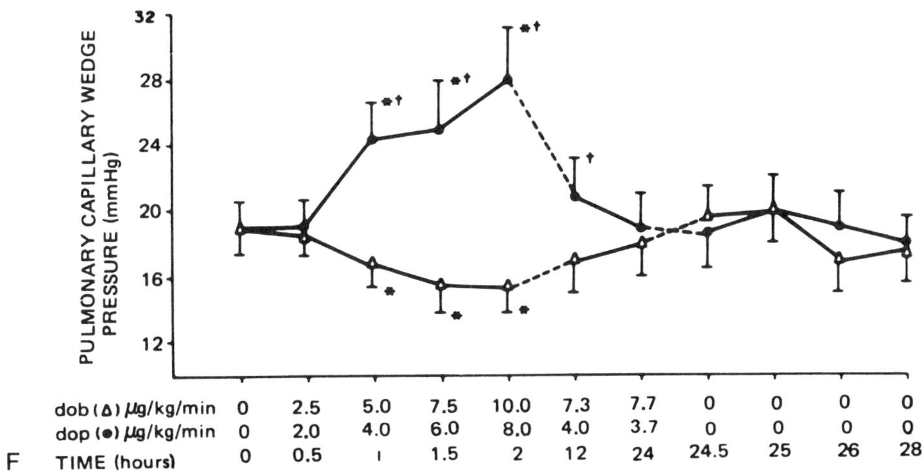

FIG. 8. *Continued.*

terenol is an ideal drug in certain situations. Bradycardia associated with third-degree heart block may respond favorably to an isoproterenol infusion while a pacemaker is being inserted. Beta-2 stimulation associated with isoproterenol produces bronchodilatation and pulmonary artery dilatation, which supports its use in patients with bronchospasm and right-sided heart failure (status asthmaticus or cor pulmonale) (16). However, agents with greater beta-2 selectivity are often used to minimize the profound tachycardia that can result with isoproterenol.

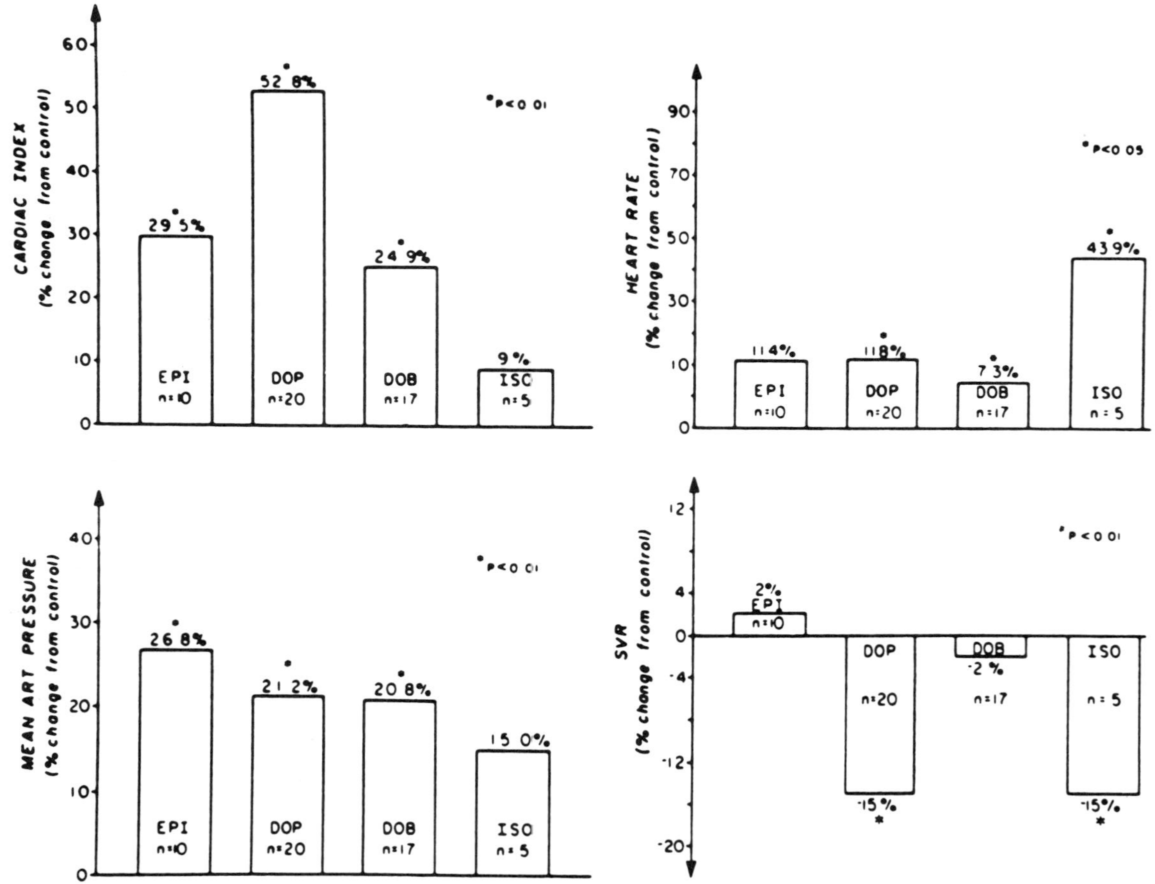

FIG. 9. Hemodynamic changes (% change from control) with four catecholamine infusions in patients after cardiopulmonary bypass. The hemodynamic changes are representative of pharmacologic changes at roughly equipotent doses ten minutes after infusions began. The data represent epinephrine 0.04 µg/kg/min, dopamine and dobutamine at 10 µg/kg/min, and isoproterenol at 0.02 µg/kg/min. (From Reves JG. Vasoactive drugs and when to use them. In: Thomas S. *Manual of cardiac anesthesia.* New York: Churchill Livingstone; 1984, with permission.) (15)

Dopexamine

Dopexamine is a synthetic analogue of dopamine with potent beta-2 adrenergic receptor and dopamine agonist properties, but little beta-1 and alpha receptor activity (17–19). As a result of its beta-2 agonist properties, dopexamine causes vasodilation, with a resultant decrease in SVR. This unloads the heart and enhances forward blood flow, particularly in patients with congestive heart failure. The beta-2 effects of dopexamine on the heart include mildly increased heart rate and positive inotropy. Blockade of norepinephrine reuptake at the nerve terminal results in some beta-1- and beta-2-mediated changes by this mechanism as well (19). Dopamine receptor activity increases renal blood flow by renal artery dilation. Although reflex tachycardia associated with vasodilation occurs with dopexamine, it is not arrhythmogenic and possibly has Class 1 antiarrhythmic properties (20).

Noncatecholamines

Amrinone

Amrinone, like aminophylline, is a phosphodiesterase inhibitor acting on the PDE_3 isoenzyme that specifically breaks down cAMP (21) (Fig. 10). Inhibition of PDE_3 by amrinone then causes cAMP levels to rise in cardiac and smooth muscle cells, ultimately increasing the level of intracellular calcium (Fig. 11) and causing increased contractility and vasodilatation. Clinical use of amrinone improves overall cardiac performance, with an accompanying decrease in pulmonary and

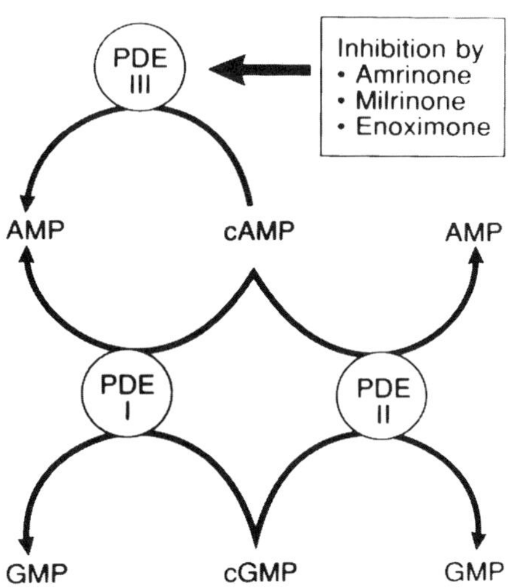

FIG. 10. Phosphodiesterase inhibitors I, II, and III and cyclic nucleotide metabolism.

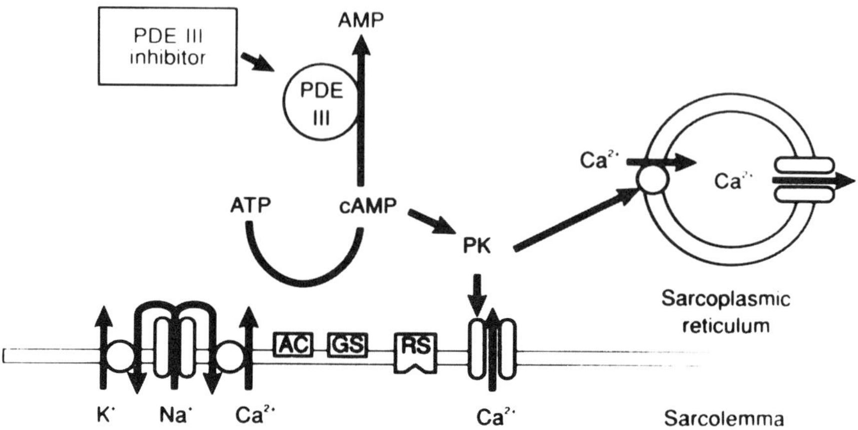

FIG. 11. Schematic representation of subcellular site of action of PDE III inhibitors. AC, adenylyl cyclase; GS, stimulatory guanine nucleotide binding protein; RS, stimulatory receptor; PK, protein kinase. (From Hnerjager P. Pharmacology of bipyridine phosphodiesterase inhibitors. In: Goenen M, ed. *Bipyridine phosphodiesterase inhibitors in clinical practice.* Cambridge, UK: Cambridge Medical Publications; 1990, with permission.) (22)

systemic vascular resistance (Fig. 12). Amrinone has no significant chronotropic effect, so tachyarrhythmias are rarely associated with its use. Because it acts directly on PDE_3 to elevate cAMP, it is an effective inotrope in the beta-blocked patient. Unlike catecholamine infusion, amrinone infusion should be preceded with a loading dose of 0.75–2.0 mg/kg over 3–5 minutes. Hypotension may develop if the drug is given at a faster rate. The maintenance infusion rate is 5–10 μg/kg/min. Thrombocytopenia, a rare side effect of amrinone therapy, responds to either dose reduction or drug discontinuation.

The concurrent administration of a catecholamine-derived inotropic agent and a phosphodiesterase inhibitor provides more effective positive inotropic support than does either agent alone (24). Catecholamine agents stimulate beta-adrenergic receptors, producing increased intracellular levels of cAMP, and phosphodiesterae inhibitors prevent cAMP breakdown, enhancing the effectiveness of the catecholamine agent. This is useful in patients with left ventricular failure after cardiopulmonary bypass (CPB).

Milrinone

Milrinone is a phosphodiesterase inhibitor that can be administered either orally or intravenously (25). Milrinone has nearly 20 times the inotropic potency of amrinone and does not cause either the fever or thrombocytopenia that can be seen with long-term amrinone infusion (26,27). Milrinone also produces significant vasodilation, and the term "inodilator" was coined to describe its effects. Despite

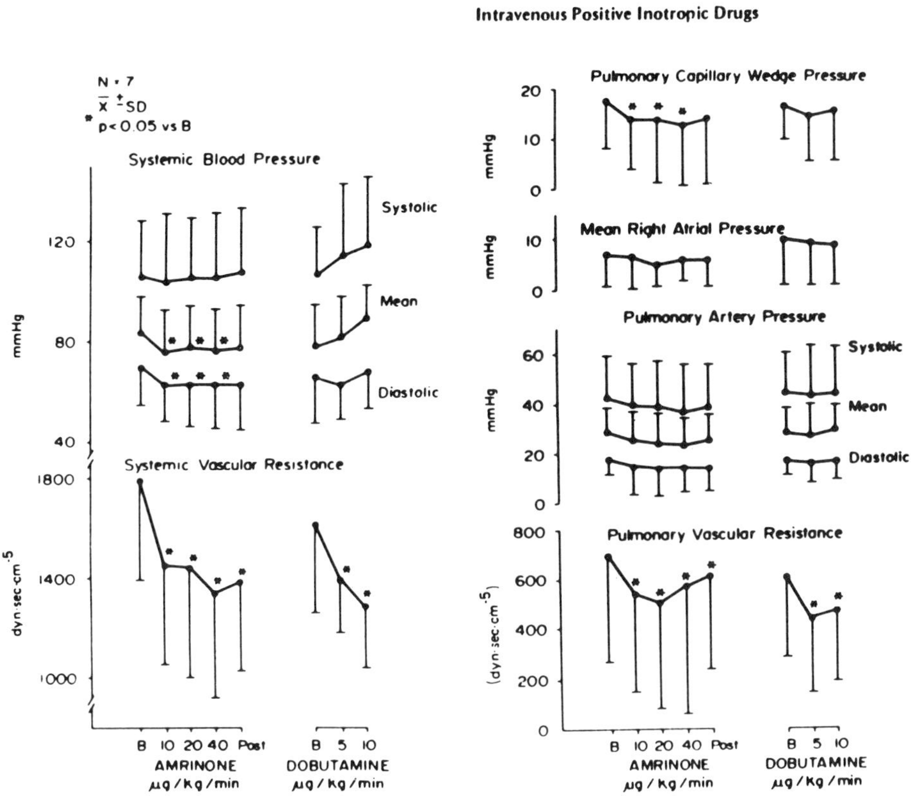

FIG. 12. Hemodynamic effects of amrinone versus dobutamine in patients with low-output congestive heart failure showing the significant decrease in systemic vascular resistance. (From Hermiller JB, et al. Amrinone in severe congestive heart failure: another look at an intriguing new cardioselective drug. *J Pharmacol Exp Ther* 1984;228: 319-326, with permission.) (23)

a significant improvement in hemodynamics and symptoms when milrinone is given orally to patients in congestive heart failure, morbidity and mortality increase (28,29). Despite these negative effects with long-term oral use, milrinone is effective when used similarly to amrinone. However, detractors of milrinone point to increased evidence of ventricular dysrhythmias as a reason to avoid its use. Milrinone is administered as an intravenous (IV) bolus of 50–75 µg/kg over 10 minutes, followed by an infusion of 0.375–0.75 µg/kg/min.

Denopamine

Denopamine is a unique noncatecholamine sympathomimetic having selective beta-1 adrenergic agonist and alpha-1 antagonist properties (30,31). Denopamine is used orally to treat congestive heart failure, producing positive inotropy by beta-

1 effects and afterload reduction through its alpha-1 effects. Although denopamine is not yet available in the United States, patients may present for surgery in the future with denopamine as a chronic oral agent for congestive heart failure.

Glucagon

Glucagon, a polypeptide released by the pancreas, was described as an inotropic agent in 1968. It is normally secreted by the pancreatic alpha cells in response to hypoglycemia and serves as a counterregulatory hormone to insulin. It activates adenyl cyclase independently of beta receptors and is effective in the presence of beta blockers. Tachydysrhythmias are uncommon during glucagon infusion, but AV conduction appears to increase, requiring caution in the presence of atrial flutter or fibrillation. Glucagon can be given in a 50-μg/kg dose, followed by an infusion of 5 μg/kg/min. The peak effect occurs in 10 minutes, and the effects will cease approximately 30 minutes after the infusion is stopped. Side effects include nausea and vomiting, hyperglycemia, hypokalemia, decreased gastric motility, and increased insulin secretion (32,33).

Digitalis Glycosides

Digitalis glycosides are among the oldest drugs used to treat congestive heart failure. Digoxin is the most common digitalis preparation used today. Inhibition of the Na-K ATPase pump, thus facilitating calcium entry into cardiac cells and augmenting contractility, is its mechanism of action. Digitalis also affects the AV node and conduction system, mimicking increased vagal tone and possibly producing AV block. Although useful for controlling the ventricular rate during atrial fibrillation, dysrhythmias are a common side effect and may be extremely difficult to treat. Because of its long elimination half-life, administration by infusion is inappropriate.

Calcium Salts

Calcium salts have long been used to augment myocardial contractility. Increasing the serum calcium level appears to augment sarcolemmal calcium flux in cardiac and smooth muscle cells. Given as a bolus, it causes a transient increase in contractile function that appears as increased cardiac output and elevated mean arterial pressure. These effects are most pronounced when calcium is used to treat hypocalcemia. Calcium may be beneficial in treating citrate toxicity secondary to massive transfusion of citrate-treated blood. Calcium is used after CPB as a temporizing measure to provide brief cardiac support during periods of hypotension and diminished cardiac function following hypothermic, hyperkalemic cardioplegia.

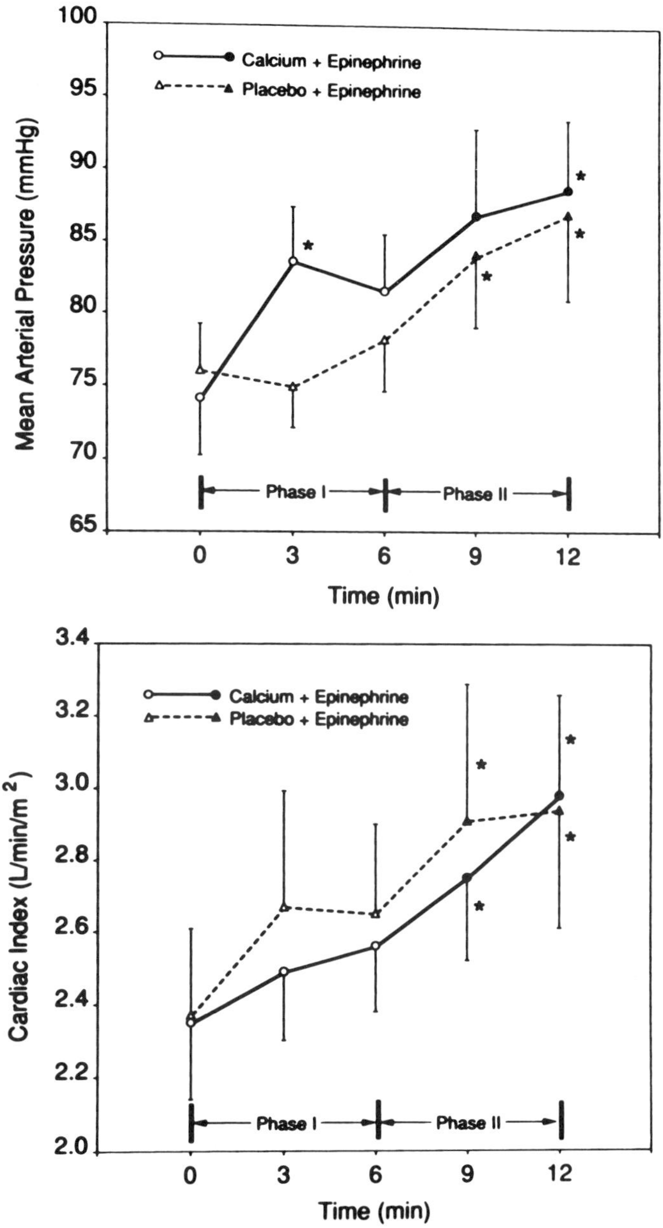

FIG. 13. Hemodynamic comparison of calcium + epinephrine and placebo + epinephrine in patients emerging from cardiopulmonary bypass. Cardiac index and mean arterial pressure were similar for the two groups, showing no significant augmentation or inhibition by calcium (5 mg/kg) of epinephrine's hemodynamic effects. (From Royster RL, et al. A randomized, blinded, placebo-controlled evaluation of calcium chloride and epinephrine for inotropic support after emergence from cardiopulmonary bypass. *Anesth Analg* 1992;74:3–13, with permission.) (35)

Epinephrine and calcium may be combined for inotropic support (34). Its proponents claim that it produces more inotropic support than does either agent given alone. However, controversy exists regarding this role of calcium for inotropic support after CPB. Conflicting data exists regarding calcium's ability to produce increases in cardiac contractility versus increases in blood pressure (35), produce added effects to those of catecholamine agents (35,36), and produce coronary artery spasm or pancreatic cellular injury in CPB patients (37,38). Recent studies show no increase in cardiac index with the administration of calcium chloride alone or in combination with epinephrine after CPB (35) (Fig. 13). The American Heart Association no longer recommends its use during advanced cardiac life support except in treating hyperkalemia, hypocalcemia, or calcium entry blocker toxicity (39).

Solutions Containing Glucose, Insulin, and Potassium

GIK solutions can support a failing heart because glucose and potassium serve as the energy substrate and insulin increases the uptake of substrate into cells, including the myocardial cells. Although physicians in some institutions continue to give this combination, clinical reports of hyperkalemic cardiac arrest after stopping the infusion explain why the practice is uncommon (40). Safer inotropic therapy with fewer side effects supplanted many of the older practices, although there is some interest in reviving this technique (41). In a recent study, a combination of 80 IU/L of insulin, 100 mEq/L of potassium in 50% intravenous glucose at a rate of 1 ml/kg/hr was effective in treating refractory heart failure after aortocoronary bypass (41).

VASOCONSTRICTORS

Studies show little correlation between blood pressure and tissue perfusion during major surgery (42). Tissue viability depends on blood flow and oxygen delivery rather than on blood pressure. A normal healthy heart can pump against increased vascular resistance and maintain adequate tissue blood flow at the expense of increased myocardial oxygen consumption. A diseased heart, however, may be unable to pump against increased vascular resistance. This may worsen tissue perfusion and increase left ventricular failure in the presence of congestive heart failure or valvular incompetence despite transient increases in blood pressure. Vasoconstrictors can maintain cerebral, myocardial, or uterine perfusion in certain situations. Without invasive hemodynamic monitors to indicate a low SVR, vasoconstrictors should be used only as a temporizing measure until appropriate therapy improves cardiac output.

The vasoconstrictors include the primarily pure alpha-1 agonists, methoxamine and phenylephrine, and the mixed alpha-1 and beta adrenergic agonist compounds shown in Fig. 4 and listed in Table 3.

TABLE 3. *Comparison of pharmacological characteristics of commonly used vasoconstrictors*

Generic name (trade name)	Receptor activity[a] Vascular Alpha	Vascular Beta-2	Cardiac Beta-1	Onset	Duration	Adult dose (IV)
Methoxamine (Vasoxyl)	++++	0	0	++	+++	Bolus, 0.2–0.5 mg
Phenylephrine (Neo-Synephrine)	++++	0	+	++	++	Infusion, 0.1–0.5 μg/kg/min
Norepinephrine (Levophed)	+++	0	++	++++	+	Infusion, 0.05–0.15 μg/kg/min
Ephedrine (Ephedrine)	+++	+	++	++	++++	Bolus, 2.5–5.0 mg

[a] The number of plus signs denotes increasing activity or time; 0 denotes no activity.

Mechanism of Hemodynamic Effects

The alpha-1 receptors regulate smooth muscle tone in resistance and capacitance vessels. Alpha-1 adrenergic stimulation increases SVR and capacitance vessel tone. Vasoconstrictive drugs vary in their specificity for adrenergic receptors and their mechanisms of action. Certain vasoactive drugs stimulate both alpha and beta receptors; others act as pure alpha agonists. Some alpha agonists cause release of norepinephrine and are considered to be indirect-acting alpha agonists. Angiotensin (not readily available in the United States) is a potent nonadrenergic vasoconstrictor that acts directly on smooth muscle, even in the presence of alpha-1 adrenergic blockade.

Hemodynamic effects of vasoconstrictors depend on two factors: the particular drug administered and the patient's cardiovascular status (vascular resistance, cardiac function, and integrity of baroreceptor reflexes). Vasoconstrictors increase vascular resistance, resulting in increased systemic and pulmonary artery pressures, particularly when systemic vascular resistance is low. Depending on the original ventricular function and the degree of beta-1 stimulation by the drug, cardiac output may decrease, increase, or remain unchanged. Although the heart rate response is variable, it primarily slows after administration of pure alpha-1 agonists. Slower heart rates are secondary to baroreceptor response to increased systemic arterial pressure.

Indications and Contraindications

Vasoconstrictors are used primarily to treat decreased SVR, often caused by administration of either general or regional anesthesia. Hypotension secondary to a high level of sympathetic blockade occurs after subarachnoid and epidural anesthesia. Venodilation decreases preload leading to decreased cardiac output. The therapeutic goals are to increase both preload by volume infusion and vascular tone. Uterine blood flow, and thus placental blood flow, decrease during hypotension associated with sympathetic blockade caused by subarachnoid or epidural anesthesia. Certain vasopressors may improve uterine blood flow during anesthesia, whereas others may decrease it despite increasing mean arterial pressure (43,44).

Vasopressors can maintain cerebral perfusion during anesthesia in patients with carotid artery stenosis who are undergoing carotid endarterectomy or other surgery. Vasoconstrictors also can be used to support blood pressure transiently in the hypovolemic patient while volume deficits are being corrected with IV fluid therapy. On rare occasions, vasoconstrictors are necessary in anaphylactic reactions or septic shock to help maintain perfusion to vital organs. However, their long-term use may result in renal damage.

Vasoconstrictors are contraindicated in left ventricular failure because, although blood pressure may transiently improve, the increased oxygen consumption associated with increased afterload will inevitably result in deterioration of cardiac function. Continued (chronic) use of vasoconstrictors in hypovolemic patients only serves to mask the degree of hypovolemia and does not improve patient outcome.

Commonly Used Agents

Phenylephrine

Phenylephrine is pure alpha-1 adrenergic agonist at clinical concentrations. At concentrations ten times greater than those used clinically, it weakly binds to alpha-2 and beta-adrenergic receptors. Phenylephrine increases arterial resistance and, as a result, blood pressure. The impact on cardiac output and tissue perfusion varies, depending on clinical circumstances. Unlike methoxamine, another alpha-1 agonist, phenylephrine appears to increase tone in venous capacitance vessels (45). This effect may augment preload and cardiac output while increasing blood pressure in the patient with a normal heart, but may worsen failure in the patient with cardiogenic shock. Although phenylephrine is commonly used to raise or maintain mean arterial pressure during CPB, no studies have evaluated the efficacy of this practice in preventing decreased organ perfusion. Phenylephrine also is used to maintain cerebral perfusion during carotid artery surgery and may be useful to maintain blood pressure during vascular access procedures. Phenylephrine, proposed as an alternative to epinephrine during cardiopulmonary resuscitation (CPR), is no longer recommended because of poor outcome (46). Hypotension during spinal or epidural anesthesia may respond appropriately to phenylephrine, but it, or any other pure alpha agonist, should be avoided in obstetric anesthesia because alpha agonists reduce uterine blood flow and promote fetal asphyxia (47,48). Phenylephrine is commonly administered either as a continuous infusion of 0.1–0.5 μg/kg/min or in repeated bolus doses of 50–100 μg.

Methoxamine

Methoxamine acts directly on alpha-1 adrenergic receptors to cause vasoconstriction. This action appears to be confined to the arterial circulation, which results in increased SVR, increased blood pressure, and decreased blood flow. At clinical concentrations, methoxamine also weakly binds to alpha-2 adrenergic receptors but is of no clinical consequence. Methoxamine, not recommended for continuous infusion, is usually given in a 2–10 mg dose. The long half-life of the drug, 60–90 minutes, limits its usefulness in the perioperative setting.

Norepinephrine

Norepinephrine, as previously mentioned, is a naturally occurring catecholamine with mixed alpha and beta agonist properties, but its alpha-1 adrenergic effect predominates. Norepinephrine infusions are occasionally used to support blood pressure in patients with low systemic vascular resistance (e.g., septic shock). Prolonged infusion of norepinephrine or any other alpha agonist is associated with decreased tissue perfusion and development of lactic acidosis. Vasopressor therapy, once more commonly used in the care of critically ill patients, has been largely supplanted by other therapy.

Metaraminol

Metaraminol, an indirect acting alpha-1 agonist, acts principally by causing norepinephrine release. A patient with a disease state associated with catecholamine depletion should not respond to an injection of metaraminol or any other indirect-acting vasopressor. Because metaraminol depletes norepinephrine at sympathetic nerve endings, tachyphylaxis occurs rapidly during repeated use. For this reason, metaraminol is not a good choice for continuous infusion.

Epinephrine

Epinephrine, a mixed alpha and beta agonist, is recommended during CPR in bolus doses. Its primary benefit during CPR is to increase aortic pressure, and thus the coronary artery perfusion pressure, as a result of its alpha-adrenergic properties. Beta stimulation increases the vigor of a fibrillating myocardium. The combination of alpha and beta effects of epinephrine during CPR increase the chance for successful defibrillation (49,50). Tachyarrhythmias are commonly produced by epinephrine, and volatile anesthetic agents lower the threshold for epinephrine-induced dysrhythmias. Therefore, epinephrine is not commonly used to increase blood pressure during general anesthesia.

Ephedrine

Ephedrine is a synthetic noncatecholamine with similar, but weaker, inotropic, chronotropic, and dromotropic properties than epinephrine. With its longer duration of action, ephedrine acts as an indirect-acting alpha agonist and thus depends on release of norepinephrine. Similar to other drugs of this type, ephedrine will eventually produce tachyphylaxis because of norepinephrine depletion. For this reason, and because of its longer duration of action, ephedrine is not administered as an infusion. Bolus doses of 5–10 mg are commonly given during anesthesia to increase blood pressure transiently. Ephedrine is the vasoconstrictor of choice when hypotension complicates regional anesthesia for obstetrics because it maintains uterine blood flow (43,44).

Mephentermine

Mephentermine, another synthetic noncatecholamine that acts as a direct beta and indirect alpha agonist, produces cardiac stimulation similar to that produced by epinephrine and ephedrine. Its alpha stimulation is the result of norepinephrine release, and tachyphylaxis to the alpha effect is observed with repeated use. Mephentermine produces some degree of cerebral stimulation in a manner similar to amphetamines. These clinical effects detract from its use under general anesthesia, thus it offers no advantage over any of the other drugs mentioned.

VASODILATORS

Vasodilators differ in their mechanism and site of action. They decrease SVR and produce varying degrees of venodilatation. Although their effects on the pulmonary circulation are not well understood, some decrease in pulmonary vascular resistance presumably occurs. Vasodilators are used to decrease blood pressure, afterload, and preload, which can decrease myocardial oxygen consumption in many cases. Because of the many vasodilators available (see Table 4), all the classes of vasodilators are mentioned, but the discussion will center primarily on those commonly given by infusion.

Mechanism of Hemodynamic Effects

Vasodilators given by infusion produce smooth muscle relaxation by a number of mechanisms. Nitrate vasodilators such as sodium nitroprusside, nitroglycerin, and hydralazine activate endothelium-relaxing factor now known to be nitric oxide (NO) (51–53). Other commonly used vasodilator groups are the calcium antagonists, alpha-1 adrenergic antagonists, alpha-2 agonists, and angiotensin-converting enzyme inhibitors. Conceptually, vasodilators lower blood pressure by reduc-

TABLE 4. *Comparison of pharmacologic characteristics of commonly used vasodilators*

Generic name (trade name)	Mode of action	Prominent vasodilation	Onset (min)	Duration	Adult dose (IV)
Sodium nitroprusside (Nipride)	Direct	Arteriovenous	0.5	2–4 min	Infusion, 0.2–8.0 μg/kg/min
Nitroglycerin (Nitrostat)	Direct	Venous	1–2	10 min	Sublingual, 0.4–0.8 mg; infusion, 0.5–5.0 μg/kg/min
Diazoxide (Hyperstat)	Direct	Arterial	1–2	4–12 hr	Bolus, 3–5 mg/kg
Trimethaphan (Arfonad)	Ganglonic blockade	Arteriovenous	1–2	4–8 min	Infusion, 10–50 μg/kg/min
Hydralazine (Apresoline)	Direct	Arterial	10–20	3–4 hr	Bolus, 5.0–7.5 mg
Labetalol (Trandate)	Alpha-1 and beta-adrenergic blockade	Arteriovenous	2–3	2–4 hr	Bolus, 0.25–1.0 mg/kg; infusion, 0.02–2.5 mg/min
Phentolamine (Regitine)	Alpha-1 and alpha-2 adrenergic blockade	Arteriovenous	1–2	20 min	Infusion, 0.5–20 μg/kg/min
Prazosin (Minipress)	Alpha-1 adrenergic blockade	Arteriovenous	Not available in a parenteral formulation		
Enalaprilat (Vasotec)	Angiotensin-converting enzyme inhibition	Arteriovenous	15	6–7 hr	Bolus, 1.25–5.0 mg
Nifedipine (Procardia)	Calcium antagonist	Arterial	5–15	2–4 hr	Sublingual, 10–20 mg
Nicardipine (Cardene)	Calcium antagonist	Arteriovenous	5–10	2–4 hr	Infusion, 4–12 mg/min
Isradipine (Dynacirc)	Calcium antagonist	Arteriovenous	5–10	5–6 hr	Bolus, 0.007–0.015 mg/kg; infusion, 8.0–40.0 μg/min

ing peripheral vascular resistance or by reducing venous return and cardiac output. Activation of guanylyl cyclase enzyme with the resultant production of cyclic guanosine monophosphate (cGMP) appears to be the common second messenger producing smooth muscle relaxation in arteries and veins (54,55).

The decrease in SVR and pulmonary vascular resistance from vasodilator therapy is accompanied by decreased right atrial and left atrial filling pressures, the degree of which depends on the agent used. A decrease in blood pressure is usually followed by a reflex increase in heart rate, an effect seen less often with labetalol and trimethaphan secondary to their beta and ganglionic blocking actions.

Vasodilators tend to increase cardiac output in the failing heart by decreasing SVR as long as preload is maintained. Because of their preload and afterload effects, they are often used in the treatment of myocardial ischemia (i.e., nitroglycerin). When using them for coronary artery disease, care must be taken to maintain preload and diastolic pressure to prevent aggravating ischemia secondary to decreased perfusion pressure and reflex tachycardia.

Indications and Contraindications

Although often used to treat myocardial ischemia, vasodilators are most frequently indicated to treat hypertension. Low cardiac-output syndromes with adequate filling pressures and valvular insufficiency also are common indications for vasodilators, which improve forward flow from the heart. Treatment of pulmonary hypertension using nitrates can be effective in some cases, but even with the use of alpha blocking agents or calcium antagonists, it is often difficult, especially when pulmonary vascular resistance is relatively fixed, such as occurs in chronic mitral valvular disease. The calcium antagonist, nimodipine, appears to improve neurologic outcome in patients with cerebral artery spasm (56,57).

Sodium nitroprusside produces hemodynamic effects similar to nitroglycerin and should be beneficial in treating myocardial ischemia. However, it may cause "coronary steal" and increase the area of damage associated with myocardial infarction (58,59). Other vasodilators, such as hydralazine, can cause reflex tachycardia, an unwanted side effect in the patient with coronary artery disease.

Hypovolemia is a relative contraindication to the use of vasodilator therapy because hypotension may be profound. Vasodilators also may increase intrapulmonary shunting with a resultant decrease in PaO_2. This effect seems to occur less often with the calcium antagonists and especially with the alpha-beta blocker labetalol. Cyanide toxicity, a potential complication of nitroprusside infusion, is extremely rare, and its incidence is unchanged by hepatic or renal dysfunction (60). Extreme care also must be taken when treating hypertension in patients with increased intracranial pressure. Pure vasodilators, such as nitroprusside and nitroglycerin, when used to treat hypertension, can significantly increase intracranial

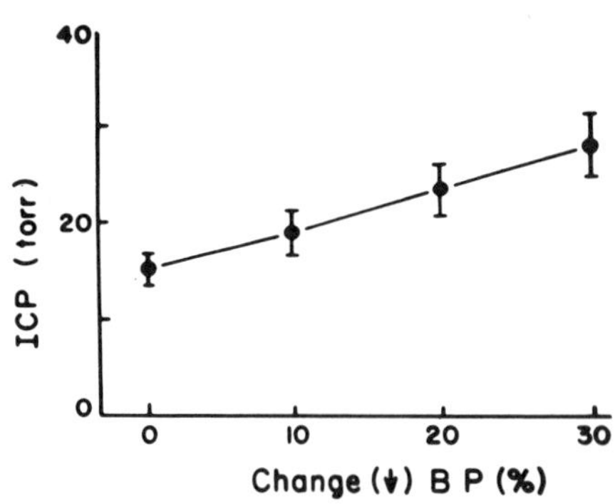

FIG. 14. Changes in intracranial pressure after nitroprusside infusion in patients with intracranial space-occupying lesions. (From Montgomery et al., ref. 39, with permission.)

pressure while decreasing mean arterial pressure, thus dangerously decreasing cerebral perfusion pressure (see Fig. 14) (61). Consideration should be given to the use of other antihypertensive medications such as labetalol or trimethaphan, which do not produce the same increase in intracranial pressure that nitroprusside and nitroglycerin do (62,63).

Commonly Used Agents

Nitroprusside

Nitroprusside causes relaxation of arterial and, to a lesser extent, venous smooth muscle by penetrating the endothelium and acting as a substrate for the formation of NO (52,53,64). NO then binds to guanylate cylase, producing configural changes that result in the production of cGMP as a second messenger in the smooth muscle cell (12). With a rapid onset, short half-life, and excellent dose response, sodium nitroprusside is an extremely effective vasodilator when used by continuous infusion. Doses of 0.2–8.0 μg/kg/min can be titrated effectively and efficiently to control hypertension in the perioperative period either by manual infusion or by computer-driven closed-loop models (65). Although cyanide toxicity and coronary steal are complications of nitroprusside therapy, the former is rare and the latter is still hotly debated, with scientific evidence supporting both sides. Nitroprusside, used frequently to induce hypotension in the perioperative period, usually requires invasive monitoring of arterial pressure because rapid pressure swings are possible.

Nitroglycerin

An organic nitrate that produces much more venodilation than arterial dilation, nitroglycerin reduces heart size and decreases left ventricular wall tension (56). Its mechanism for producing vasodilation is similar to that described for nitroprusside in the previous section (53,12). Nitroglycerin is an effective vasodilator for administration by continuous infusion because of its rapid onset of action and short elimination half-life (see Table 4). However, large doses may be required to treat severe hypertension because of its predominant venodilation. Nitroglycerin is often used to treat myocardial ischemia because it reduces preload and afterload without causing coronary steal. Nitroglycerin improves the washout of radioactive materials from ischemic areas of myocardium, indicating redistribution of flow to these ischemic areas (66). When nitroglycerin is used to treat acute myocardial infarction, morbidity and mortality are reduced (67). However, hypovolemic patients should have adequate fluid-volume replacement before treatment.

Trimethaphan

Trimethaphan is a peripheral vasodilator and ganglionic blocker that has a rapid onset and offset of effect when given by continuous infusion (68). Because it blocks the autonomic nervous system and causes peripheral vasodilatation, trimethaphan decreases blood pressure by reducing cardiac output and SVR (69). Increases in heart rate associated with its use are usually from parasympathetic ganglionic blockade. Trimethaphan is used as a continuous infusion at rates of 10–200 µg/kg/min to produce controlled hypotension or to achieve autonomic control during nitrous-narcotic or neuroleptic anesthesia. Desensitization limits the duration of effective ganglionic blockade. Mydriasis, ileus, and urinary retention are ganglionic blocking side effects of trimethaphan that limit its usefulness. As a potent inhibitor of plasma cholinesterase, trimethaphan can prolong the action of succinylcholine (70). Because of their many side effects, trimethaphan and other ganglionic blockers are seldom used in the perioperative period.

Phentolamine

Phentolamine, an imidazole derivative that produces nonselective alpha-adrenergic blockade, decreases both SVR and blood pressure within 2 minutes and lasts 10–15 minutes. The alpha-2 blockade of phentolamine increases the release of norepinephrine, resulting in an increased heart rate and cardiac output. This increase in norepinephrine is manifested by cardiac arrhythmias and angina pectoris. Because of these side effects, phentolamine has largely been replaced by newer medications. Intraoperative management of pheochromocytoma or autonomic hyperreflexia is its primary use. Some physicians also combine norepinephrine and phentolamine for inotropic support status post-CPB, but this, too, has largely been replaced by newer, more selective agents. The usual infusion rate for phentolamine is 0.5–20 µg/kg/min (see Table 4).

Hydralazine

Hydralazine, a phthalazine derivative, decreases blood pressure by vascular smooth muscle relaxation by a mechanism similar to that described for nitroprusside and nitroglycerin. Arteriolar vasodilation is significantly greater than venous dilation, causing a decrease in SVR and an associated increase in heart rate, stroke volume, and cardiac output. The baroreceptor stimulates an increase in sympathetic output. The tachycardia associated with the administration of hydralazine is significantly greater than would be expected from reflex mechanisms, but its etiology is unknown. This tachycardia, along with the preferential decrease in diastolic pressure, could place patients with coronary artery disease at risk for ischemia. The onset of action of hydralazine is 15–20 minutes, with an elimination half-life averaging 3 hours. The usual IV bolus dose is 2.5–10 mg. Infusions are not used secondary to its long half-life.

Labetalol

Labetalol, a selective alpha-1 and nonselective beta antagonist, produces dose-dependent decreases in SVR and, to a lesser extent, cardiac output. The ratio of beta blockade to alpha blockade from parenteral administration is approximately 7:1. The usual dose of labetalol is 0.25 to 1.0 mg/kg given over 2 minutes, but a 5–10 mg dose is often effective to control perioperative hypertension. The peak effect occurs 5 minutes after IV administration, which makes dose titration relatively easy. In patients with coronary artery disease, labetalol decreases blood pressure without reflex tachycardia. The infusion dose rate of labetalol is 0.02 to 2.5 mg/min to control hypertension in the operating room and the intensive care unit. Labetalol infusions produce stable blood-pressure control, but because of labetalol's half-life of 3–4 hours, discontinuing the drug will not eliminate undesired effects. Common side effects are orthostatic hypotension and bradycardia.

Diazoxide

Diazoxide, a benzothiadiazene derivative, decreases blood pressure by direct action on smooth muscle. Treatment of accelerated or severe hypertension is its primary use. A single injection of 1 mg/kg to 3 mg/kg reduces systolic and diastolic blood pressure within 1–2 minutes and lasts 6 to 7 hours. Its disadvantages include inability to carefully titrate the drug, long half-life, and propensity for hypotension. The reflex increase in cardiac output, heart rate, and left ventricular ejection velocity make diazoxide unsuitable for the treatment of hypertension associated with dissecting aortic aneurysm or significant coronary artery disease.

Enalaprilat

Enalaprilat is an intravenously administered angiotensin-converting enzyme (ACE) inhibitor, with enalapril being the oral forrn. In single doses of 1.25–5.0 mg, enalaprilat reduces mean arterial pressure, pulmonary capillary wedge pressure, and systemic vascular resistance (71). This indicates an improvement in left ventricular function without a change in coronary sinus blood flow or myocardial oxygen consumption (71). This medication is indicated for patients with hypertension and congestive heart failure. Its 15-minute onset of effect is valuable in the perioperative period, but its 6–7-hour half-life makes titration by infusion difficult. Chronic oral ACE inhibitors improve long-term outcome in patients with congestive heart failure (72).

Calcium Channel Antagonists

Nifedipine, nicardipine, and isradipine are examples of calcium channel antagonists that produce significant vasodilation with minimal negative inotropic effects. Nicardipine and isradipine are similar in structure to nifedipine but produce fewer negative inotropic effects and less reflex tachycardia (73,74). Infusions of nicardipine or isradipine produce rapid but controlled decreases in blood pressure secondary to decreased SVR (74,75). Because they produce less reflex tachycardia, improve coronary blood flow, decrease capillary wedge pressure, and reduce myocardial oxygen consumption, both drugs can be used to treat postoperative hypertension in the patient with coronary artery disease. The recommended dose to treat hypertension is 4–7.5 mg/hr as an infusion.

NEGATIVE INOTROPIC AND CHRONOTROPIC DRUGS

Despite a decrease in the incidence of coronary artery diseases associated with improved diet, exercise, and life-style, the number of patients at risk for coronary artery disease remains high. Approximately 10% of the more than 2 million patients who undergo surgery each year have significant coronary artery disease. However, many patients and their physicians are unaware of the progress of their disease. Therefore, research in the prevention of myocardial ischemia or infarction in the perioperative period continues. Multiple studies show an improved tolerance for and prevention of myocardial ischemia in patients treated chronically or perioperatively with beta-adrenergic antagonists (76). Calcium antagonists also can provide protection by decreasing myocardial oxygen consumption. The characteristics and dosing of these drugs are compared in Table 5 and in the following section.

Mechanism of Hemodynamic Effects

The negative inotropic and chronotropic drugs are primarily the beta-adrenergic antagonists, calcium antagonists, and inhalational anesthetics. Beta-adrenergic antagonists exert their effects by binding selectively to beta-adrenergic receptors and by interfering with the ability of catecholamines' or other sympathomimetics to provoke beta-adrenergic responses. Patients receiving beta-adrenergic antagonists should have them continued through the perioperative period to avoid the risk of hyperactivity of the sympathetic nervous system.

Calcium antagonists selectively interfere with the inward transfer of calcium ions through slow calcium channels (77). Verapamil and diltiazem, two calcium antagonists, also may have some blocking activity at the fast calcium channels. Calcium-channel antagonists exert their effects by decreasing myocardial contractility, heart rate, conduction through the AV node, and SVR (78).

The exact hemodynamic effects exerted by the negative inotropic and chronotropic agents depend on the particular drug used and the cardiovascular status of the

TABLE 5. *Comparison of the pharmacologic characteristics of negative inotropic and chronotropic drugs*

Generic name (trade name)	Negative inotropic effect[a]	Negative chronotropic effect[a]	Mechanism of action	Adult dose[b]	Comments[c]
Halothane (Fluothane)	++	0	Direct	0.5–1.0 vol % (inhalation)	
Enflurane (Ethrane)	+++	0	Direct	1.0–1.5 vol % (inhalation)	
Propranolol (Inderal)	++	++++	Beta-1 adrenergic	0.25–0.5 mg (IV)	Used primarily to reduce HR and treat arrhythmias
Metoprolol (Lopressor)	++	++++	Beta-1 adrenergic blockade	50–100 mg (PO); 5–10 mg (IV)	Used primarily for medical therapy of hypertension.
Esmolol (Brevibloc)	++	++++	Beta-1 adrenergic blockade	500 μg/kg/min x 1 min, then 50–300 μg/kg/min (IV)	To decrease HR, treat SVT or hypertension
Labetalol (Trandate)	+	++	Beta and alpha-1 adrenergic blockade	0.02–2.5 mg/min infusion	Primarily for treatment of hypertension
Verapamil (Isotopin)	+	+	Calcium antagonist	0.1 mg/kg (IV)	Used primarily for supraventricular arrhythmias
Diltiazem (Cardizem)	+	+	Calcium antagonist	75–150 mg/kg (IV)	Used primarily for treatment of angina pectoris

[a] The number of plus signs denotes increasing activity; 0 denotes no activity.
[b] IV, intravenous administration; PO, oral administration.
[c] HR, heart rate; SVT, supraventricular tachycardia.

patient. Generally, these agents reduce cardiac contractility and heart rate. Secondarily, there is a decrease in both cardiac output and blood pressure and an increase in right atrial and left atrial pressure—an increase in filling pressure not seen with the newer calcium antagonists. Calcium antagonists decrease SVR, whereas, with the exception of the mixed alpha-beta antagonist, labetalol, the beta-adrenergic antagonists do not.

Indications and Contraindications

Negative inotropic and chronotropic drugs are used to treat hypertension, myocardial ischemia, tachycardia or arrhythmias. Verapamil and esmolol, a selective beta-1 antagonist, are used to treat supraventricular dysrhythmias. Beta-adrenergic antagonists and, to a lesser extent, calcium antagonists also prevent perioperative hypertension, tachycardia, and myocardial ischemia (Fig. 15) (76,79,80).

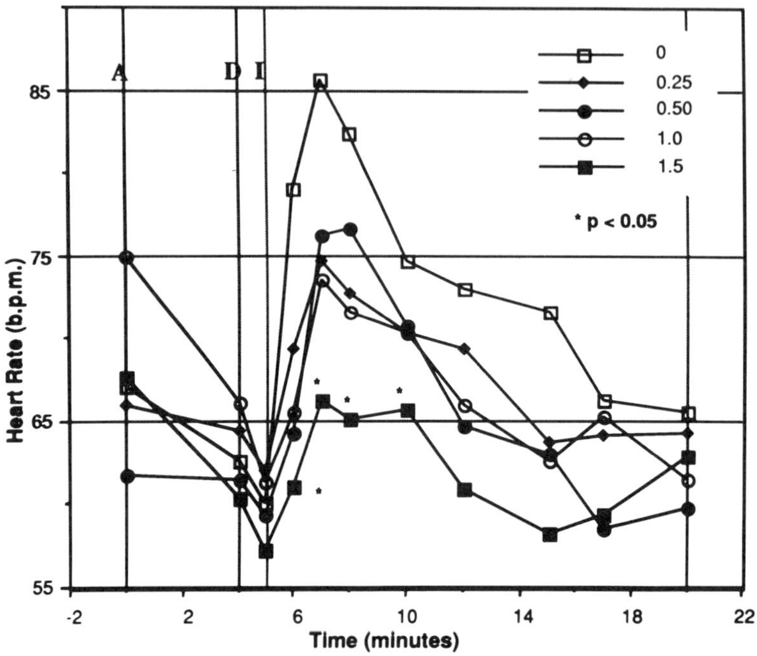

FIG. 15. Esmolol bolus-dose heart rate responses. Comparative hemodynamic (heart rate) changes with varying doses of esmolol in patients with coronary artery disease undergoing induction and intubation for coronary artery bypass grafting. A, anesthesia induction; D, drug (esmolol) bolus; I, intubation. (From Welty, ref. 56, with permission.)

Negative inotropic drugs are used in the treatment of hyperdynamic hypertension associated with pheochromocytoma. Coronary artery vasospasm is a major indication for their use.

Low cardiac-output syndromes are a relative contraindication to the use of these drugs. Bronchospastic pulmonary diseases, including asthma and chronic obstructive pulmonary diseases, are relative contraindications to the use of nonselective beta adrenergic antagonists, but the beta-1 selective agents metoprolol and esmolol, in addition to the weaker beta-antagonist labetalol, can be used cautiously (81,82). Second-degree AV block may progress to complete heart block with the use of beta blockers or verapamil.

Commonly Used Agents

Propranolol

Propranolol, a nonselective beta-adrenergic antagonist that produces approximately equal beta-1 and beta-2 antagonism, is the standard by which other beta-adrenergic antagonists are measured. Propranolol decreases heart rate and contractility, increases airway resistance in patients with reactive airway disease, causes arterial vasoconstriction, and blunts the response to hypoglycemia. These side effects prompted the search for more selective beta-adrenergic agents.

Metoprolol

Metoprolol, a beta-1 selective adrenergic antagonist, is less likely than propranolol to cause adverse effects in patients with chronic obstructive pulmonary disease, peripheral vascular disease, or vulnerable hypoglycemia. At higher doses, metoprolol produces more beta-2 blockade. Metoprolol has an elimination half-life of 3–4 hours and is usually given in 5 mg to 10 mg IV doses to treat tachycardia or ischemia. Metoprolol is not given by infusion.

Esmolol

Esmolol, an ultrashort-acting beta-1 selective beta adrenergic antagonist with an elimination half-life of 9 minutes, is efficacious in the perioperative period for both treatment and prevention of hypertension and tachycardia (79). Because esmolol decreases heart rate and myocardial oxygen consumption, it is also effective in the treatment of myocardial ischemia. Its extremely short duration of action and beta-1 selectivity allows its cautious use in patients with reactive airway disease. Doses of 0.25–1.5 mg/kg, followed by an infusion of 50–300 μg/kg/min, effectively control heart rate and blood pressure. Esmolol blunts the hemodynamic response to intubation better than do typical adjuvant doses of lidocaine or fentanyl.

Labetalol

Labetalol, a weak nonselective beta-adrenergic antagonist and alpha-1 antagonist, was discussed with the vasodilators. It also possesses some properties of a beta-2 agonist, which allows it to be used cautiously in patients with reactive airway disease.

Verapamil

Verapamil, a calcium antagonist, is a synthetic derivative of papaverine that directly depresses the sinoatrial node and delays antegrade conduction through the AV node (83). Negative inotropic effects of verapamil, although present, are unimportant except in preexisting left ventricular dysfunction. Verapamil produces less vascular smooth muscle relaxation than nifedipine does and, secondarily, less decrease in blood pressure. Care must be taken when verapamil is used with beta-adrenergic antagonists because AV block may occur (84). Verapamil is used primarily in the treatment of acute supraventricular tachydysrhythmias and is used less often to treat angina pectoris. The usual antiarrhythmic dose is 5 mg intravenously. Its elimination half-life is 3 hours, and it is not given by infusion. Because verapamil is highly protein bound, care must be taken when used with drugs such as lidocaine and propranolol because the active unbound portion of the drug may increase (85).

Nifedipine

Nifedipine, a calcium antagonist with greater coronary and peripheral artery vasodilatory properties than verapamil (83), possesses little of verapamil's depressant effect on the sinoatrial or AV node. The negative inotropic and chronotropic effects appear to be greater with nifedipine, although reflex sympathetic responses to increased heart rate counter these effects to some degree. Nifedipine also is given sublingually in doses of 10–20 mg to treat hypertension, but no IV preparation is currently available in the United States. A parenteral preparation is forthcoming.

Diltiazem

Diltiazem is a calcium antagonist that produces cardiovascular effects similar to verapamil (83). It often decreases heart rate and dilates peripheral and coronary arteries. Like the other calcium antagonists discussed, diltiazem produces a greater direct inotropic depression in patients who have reduced left ventricular function or are receiving concomitant beta-antagonist therapy. The primary use of diltiazem is treatment of angina pectoris. The usual IV dose is 75–150 μg/kg, and the elimination half-life is 4–6 hours.

DECISION MAKING

The decision to intervene or, more importantly, not to intervene with the many vasoactive drugs is crucial to good management. The previous sections discussed the pertinent hemodynamic effects and side effects of the vasoactive drugs that are currently available. Even with this information, always making correct decisions is difficult under ideal conditions and is impossible under suboptimal conditions. Decision making is suboptimal when the physician lacks the pertinent physiological data describing the patient's condition. When this data becomes available from the patient's history, physical examination, and noninvasive or invasive monitoring, the physician, through personal experience and reading of scientific literature, can determine the probability of success of a given intervention

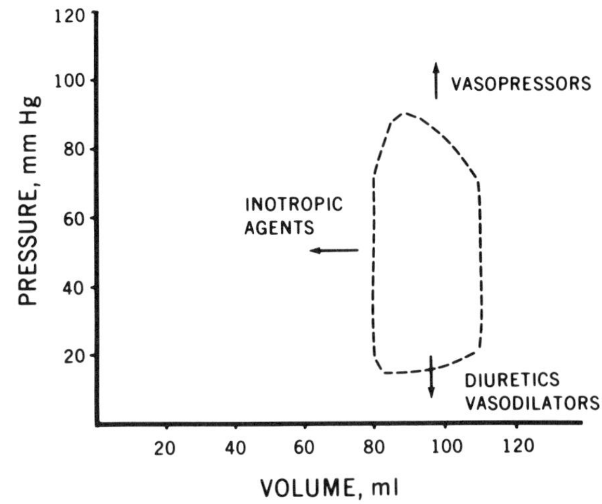

FIG. 16. Pressure-volume loop demonstrating the impact of various pharmacologic interventions during cardiogenic shock. The changes produced by the various interventions demonstrate the importance of monitoring in obtaining baseline information and evaluating the consequences of therapeutic interventions. (From Rackley CE, et al. Cardiogenic shock. In: Rackley CE, ed. *Critical care cardiology.* Philadelphia: FA Davis; 1981, with permission.) (86)

for a particular clinical scenario (Fig. 16). Although all untoward events cannot be predicted, the patient's history can help predict a possibility of interventions producing a low output state, hypotension or hypertension, and tachycardia. Preoperative preparation, calm and efficient management during the period of hemodynamic abnormality, and a thorough understanding of the patient's clinical pathophysiology and the pharmacodynamic effect of the drugs will make decision making more precise and less stressful. An example of a logical progression of decision making is presented below and in Fig. 17.

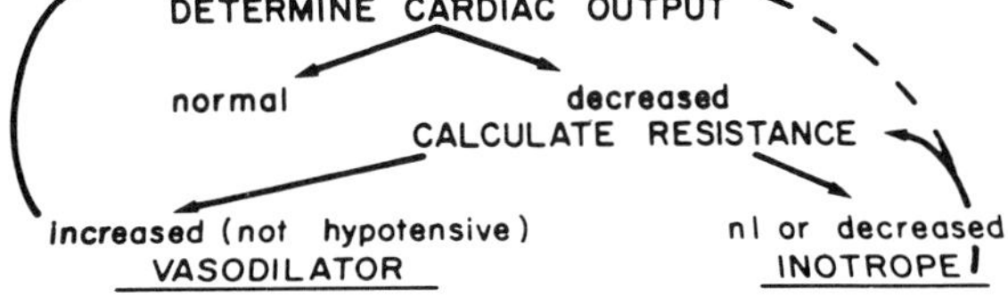

FIG. 17. Schematic for the treatment of low cardiac-output syndrome. (From Reves JG. Vasoactive drugs and when to use them. In: Thomas S. *Manual of cardiac anesthesia.* New York: Churchill Livingstone; 1984, with permission.) (15)

TABLE 6. *Concentrations of vasoactive drugs used at Duke University Medical Center*[a]

		For infusion IV	
Drug	For bolus IV	Infants and children[b]	Adults
Calcium	1 g/10 ml (100 mg/ml)	—	—
Dobutamine	—	60 mg/100 cc	500 mg/250 ml (2 mg/ml)
Dopamine	—	60 mg/100 cc	800 mg/250 ml (3.2 mg/ml)
Ephedrine	50 mg/100 ml (5 mg/ml)	—	—
Epinephrine	0.1 mg/10 mg (10 μg/ml)	0.6 mg/100 cc	5 mg/250 ml (20 μg/ml)
Isoproterenol	—	0.6 mg/100 cc	1.0 mg/250 ml (4 μg/ml)
Methoxamine	20 mg/10 ml (2 mg/ml)	—	—
Nitroglycerin	—	—	50 mg/250 ml (200 μg/ml)
Nitroprusside	—	—	50 mg/250 ml (200 μg/ml)
Norepinephrine	—	—	4 mg/250 ml (16 μg/ml)
Phenylephrine	1 mg/10 ml (100 μg/ml)	—	20 mg/250 ml (80 μg/ml)

[a] Other institutions may have different concentrations, but institutional practices regarding drug dilutions are strongly recommended so that inadvertent over- or underdosages do not occur because mistaken concentrations are administered at a given infusion rate.

[b] Pediatric advanced life-support recommendations: Infuse at 1 ml/kg/hr to give 0.1 μg/kg/min isoproterenol or epinephrine and 10 μg/kg/min of dopamine or dobutamine.

The steps for increasing low cardiac output are as follows (15):

1. Simultaneously optimize the heart rate (70–90 bpm) and preload (left atrial pressure or pulmonary capillary wedge pressure, 10–15 mmHg).
2. Compute the cardiac output and, if still low (less than 1.8–2.0 L/min/m^2), do the following:
   - Use a vasodilator to reduce systemic vascular resistance (if elevated) and reoptimize preload if necessary with this intervention.
   - Use an inotropic drug if SVR is low or normal and if the patient is hypotensive with reduced output.
3. Use a vasoconstrictor if systemic vascular resistance is low and cardiac output is normal or elevated and the patient is hypotensive. (Remember that chronic support with a vasoconstrictor may decrease renal perfusion and endanger renal function.)
4. Then remeasure cardiac output and institute appropriate pharmacologic (additional inotropes or vasodilators) or mechanical support (intraaortic balloon pump) according to heart rate, systemic vascular resistance, and cardiac output.

This description and the accompanying figure show a logical progression from problem, to solution, or at least to temporization. Adequate preoperative planning and the availability of adequate equipment is essential. The availability of drug infusions and a standardized mixing scheme will save time and minimize errors (see standard mixing scheme for Duke University Medical Center in Table 6). Drug infusion nomograms (Fig. 18), computer facilitated drug-infusion schemes

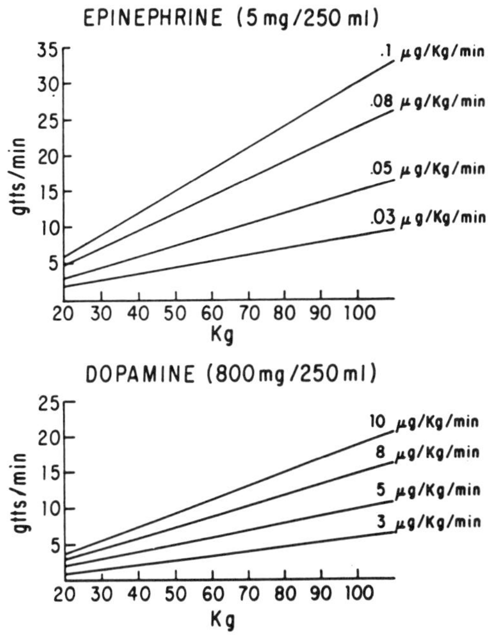

FIG. 18. Nomograms for the infusion of epinephrine and dopamine at the specified dilutions. Following the desired dosage rate to the patient's weight, the number of drops/min or cc/hr can be determined.

NAME: PATIENT HT: 175 CM.
WT: 85KG.
BSA=2 SQUARE METERS
DOSAGES IN MICROGRAMS/KILOGRAM/MIN.

GTTS:	DOBU	DOPA	SNP	NTG	EPI	ISUP	LIDO	NEO	NREP	AMNPH
	500	800	100	400	5	2	2000	40	4	1000
	---	---	---	---	---	---	----	---	---	----
	250	250	250	500	250	250	250	250	250	500
1:	.392	.627	.078	.157	4E-03	2E-03	1.6	.031	3E-03	.392
2:	.784	1.3	.157	.314	8E-03	3E-03	3.1	.063	6E-03	.784
3:	1.2	1.9	.235	.471	.012	5E-03	4.7	.094	9E-03	1.2
4:	1.6	2.5	.314	.627	.016	6E-03	6.3	.125	.013	1.6
5:	2	3.1	.392	.784	.02	8E-03	7.8	.157	.016	2
6:	2.4	3.8	.471	.941	.024	9E-03	9.4	.188	.019	2.4
7:	2.7	4.4	.549	1.1	.027	.011	11	.22	.022	2.7
8:	3.1	5	.627	1.3	.031	.013	12.5	.251	.025	3.1
9:	3.5	5.6	.706	1.4	.035	.014	14.1	.282	.028	3.5
10:	3.9	6.3	.784	1.6	.039	.016	15.7	.314	.031	3.9

FIG. 19. Computer-generated infusion sheet giving dosage of vasoactive drugs in relation to infusion rates for standard concentrations.

(Fig. 19), or automated infusion pumps (smart pumps) should be used to free the physician from time-consuming calculations (needless diversions) and allow him or her to concentrate on solving clinical problems.

When making clinical decisions, vasoactive drugs can be life threatening as well as life saving. Familiarity with their use brings confidence and improved clinical understanding. The newest vasoactive drug will perform only as well as clinicians understand its use, and possibly not as well as one they are comfortable using. To reiterate a point, it is crucial to know when or when not to intervene with vasoactive drugs.

REFERENCES

1. Mason et al. Vasodilator therapy of congestive heart failure. *Drug Ther* 1978.
2. Schwinn DA. Cardiac pharmacology. In: Estafanous FG, et al., eds. *Cardiac anesthesia: principles and clinical practice;* 1994.
3. Rasmussen H, Barret PO. Calcium messenger system: an integrated view. *Pharmacol Rev* 1984;64: 938–984.
4. Newfield P, Cottrell JE, eds. *Handbook of Neuroanesthesia* Boston: Little Brown and Copany. 1983;126.
5. Gilman AG, Goodman LS, Gilman A. *The pharmacological basis of therapeutics*. New York: Macmillan; 1980:138–175.
6. Zaritsky AL, Chernow B. Catecholamines, sympathomimetics. In: Zieglar MG, Lake CR, eds. *Frontiers of clinical neuroscience*. Vol. 2. *Norepinephrine*. Baltimore: Williams & Wilkins; 1984:481.
7. Smith NT, Corbascio AN. Thc usc and misusc of pressor agents. *Anesthesiology* 1970;8:58–59.
8. Hilberman M, Maseda J, Stinson EB, et al. The diuretic properties of dopamine in patients following open heart operations. *Anesthesiology* 1984;61:481.
9. Miller ED Jr. Renal effects of dopamine. *Anesthesiology* 1984;61:487.
10. Schaer GL, et al. Norepinephrine infusion alone versus norepinephrine plus low dose dopamine: enhanced renal blood flow with combination pressor therapy. *Crit Care Med* 1985;13:492.
11. Park JR, Tinker JH. Cardioactive drugs and their monitorable effects. *Semin Anesth* 1983;11:268.
12. Snyder SH, Bredt DS. Biological roles of nitric oxide. *Sci Am* 1992;68.
13. Leier CV, et al. Comparitive systemic and regional hemodynamic effects of dopamine and dobutamine in patients with cardiomyopathic heart failure. *Circulation* 1978; 58: 466–475.
14. Chernow B, Rainey TG, Lake CR. Catecholamines in critical care medicine. In: Zieglar MG, Lake CR, eds. *Frontiers of clinical neuroscience*. Vol 2. *Norepinephrine*. Baltimore: Williams & Wilkins, 1984:381.
15. Reves JG. Vasoactive drugs and when to use them. In: Thomas S. *Manual of cardiac anesthesia* New York: Churchill Livingstone; 1984.
16. Waller JC. Inotropes and vasopressors. In: Kaplan JA, ed. *Cardiac anesthesia. Vol. 2. Cardiovascular pharmacology*. New York: Grune & Stratton; 1983:273.
17. Ghosh S, Gray B, Oduro A, Latimer RD. Dopexamine hydrochloride: pharmacology and use in low cardiac output states. *J Cardiothorac Vasc Anesth* 1991;5:382.
18. Gray PA, Bodenham AR, Park GR. The pharmacokinetics of dopexamine hydrochloride in patients undergoing orthotopic liver transplantation. *Intensive Care Med* 1990;16:A143.
19. Foulds RA. Clinical development of dopexamine hydrochloride and an overview of its hemodynamic effects. *Am J Cardiol* 1988;62:41C.
20. Boachie-Ansa G, Kane KA, Parat JR. The cardiac electrophysiologic effects of dopexamine under normal and stimulated ischaemic conditions. *J Mol Cell Cardiol* 1989;21:S23.
21. A Symposium. Amrinone. Braunwald E (ED) *Am J Cardiology*, July 1985.
22. Hnerjager P. Pharmacology of bipyridine phosphodiesterase inhibitors. In: Goenen M, ed. *Bipyridine phosphodiesterase inhibitors in clinical practice*. Cambridge,UK: Cambridge Medical Publications; 1990.
23. Hermiller JB, et al. Amrinone in severe congestive heart failure: another look at an intriguing new cardioselective drug. *J Pharmacol Exp Ther* 1984; 228:319–326.
24. Royster RL, Butterworth JF, Prielipp RC, et al. Combined inotropic effects of amrinone and epinephrine after cardiopulmonary bypass in humans. *Anesth Analg* 1993;77:662.

25. Makela VHM, Kapur PA. New drugs for the treatment of heart failure: amrinone and milrinone. *Semin Anesth* 1988;7:92.
26. Baim DS, McDowell AV, Cherniles J. Evaluation of a new bipyridine inotropic agent—milrinone—in patients with severe congestive heart failure. *N Engl J Med* 1983;309:748.
27. Colucci WS. Myocardial and vascular actions of milrinone. *Eur Heart J* 1989;10:32.
28. Packer M, Carver JR, Rodeheffer RJ, et al. Effect of oral milrinone on mortality in severe chronic heart failure. *N Engl J Med* 1991;325:1468.
29. Curfman GD. Inotropic therapy for heart failure—an unfulfilled promise. *N Engl J Med* 1991;325:1509.
30. Aikawa J, Koike K, Takayanagi I. Vascular smooth muscle relaxation by a_1-adrenoreceptor blocking action of denopamine in isolated rabbit aorta. *J Cardiovasc Pharmacol* 1991;17:440.
31. Inamasu M, Totsuka T, Ikeo T, Nagao T, Takeyama S. Beta$_1$-adrenergic selectivity of the new cardiotonic agent denopamine in its stimulating effects on adenylate cyclase. *Biochem Pharmacol* 1987;36:1947.
32. Carlucci WS, Wright RF, Braunwald E. New positive inotropic agents in the treatment of congestive heart failure: part 1. *N Engl J Med* 1986;314:290.
33. Zaloga GP, Chernow B. Insulin, glucagon, and growth hormone. In: Chernow B, Lake CR, eds. *The pharmacologic approach to the critically ill patient.* Baltimore: Williams & Wilkins; 1983:562.
34. Sladen RN. Management of the adult cardiac surgical patient in the intensive care unit. In: Ream AK, Fogdal RP, eds. *Acute cardiovascular management.* Philadelphia: JB Lippincott; 1982:506.
35. Royster RL, Butterworth JF, Prielipp RC, et al. A randomized, blinded, placebo-controlled evaluation of calcium chloride and epinephrine for inotropic support after emergence from cardiopulmonary bypass. *Anesth Analg* 1992;74:3.
36. d'Hollander A, Primo G, Hennart D, et al. Compared efficacy of dobutamine and dopamine in association with calcium chloride on termination of cardiopulmonary bypass. *J Thorac Cardiovasc Surg* 1982;83:264.
37. Buxton AE, Goldberg S, Harken A, et al. Coronary artery spasm immediately after myocardial revascularization. *N Engl J Med* 1981;304:1249.
38. Boulanger M, Maille JG, Pelletier GB, et al. Vasospastic angina after calcium injection. *Anesth Analg* 1984;63:1124.
39. Montgomery WH, Donegan JD, Mcintyre KM. Standards and guidelines for cardiopulmonary resuscitation and emergency cardiac care: Pt 3. Adult advanced cardiac life support. *JAMA* 1986;255:2933.
40. Bohrer H, Fleischer F, Krier C. Hyperkalemic cardiac arrest after cardiac surgery following high dose glucose insulin potassium for inotropic support. *Anesthesiology* 1988;69:949–953.
41. Gradinac S, Coleman GM, Taegtmeyer H, et al. Improved cardiac function with glucose insulin potassium after aortocoronary bypass. *Ann Thorac Surg* 1989;48:484–489.
42. Reinhart, K. *Principles and practice of SVO$_2$ monitoring: intensive care.* Vol. 5. London, UK: World, King and Worth; 1988:121–124.
43. Schnider SM, deLorimer AA, Hall JW, Chapler FK, Morishima HO. Vasopressors in obstetrics: correction of fetal acidosis with ephedrine during spinal hypotension. *Am J Obstet Gynecol* 1968;102: 911–919.
44. James FM, Greiss FC, Kemp RA. An evaluation of vasopressor therapy for maternal hypotension during spinal anesthesia. *Anesthesiology* 1970;33:25–34.
45. Schmid PG, Eckstein JW, Abboud FM. Comparison of the effects of several sympathomimetic amines on resistance and capacitance vessels in the forearm of man. *Circulation* 1966;34:209.
46. Livesay JJ, Follette DM, Fey KH, et al. Optimizing myocardial supply/demand balance with alpha-adrenergic drugs during cardiopulmonary resuscitation. *J Thoracic Cardiovasc Surg* 1978;76: 244–251.
47. Schnider SM, deLorimer AA, Ashling JW, Morishima HO. Vasopressors in obstetrics: fetal hazards of methoxamine administration during obstetric spinal anesthesia. *Am J Obstet Gynecol* 1970;106: 680–686.
48. Greiss FC, Van Wilkes D. Effects of sympathomimetic drugs and angiotensin on the uterine vascular bed. *Obstet Gynecol* 1964;23:925–930.
49. Yakaitis RW, Otto CW, Blitt CD. Relative importance of alpha and beta adrenergic receptors during resuscitation. *Crit Care Med* 1979;7: 293–296.
50. Brown CG, Birinyi F, Werman HA, et. al. The comparative effects of epinephrine versus phenylephrine on regional cerebral blood flow during cardiopulmonary resuscitation. *Resuscitation* 1986;3:171.
51. Grueter CA, Barry BK, McNamara DB, Gruetter DY, Kadowitz PJ, Ignarro LJ. Relaxation of bovine coronary artery and activation of coronary arterial guanylate cyclase by nitric oxide, nitroprusside and a cardiogenic nitrosoamine. *J Cyclic Nucl Res* 1979;5:211.
52. Gruetter CA, Gruetter DY, Lyon JE, Kadowitz PJ, Ignarro LJ. Relationship between cyclic guanosine

3:5-monophosphate formation and relaxation of coronary arterial smooth muscle by glyceryl trinitrate, nitroprusside, nitrite and nitric oxide: effects of methylene blue and methemoglobin. *J Pharm Exp Ther* 1981;219:181.

53. Moncada S, Palmer RMJ, Higgs EA. Nitric oxide: the endogenous regulator of vascular tone. In: Warren JB, ed. *The endothelium: an introduction to current research.* New York: Wiley-Liss, 1990;1.
54. Rapoport RM, Murad F. Agonist-induced endothelium-dependent relaxation in rat thoracic aorta may be mediated by cGMP. *Circ Res* 1983; 52:352–357.
55. Stoelting RK. *Pharmacology and physiology in anesthetic practice.* Philadelphia: JB Lippincott: 1987:308.
56. Welty TE. Use of nimodipine for prevention and treatment of cerebral arterial spasm in patients with subarachnoid hemorrhage. *Clin Pharmacy* 1987;6:940.
57. Gelmers HJ, Gorter K, deWeerdt CJ, et al. A controlled trial of nimodipine in acute ischemic stroke. *N Engl J Med* 1988;318:203.
58. Chiariello M, Gold HK, Leinbach RC, Davis MA, Maroko PR. Comparison between the effects of nitroprusside and nitroglycerin on ischemic injury during acute myocardial infarction. *Circulation* 1976;54:766–773.
59. Becker LC. Conditions for vasodilator-induced coronary steal in experimental myocardial ischemia. *Circulation* 1978;57:1103–1110.
60. Tinker JH, Michenfelder JD. Sodium nitroprusside: pharmacology, toxicology and therapeutics. *Anesthesiology* 1976;45:340–354.
61. Cottrell JE, Patel K, Turndorf H, Ranschoff J. Intracranial pressure changes induced by sodium nitroprusside in patients with intracranial mass lesions. *J Neurosurg* 1978;48:329–331.
62. Turner JM, Powell D, Gibson RM, McDowell DG. Intracranial pressure changes in neurosurgical patients during hypotension induced with sodium nitroprusside or trimethaphan. *Br J Anaesth* 1977; 49:419–424.
63. Orlowski JP, Shiesley D, Vidt DG, et. al. Labetalol to control blood pressure after cerebrovascular surgery. *Crit Carc Mcd* 1988;16:765.
64. Kaplan JA, Finlayson DC, Woodward S. Vasodilator therapy after cardiac surgery: a review of the efficacy of and toxicity of nitroglycerine and nitroprusside. *Can Anaesth Soc J* 1980;27:154–158.
65. Reves JG, Sheppard LC, Wallach R, Lell WA. Therapeutic uses of sodium nitroprusside and an automated method of administration. *Int Anesthesiol Clin* 1978;16:51.
66. Horwitz LD, Garlin R, Taylor WJ, Kemp HG. Effects of nitroglycerin on regional myocardial blood flow in coronary artery disease. *J Clin Invest* 1971;50:1578–1584.
67. Yusuf F, Collins R, MacMahon S, Peto R. Effect of intravenous nitrates on mortality in acute myocardial infarction: an overview of the randomized trial. *Lancet* 1988;1(8549):1088–1092
68. Vickers MD, Schneiden H, Wood-Smith FG. *Cardiovascular drugs (trimethaphan camsylate): drugs in anesthesia practice.* 6th ed. London, UK: Butterworths; 1984:344.
69. Harioka T, Hatano Y, Mori K, Toda N. Trimethaphan is a direct arterial vasodilator and an alpha-adrenoreceptor antagonist. *Anesth Analg* 1984;63:290–296.
70. Sklar GS, Lanks KW. Effects of trimethaphan and sodium nitroprusside on hydrolysis of succinylcholine in vitro. *Anesthesiology* 1977;47:31–33.
71. DeMarco T, Daly PA, Liu m, Kayser S, Parmley WW. Enalaprilat, a new parenteral angiotensin-converting enzyme inhibitor: rapid changes in systemic and coronary hemodynamics and humoral profile in chronic heart failure. *J Am Coll Cardiol* 1987;9:1131–1138.
72. Ramahi TM, Lee FA, Medical therapy and prognosis in congestive heart failure: lessons from clinical trials. *Cardiol Clin* 1995;13:5–26.
73. Mauser M, Voelker W, Karsch KR. Isradipine (PN200-110): a new dihydropyridine calcium antagonist produces less negative inotropic effect than nifedipine. *Z Kardiol* 1988;77:373–377.
74. Wallin JD, et. al. Intravenous nicardipine for the treatment of severe hypertension. *Am J Med* 1988; 85:331–338.
75. vandenBerg EK, Dehmer GJ. Acute hemodynamic effects of intravenous isradipine. *Am J Cardiol* 1988;61:1102–1105.
76. Chung F, et al. Calcium channel blockade does not offer adequate protection from perioperative myocardial infarction. *Anesthesiology* 1988;69:343–347.
77. Fleckenstein. Specific pharmacology of calcium in myocardium, cardiac pacemakers, and vascular smooth muscle. *Ann Rev Pharmacol Toxicol* 1977;17:149–166.
78. Reves JG, Kissin I, Lell WA, Tosone S. Calcium entry blockers: uses and implications for anesthesiologists. *Anesthesiology* 1982;57:504–518.

79. Newman MF, Leslie JB, Macciolli GA, Reves JG. Determination of optimal bolus esmolol for prevention of intraoperative hypertension and tachycardia. *Anesthesiology* 1989;71:A145(abst).
80. Stone JG, Foex P, Sear JW, et al. Myocardial ischemia in untreated hypertensive patients: effect of a single oral dose of beta-adrenergic blocking agent. *Anesthesiology* 1988;68:495–500.
81. Sheppard D, DiStefano F, Byrd RC, et. al. Effects of esmolol on airway function in patients with asthma. *J Clin Pharmacol* 1986;26:169–174.
82. George RB, Light RW, Hudson L, et. al. The use of labetalol for the treatment of hypertension in patients with reversible airway obstruction. *J Clin Hypertens* 1985;1:80–83.
83. Reves JG. The relative hemodynamic effect of Ca-entry blockers. *Anesthesiology* 1984;61:3–5.
84. Benaim ME. Asystole after verapamil. *Br Med J* 1972;2:169–170.
85. Yong CL, Kunka RL, Bates TR. Factors affecting the plasma protein binding of verapamil and norverapamil in man. *Res Commun Chem Pathol Pharmacol* 1980;30:329–479.
86. Rackley CE, et al. Cardiogenic shock. In: Rackley CE ed. *Critical care cardiology.* Philadelphia: FA Davis; 1981.

Drug Infusions in Anesthesiology, Second Edition,
edited by R. J. Fragen. Lippincott-Raven Publishers,
Philadelphia © 1996.

Appendix

This appendix is provided as a ready reference to drug doses. they are really dose ranges and should be used as guidelines or starting points for bolus and infusion doses. Eventually the doses should be titrated to the patient's needs, always aiming for the lowest effective dose to reduce the incidence and severity of side effects. There is also a table of available blood concentration ranges. Titration to blood concentrations will be useful as "smart" infusion pumps become available.

Table 1. Doses of hypnotic drugs for anesthesia and sedation
Table 2. Doses of opiates for anesthesia and analgesia
Table 3. Doses of muscle relaxants
Table 4. Doses of positive ionotropes and chronotropes
Table 5. Doses of negative inonotropes and chronotropes
Table 6. Doses of opiates for administration of patient-controlled anesthesia (PCA)
Table 7. Recommended drug doses for epidural administration: opiates and combinations of local anesthetics and opiates
Table 8. Approximate plasma drug levels required for various stimuli

TABLE 1. *Doses of hypnotic drugs for anesthesia and sedation*

Drug	Loading dose (μg/kg)	Maintenance dose (μg/kg/min)
	Anesthesia	
Etomidate a)	200–300	20 for 27 min, then 10
b)	100 for 10 min	10
Ketamine	1500–2500	25–75
Methohexital	1500–2500	50–150
Midazolam	50–150	0.25–1.5
Propofol	1000–2500	50–150
	Sedation	
Etomidate	–	–
Ketamine	500–1000	10–20
Methohexital	250–1000	10–50
Midazolam	25–100	0.25–1.0
Propofol	250–1000	10–50

TABLE 2. *Doses of opiates for anesthesia and analgesia*

Drug	Loading dose (μg/kg)	Maintenance dose (μg/kg/min)
	Anesthesia	
Alfentanil	50–150	0.5–3.0
Fentanyl	5–15	0.03–0.1
Remifentanil[a]	0.5–2.0	0.25–0.5
Sufentanil	1–3	0.01–0.05
	Analgesia	
Alfentanil	10–25	0.25–1.0
Fentanyl	1–3	0.01–0.03
Remifentanil[a]	–	0.025–0.2

[a]Proposed dose.

TABLE 3. *Doses of muscle relaxants*

Drug	Loading dose (μg/kg)	Maintenance dose (μg/kg/min)
Atracurium	200–400	4.0–8.4
Mivacurium	150–250	6.0–8.3
Rocuronium	600–1200	9.8–11.2
Succinylcholine	500–1000	60–120
Pancuronium	70–100	0.4–0.6
Vecuronium	40–80	1.0–1.7

TABLE 4. *Doses of positive ionotropes and chronotropes*

Drug	Bolus dose	Maintenance dose
Epinephrine	–	0.05–0.2 μg/kg/min
Amrinone	500–2000 μg/kg	5–10 μg/kg/min
Dobutamine	–	5–20 μg/kg/min
Dopamine, beta effect	–	3–7 μg/kg/min
Dopamine, alpha effect	–	7–20 μg/kg/min
Dopexamine	–	1–10 μg/kg/min
Glucagon	50 mg/kg	5 mg/kg/hr
Glucose-insulin-potassium (GIK) solution	–	1 ml/kg/hr
Isoproterenol	–	0.025–0.05 μg/kg/min
Milrinone	50–75 μg/kg	0.375–0.75 μg/kg/min
Norepinephrine	–	0.05–0.15 μg/kg/min
Phenylephrine	–	0.1–0.5 μg/kg/min

TABLE 5. *Doses of negative ionotropes and chronotropes*

Drug	Bolus dose	Maintenance dose
Esmolol	250–1000 μg/kg, over 1 min	50–300 μg/kg/min
Isradipine	7–15 μg/kg	8–40 μg/min
Labetalol	250–1000 μg/kg, over 2 min	20–2500 μg/min
Nicardipine	–	4–12 mg/min
Nitroglycerine	–	0.5–5.0 μg/kg/min
Nitroprusside	–	0.2–8.0 μg/kg/min
Phentolamine	–	0.5–20.0 μg/kg/min
Trimethaphan	–	10–50 μg/kg/min

TABLE 6. *Doses of opiates for administration of patient-controlled analgesia (PCA)*

Drug	Bolus dose (mg)	Lockout interval (min)	Continuous infusion ($mg \cdot hr^{-1}$)
	Agonists		
Fentanyl citrate	0.015–0.05	3–10	0.02–0.1
Hydromorphone hydrochloride	0.10–0.5	5–15	0.2–0.5
Meperidine hydrochloride	5–15	5–15	5–40
Methadone hydrochloride	0.50–3.0	10–20	–
Morphine sulphate	0.50–3.0	10–20	1–10
Oxymorphone hydrochloride	0.2–0.8	5–15	0.1–1.0
Sufentanil citrate	0.003–0.015	3–10	0.004–0.03
	Agonist-antagonists		
Buprenorphine hydrochloride	0.03–0.2	10–20	–
Nalbupine hydrochloride	1–5	5–15	1–8
Pentazocine hydrochloride	5–30	5–15	6–40

TABLE 7. *Recommended drug doses for epidural administration*

Drug	Opiates Alone Drug concentration (μg/ml)	Infusion rate[a] (ml/hr)
Fentanyl	2.5–10.0	4–12
Hydromorphone	50	6–8
Morphine	100–250	1–6
Meperidine	2000–5000	4–6
Sufentanil	1	10

[a]Best results when the epidural catheter is positioned in the middle of the involved dermatome(s).

Procedure	Catheter site	Combinations of Local Anesthetics and Opiates Drugs[a]	Infusion rate (ml/hr)
Lower extremities	Lumbar	Bup. 0.25% + fent. 5 μg/ml	6–8
		Bup. 0.125% + fent. 5 μg/ml	6–8
		Bup. 0.125% + mep. 2.5 mg/ml	6–8
Major abdominal	Lumbar	Bup. 0.125% + fent. 5 μg/ml	6–8
		Bup. 0.125% + morp. 0.1 mg/ml	6–8
	Thoracic	Bup. 0.125% + fent. 5 μg/ml	4–6
		Bup. 0.125% + morp. 0.1 mg/ml	3–4
Thoracotomy	Thoracic	Bup. 0.125% + fent. 5 μg/ml	3–4
		Bup. 0.125% + morp. 0.1 mg/ml	3–4

[a]Bup., bupivacaine; fent., fentanyl; mep., meperidine; morp., morphine.

TABLE 8. Approximate plasma drug levels required for various stimuli[a]

Drug	Skin incision	Major surgery	Minor surgery	Spontaneous ventilation	Analgesia and/or awakening*	Sedation
Alfentanil (ng/ml)	200–300	250–450	100–300	<200–250	50–100	50–200
Etomidate (ng/ml)	400–600	500–1000	300–600	–	200–350*	100–300
Fentanyl (ng/ml)	3–6	4–8	2–5	<1–3	1–2	–
Ketamine (μg/ml)	?	?	1–2	–	0.1–1.0	0.5–2.0
Methohexital (mg/ml)	5–10	5–15	5–10	–	1–3*	2–5
Midazolam (ng/ml)	–	50–250 (when combined with an opiate)	50–250 (when combined with an opiate)	– –	150–200* (reduced to 50–100 in presence of an opiate)	40–100
Propofol (μg/ml)	2–6	2.5–7.5	2–6	–	0.8–1.8*	1.0–3.0
Sufentanil (ng/ml)	1–3	2–5	1–3	<0.5	?	–
Thiopental (μg/ml)	7.5–12.5 (with N_2O) 35–45 (without N_2O)	10–20	10–20	–	4–8*	7.5–15.0

[a]The above drug levels represent those when combined with 65–70% N_2O unless otherwise stated. Effective plasma concentrations may differ markedly, depending on premedication and intraoperative drug combinations.

Index

ISBN 0-7817-0265-8